Drug-Dependent Mothers and Their Children

Mary Haack, Ph.D., F.A.A.N., joined The George Washington University Center for Health Policy Research in 1990 as a Senior Research Staff Scientist. She is also Adjunct Associate Professor of Psychiatry and Behavioral Science and Associate Research Professor of Health Services Management and Policy, The George Washington University School of Medicine and Health Sciences.

Dr. Haack specializes in health policy analysis and research, with a focus on substance abuse and mental health, state regulatory policy concerning impaired nursing practice, and public health workforce training issues.

Dr. Haack's background includes several years as a nurse clinician, five years as a Visiting Associate at the National Institutes of Health and the National Institute on Alcohol Abuse and Alcoholism, as well as faculty positions at the University of Illinois School of Nursing, Northwestern University Center for Nursing, and the University of Maryland School of Nursing.

Dr. Haack co-chairs the Primary Health Providers Section of the International Council on Alcohol and Addictions, and is a member of the Department of Health and Human Services Subcommittee on Public Health Workforce, Training, and Education. She is a Fellow of the American Academy of Nursing.

Drug-Dependent Mothers and Their Children

Issues In Public Policy and Public Health

Mary R. Haack, PhD, FAAN
Editor

 Springer Publishing Company

Springer Publishing Company, Inc.
536 Broadway
New York, NY 10012–3955

Cover design by Stephen Haack and Margaret Dunin
Cover photograph by Eugene Richards from *Cocaine True,
Cocaine Blue* (Aperture, 1994). Reprinted with permission.
Acquisitions Editor: Matt Fenton
Production Editor: Jeanne Libby

97 98 99 00 / 5 4 3 2 1

Library of Congress Cataloging-in-Publication Data

Drug dependent mothers and their children: issues in public policy
  and public health / Mary R. Haack, editor.
      p. cm.
    Includes bibliographical reference and index.
    ISBN 0-8261-9630-6
    1. Pregnant women—Drug use—Government policy—United
  States. 2. Drug abuse in pregnancy—Government policy—United
  States. 3. Children of narcotic addicts—United States. 4. Children
  of narcotic addicts—Services for—United States. 5. Maternal
  health services—United States. I. Haack, Mary R.
  HV5824.W6D78 D1997
  362.29'085'20973—dc21   97-3391
                                                                 CIP

For

Peter, Barbara, Jackson, Stephen, Wendy, and Jennifer

For teaching me the power and joy of family

Contents

PART II   Issues in Public Policy

PART III   Contrasts and Conclusions

PART IV   Appendixes

Contributors

Jane B. Atwater, Ph.D.
Assistant Research Professor
Juniper Gardens Children's
    Project
University of Kansas

Kathleen M. Baggett
Research Assistant
Juniper Gardens Children's
    Project
University of Kansas

Peter P. Budetti, M.D., J.D.
Professor of Health Services
    Management, Preventive
    Medicine and Law
Director, Institute for Health
    Services Research and Policy
    Studies
Northwestern University

Judith J. Carta, Ph.D.
Senior Scientist
Juniper Gardens Children's
    Project
University of Kansas

Julie Darnell, M.H.S.A.
Research Scientist
Center for Health Policy Research
The George Washington University

**Janet A. Deatrick, Ph.D.,
    F.A.A.N.**
Associate Professor
Program Director, Acute-Chronic
    Care Nurse Practitioner Program
Co-Director, International Center
    for Research of Women,
Children, and Families
University of Pennsylvania, School
    of Nursing

Laura Feig, M.P.P.
Social Science Analyst
US Department of Health and
    Human Services
Office of the Assistant Secretary
    for Planning and Evaluation

Charles R. Greenwood, Ph.D.
Senior Scientist
Juniper Gardens Children's
    Project
University of Kansas

Mary R. Haack, Ph.D., F.A.A.N.
Senior Research Staff Scientist
Center for Health Policy Research
Adjunct Associate Professor of
    Psychiatry and Behavioral
    Science
Associate Research Professor of
    Health Services Management
    and Policy
The George Washington University
    School of Medicine and Health
    Sciences

Paul Jellinek, Ph.D.
Vice President
The Robert Wood Johnson
    Foundation

Leslie L. Jordan
Vice-President Policy & Program
Missouri Coalition of Community
    Mental Health Centers

Philip H. Jos, Ph.D.
Associate Professor
Department of Political Science
College of Charleston
Charleston, SC

Ted Lardner, Ph.D.
English Department
Cleveland State University
Cleveland, OH

Judith Larsen, J.D.
Trial Attorney
Counselor to national organizations
    on issues of substance use in
    family law cases

Mary Faith Marshall, Ph.D.
Director
Program in Bioethics
Medical University of South
    Carolina

Scott R. McConnell, Ph.D.
Director
Institute on Community Integration
University of Minnesota

Charlotte McCullough, M.Ed.
Director, Managed Care Institute
    for Children's Services
Child Welfare League of
    America

Mary A. McEvoy, Ph.D.
Director
Center for Early Education and
    Development
University of Minnesota

Roger Meyer, M.D.
Senior Scholar in Residence
Association of Academic Health
    Centers
Clinical Professor of Psychiatry
Georgetown University

Ann Marie Pagliaro, R.N.
Professor and Director, Substance
    Abusology Research Unit
Faculty of Nursing
University of Alberta

Louis A. Pagliaro, Ph.D.
Professor, Faculty of
    Pharmacology
University of Alberta

Martin Perlmutter, Ph.D.
Associate Professor
Department of Philosophy
College of Charleston
Charleston, SC

Sidney Schnoll, M.D., Ph.D.
Professor and Chair
Division of Substance Abuse
    Medicine
Medical College of Virginia
Virginia Commonwealth University

Bonnie B. Wilford, M.S.
Center for Health Policy Research
The George Washington University

Peter Weilenmann, M.A.
Acting Preschool Coordinator
Arlington Public Schools
Arlington, VA

Rosanne C. Williams, Ph.D.
Associate Professor
Early Childhood Research
    Institute on Substance Abuse
University of South Dakota

Foreword

TOWARD A MODEL OF COMPREHENSIVE CARE

If a society is to be judged by how it responds to the needs of its most vulnerable citizens, then it is difficult to imagine a more stringent test than that posed by this book: the challenge of caring for drug-exposed children and their families. Few in our society are more vulnerable or more in need of assistance. And certainly, when we hear or read the stories of these children and their families, our impulse to respond—to do *something* to help—is strong.

Yet as we begin to understand the full scope of the clinical, social, and emotional problems confronting these children and their families, we may feel overwhelmed. Where do we start? Where does it end? And who is responsible for what?

In the 1980s, as a byproduct of the crack cocaine epidemic, there was a sudden surge in the number of drug-exposed newborns. As these children approached preschool and school age, this wave of drug-exposed children came as a major shock to our health, social service, educational and legal systems. Although drug-exposed children were not unknown to the professionals in these systems, the severity of the problems confronting this new wave of children and their families—as well as the sheer number of children involved—was utterly unprecedented. The questions of where to start, what to do, and who was responsible for what suddenly assumed a new urgency.

This important book edited by Dr. Mary Haack has been prepared in response to that urgency. With contributions from leading thinkers and practitioners in the field, it provides a wealth of much-needed practical information to those charged with responding to the needs of these children and their families—policymakers as well as service providers.

In addition to its obvious practical value, however, as one reads through these chapters it becomes increasingly clear that the book has another kind of value as well. On the one hand, the crisis posed by drug-exposed children and their families clearly illuminates some of the most serious weaknesses and limitations of our existing health and social systems. On the other hand, it is often only under crisis conditions such as these that one can hope to bring about truly meaningful improvements in these large and complex systems, improvements that could affect not only drug-exposed children and their families, but all of us who must turn to these systems in our own hour of need. In chapter after chapter, this book points to what some of those improvements might be.

Thus, I believe this book can and should be read at more than one level—the conceptual as well as the practical. For it is only if we do our best at both levels—doing everything we can within our existing systems, while at the same time doing everything we can to improve those systems—that we will be able to meet the tremendous social and moral challenge of caring for drug-exposed children and their families.

Paul Jellinek, Ph.D.
Vice President
The Robert Wood Johnson Foundation
Princeton, New Jersey
April 26, 1996

Preface

In the mid-1970s when I first entered the substance-abuse treatment field, I became acutely aware of how few women with alcohol and drug problems had access to treatment. In the hundred-bed program where I worked, it was not uncommon for men to outnumber women by twenty to one. We believed many more women needed help, but they were out "there" somewhere—their names and faces shrouded in the secrets and pain that permeate the illness.

It was during the 70s that Betty Ford disclosed her drug dependence. Through her courage and that of other valiant women like her, the faces of drug-dependent women gradually came into focus and conformed what we already knew—that drug dependence affects every strata of society—including the wife of the President of the United States. Betty Ford's honesty and subsequent contributions to improving treatment for women will be among her most important legacies. But not all women have been reached by her contribution. This book is about those women; they are the urban mothers who struggle with drug dependence, mental illness, HIV infection, poverty, and a lack of education—under conditions that would challenge even the most robust in society.

In compiling the chapters of this book, I have chosen authors who can provide a cool analytic perspective to assist the reader in separating scientific and legal facts from popular myths. By necessity, such a book is rather dry and scholarly. It may even seem cold. To put a human face on this work, I have included a photograph from Eugene Richard's widely acclaimed photo essay, "Cocaine Blue, Cocaine True."

The woman on our cover is a poor woman with a drug problem. Her young son watches over and cares for her. The bond between this mother and child is the most important thing in their lives; indeed, they have little else. Typical of the drug-dependent mothers who are identified by the child welfare system or who enter treatment programs through court referral, her history includes physical abuse, family violence, HIV infection, and clinical depression. And because poor minority women are more likely to be found in these systems, she is Black.

Certainly most minority women do not fit this profile. Epidemiological data clearly demonstrate that minority women in general use alcohol and drugs to a lesser extent than White women. However, minority women who have drug problems rarely benefit from the scientific advancements of drug research in this country or from the heavily funded "War on Drugs." In fact these women and their children have very limited access to adequate drug treatment, access that could be extinguished with the implementation of the Personal Responsibility and Work Opportunity Act of 1996 (the Welfare Reform Bill).

Ironically, without appropriate treatment, these mothers will never achieve the independence envisioned by the drafters of the welfare reform legislation. And tragically, the chance to prevent prenatal drug-exposure and HIV transmission to their future children will be forever lost. The scarcity of treatment services for poor women with drug problems is sometimes based on the assumption that addicted pregnant women will not respond to treatment and that drug-exposed children will have prolonged and chronic health problems regardless of what services are provided. This assumption, perpetuated by the media, has led the public to believe that these children are "throwaway" kids. The assumption is, however, largely unfounded—these mothers and their children have a remarkable capacity to recover if they are given the chance.

Although the life circumstances of poor drug-dependent women may be very different from those of Betty Ford, their need for health care and drug treatment is no less. They and their children suffer from the same illness that Betty Ford has, an illness we know to be a widely studied public health problem, an illness we know how to treat. But instead of using that knowledge to benefit these women and their children, we, through our public policies, choose to withhold our precious health care resources. And more often than not, we choose to punish them. My hope is that this book will help us to reconsider these choices.

Mary Haack, Ph.D., FAAN
Senior Research Staff Scientist
Center for Health Policy Research
The George Washington University
Washington, DC

Acknowledgments

This book would not be possible without the invaluable assistance of many people. I am indebted to:

The Robert Wood Johnson Foundation for the grants that supported the groundwork for this book and that funded the development of the book itself—especially to Foundation Vice President, Paul Jellinek, for making it all possible;

to Peter Budetti for leading me to this project and for being a critical force in shaping the work as it evolved;

to Matt Fenton, my editor at Springer, for his encouragement and guidance;

to Bonnie Wilford for providing technical assistance in editing the book and for being a constructive sounding board in times of desperate need;

to Eugene Richards for the extraordinary photograph on the cover;

to Steve Haack for designing of the cover;

to Arthur Content for his unwavering belief that the book was worth the effort.

Introduction

Peter Budetti, M.D., J.D.

DEFINING THE ISSUES

News reports depicting an epidemic of drug abuse by pregnant women in this country—and the legions of violent, mentally defective, welfare-bound children it allegedly is producing—abound. Schools are said to be falling apart because teachers and good students cannot possibly deal with the disruptive, irascible products of *in utero* addiction in their classrooms. Inner cities are portrayed as the breeding grounds for multiple generations of dependent, crime-prone parents who abuse drugs and children alike. Cash assistance and medical assistance programs are characterized as bankrupting states and cities that cannot keep up with this epidemic. Worst of all, it is said, nothing can be done—treatment programs may suck up resources, but they are futile, since chemically damaged children cannot be salvaged, let alone repaired.

This book tests these assertions and puts them in perspective. Chapter authors summarize the available literature to identify how much is actually known about the extent of damage produced by fetal exposure to illicit drugs and the prospects for overcoming the injury that does occur. Beyond a synthesis of the state of the relevant science, the book also develops the public health and public policy implications of that knowledge. A comprehensive model for services to address these problems is presented, together with approaches to training necessary personnel and organizing the public and private resources to deliver those services.

Certain themes emerge across the different chapters. One is the complexity of trying to specify the causal chain between *in utero* drug exposure and subsequent behavioral, social, or educational difficulties; the same children who are subjected to maternal drugs as fetuses also experience multiple other risk factors after they are born, including low socioeconomic status and abuse and neglect. A second theme, which is a corollary of the multifactorial character of the problem, is that drug-exposed children and their families have a great diversity of support and service needs. The programs and agencies that have been created to meet some or many of those needs do not generally coordinate their activities, or in some cases, even share the same goals. A serious conundrum is that in many cases the necessary treatments and social services may not be available in the local area—even when women are ordered by the courts to use those services. Fortunately, an optimistic conclusion can be fashioned: when programs, agencies, and professionals do cooperate in specially structured comprehensive service delivery models, the prospects for producing well-functioning children are very encouraging.

Mary Haack (Chapter One) has integrated knowledge about the needs of drug-exposed children and their families and the options for delivering services to meet those needs into a model of comprehensive care. The array of diverse needs and services is organized into a systematic matrix that portrays them according to a distinct hierarchy. This extensive theoretical construct is then made practical, by identifying comprehensive approaches that have actually been put in place to deliver and fund many of the needed services. The matrix also serves to illustrate the scope of the public policy issues stemming from this analysis, as well as a framework for analyzing those issues.

Anne Marie Pagliaro and Louis A. Pagliaro (Chapter Two) assess the ability of psychotropic drugs to cause physical or mental fetal abnormalities when they are abused during pregnancy. These effects are heavily dependent on the frequency, timing, type and variety of drugs abused, as well as a range of maternal and environmental factors. As is true throughout the book, the Pagliaros stress the interactive effects of such factors, especially multiple drug exposure, as well as the unique response of humans compared with other animals. They pay particular attention to alcohol, because it is so frequently abused and its adverse effects have been so well studied. Cocaine, by comparison, has been inadequately studied, but appears to have a significant, but low, teratogenic potential.

Judith Carta and colleagues (Chapter Three) analyze the effects of *in utero* drug exposure on the neurological and behavioral development of children. Echoing the theme noted above, they discuss both the earlier literature, which studied the effects of "single drug" abuse, and the more recent analytic techniques that seek to assess the interactive consequences of multiple drug use and other risk factors for developmental impairment. In addition, they point out the distinction between the relatively rich data on short-term outcomes and the paucity of long-term measurements. The longer-term studies that do exist illustrate the potential for both transient adverse consequences that diminish over time and the late appearance of other developmental problems. Finally, the most recent studies and ones in progress are designed to identify positive, protective factors, as well as harmful ones.

Philip Jos, Mary Faith Marshall, and Martin Perlmutter (Chapter Four) analyze the legal and ethical considerations of trying to strike a balance between protecting fetuses and permitting adults—albeit pregnant ones—to engage in behaviors of their own choosing. They trace the rise and fall of a single medical center's approach, which led to criminal prosecution of pregnant women who were diagnosed as illicit drug users but did not undergo recommended treatment, or who delivered a baby who tested positive for drugs. The intrusiveness and punitive character of this approach—and its selective application to predominantly low-income, African-American patients in the hospital's obstetrics clinic—raised questions of violations of the women's rights to privacy, to refuse treatment, to procreate, to give informed consent for experimentation, and to equal protection under the law. A serious conundrum, as noted elsewhere in this book, is that in many cases the treatments and social services the women failed to use may not, in fact, have been available in the local area.

Sidney H. Schnoll (Chapter Five) outlines the measures that should be taken by primary care practitioners to diagnose, prevent, and treat illicit drug use, with particular attention to the special considerations raised during pregnancy. Since the signs and symptoms may be subtle, and the likelihood of concealment high, the practitioner needs to be alert to the specific diagnostic tools that are likely to detect abuse — beginning with an appropriately high index of suspicion, and including a comprehensive history and physical exam that applies screening techniques targeted toward substance abuse. Pregnancy may offer a window of receptivity for preventive measures, but such activities need to address the multifactorial character of abuse, and comprise social and educational as well as medical interventions. Treatment of both the addicted mother and drug-exposed neonate similarly includes a range of medical and supportive services, and a time frame extending well beyond pregnancy.

Mary Haack and Janet Deatrick (Chapter Six) outline the extensive content areas in which health professionals must be trained to provide adequate care for drug-exposed babies and their families. These include specific topics in medical and nursing care, as well as a range of legal, social, management, and interactive knowledge and skills. The authors illustrate how this has been done through a comprehensive curriculum developed and used at the University of Pennsylvania School of Nursing, and demonstrate how this prepares practitioners to meet many of the needs identified in Haack's Model of Comprehensive Care. Because specialized comprehensive training programs require financial support, they caution that loss of such funding threatens to restrict both the numbers of specialists in substance-related disorders and the adequacy of training of generalists in this content area.

The book moves from health policy to public policy as Bonnie Wilford (Chapter Seven) discusses legislative responses to the stresses that substance abuse has placed on social services, education, and medical care programs. Our complex system of federal-state-local governmental authorities greatly complicates addressing the multifactorial character of the problem of substance abuse in pregnancy. The result is a series of laws that vary from highly punitive to rehabilitative, depending on whether the problem is predominantly viewed as a criminal or medical one in the respective jurisdiction. Legal strategies thus range from criminal or civil incarceration and separation of mother from infant to prevention, treatment, and education. The consequences for training and use of health professionals are very different across such diverse areas.

Julie Darnell (Chapter Eight) completes the picture of diverse services to meet diverse needs by describing the federal programs, with a particular emphasis on the role of Medicaid, available for funding comprehensive services for drug-exposed infants and their families. These sources are characterized by fluctuations in funding, varying but often extensive federal controls, and recurrent proposals for dramatic change in their operations. Particularly with welfare and health care programs, the likely trend seems to be toward increased state flexibility in the use of funds, with federal payments to the states not increasing at the rates experienced in recent years.

Judith Larsen (Chapter Nine) focuses on social policy from the perspective of courts that are faced with substance-abusing parents and drug-exposed children. Many cases are treated under general abuse and neglect laws, with judges having great leeway to determine what services, if any, will be made available to the family, and whether the emphasis will be on removing and protecting the child or reunifying and preserving the family. A recent trend is for such laws to have specific references to drug abuse, with consequent limitations on court discretion. A tidal wave of maternal prosecutions for exposing newborns to drugs was predicted a few years ago, but has not materialized. Future directions for the courts now appear to favor early identification and early separation of children from drug-involved parents, stricter compliance of parents with treatments if they are to get their children back, and further development of out-of-court mediation.

Charlotte McCullough and Laura Feig (Chapter Ten) describe the front lines of the child welfare system—the societal effort to protect children from substance-abusing parents while trying to strengthen and support families when possible. Reports of child abuse and neglect are on the increase, with some 700,000 substantiated cases handled by child protective services in 1993; of these, one-third to two-thirds or even more are related to parental drug or alcohol abuse. The growing number of infants needing placements and other services raises particular challenges for child welfare agencies. The diversity of needs of substance-abusing parents and their children is best addressed by comprehensive, well-coordinated services, but instead may lead to conflict between professionals with different perspectives. For example, those emphasizing substance-abuse treatment may view the child's presence in the home as part of the recovery plan, while child welfare agencies may see recurring drug use as a threat to the child's safety and development. Future challenges include incorporating managed care into child welfare services, and maintaining the capacity to serve these families in the face of budget-driven welfare reforms.

Ted Lardner (Chapter Eleven) lays out the two principal issues confronting the educational system: the multifactorial relationships linking prenatal drug exposure to poor school performance, and the presumed self-fulfilling consequences of reduced teacher expectations when children are labeled as "crack babies." Two case studies suggest approaches to overcoming these problems: support systems extending beyond the schools for meeting the diverse educational needs of children with such a variety of factors threatening their educational progress, and intensive, small-group educational programs with appropriately prepared teachers. The hope is that these approaches can capitalize on the apparent resilience of children, and sustain their developmental potential even as they face compromising factors long after the immediate effects of prenatal drug exposure.

Leslie Jordon (Chapter Twelve) describes a model of comprehensive alcohol and drug treatment that consolidated and coordinated a wide range of services for drug-exposed children and their families in the State of Missouri. This model was in large part made possible by new flexibility in the use of what had been program-specific funds. Interdisciplinary teams work to enhance access to individualized services, and providers must meet comprehensive standards and regulations for core services. Building and sustaining cooperative linkages across numerous social, medical, criminal justice, and other agencies remains a continuing issue in implementing such a multifaceted approach. Concerns for the future include uncertainty over whether managed care contractors may recapture health care funds that have been available to the program.

Roger Meyer, in his Afterword, sums up the challenges of understanding and designing ways to alleviate the consequences of the multiple risk factors faced by drug-exposed children and their families. Maternal drug abuse cannot be separated from alcohol abuse, neglect, violence, and the many forms of deprivation that these children experience—and, consequently, an exclusive focus on maternal behavior during pregnancy will not make the problem disappear. Beyond all the research that has been done and should be undertaken, however, is the real challenge of how to get society to care about these problems sufficiently to craft real solutions.

Peter P. Budetti, M.D., J.D.
Professor of Health Services Management,
Preventive Medicine, and Law
Director, Institute for Health Services
Research and Policy Studies
Northwestern University
Evanston, IL 60208-4170

1

Comprehensive Community-Based Care: The Link between Public Policy and Public Health

Mary R. Haack, Ph.D., F.A.A.N.

P regnancy-related substance abuse and its consequences are among the most complex health problems confronting policymakers and public health officials. Manifestations of the problem touch every part of the community: city hospitals, prenatal care clinics, drug treatment centers, courts, child welfare services, schools, and prisons.

This chapter lays the groundwork for a model of comprehensive care that represents a standard by which public health services for this population can be judged. In light of today's rapidly changing health care environment and the contemporary focus on meeting primary health care needs of underserved populations, such a model offers a starting point for discussing the policy dilemma surrounding this public health problem.

What follows is a description of the problem, a model of community-based care relevant to public health practice, a discussion of relevant public policies, and an analysis of barriers that prevent communities from addressing the problem. The chapter follows the Patton and Sawicki (1993) policy analysis process, which involves:

1. defining the problem;
2. identifying alternative policies;
3. determining evaluation criteria;
4. evaluating alternative policies;

5. selecting the preferred policy; and
6. implementing the preferred policy.

STEP 1: DEFINING THE PROBLEM

Mother-to-infant drug exposure is rising in the United States, with some estimates showing as many as 375,000 children affected annually (Chasnoff, Landress, & Barrett, 1990). The phenomenon comes at great economic and social cost to the nation. The national price tag for treating drug-exposed infants is estimated at up to $3 billion annually. Short-term human costs are evidenced by premature and low-birthweight infants, while long-term costs include chronic illness and learning disabilities.

From an international perspective, the U.S. infant mortality and infant low-birthweight rates rank poorly among other Western countries. Maternal use of alcohol, tobacco, and other drugs is thought to be a contributing factor.

- The U.S. ranks 20th in infant mortality, and 31st in infant low-birthweight. Even Romania, Iran, and Russia have higher birthweights than the U.S. (United Nations International Children's Educational Fund [UNICEF], 1992). Prenatal use of cocaine and cigarettes as well as lack of access to prenatal care contribute to the U.S. rankings (Racine, Joyce, & Anderson, 1993).
- Twenty-two thousand babies are abandoned each year at the time of birth; eight out of ten test positive for drugs (Shalala, 1993).
- In 1993 (the most recent year for which complete data are available), an estimated 7,000 HIV-infected women gave birth in the United States. Assuming an HIV transmission rate from mother to infant of about 15%–30%, about 1,000–2,000 HIV-infected infants were born in 1993. Most maternal HIV infection is the result of the mother's IV drug use or that of her partner (Centers for Disease control [CDC], 1993).
- Median hospital costs for drug-exposed babies range from $1100 to $8450 higher than for normal babies (General Accounting Office [GAO], 1990).
- Medicaid costs per beneficiary with AIDS range from $9,516 to $43,224 (Conners, 1992–93).

EPIDEMIOLOGY

Of the 59.2 million women of childbearing age (15–44) in the U.S., over 4.5 million are current users of illegal drugs, 5.6% use marijuana and 1% use cocaine. Estimates of use during pregnancy are not available (National Institute on Drug Abuse [NIDA], 1991).

Approximately 59 to 73% of women between the ages of 12–34 drink alcohol during pregnancy (Frank et al., 1988; NIDA, 1991; Zuckerman et al., 1989). At least 30% of all women in the U.S. smoke at the time they conceive and 25% continue to smoke during pregnancy (U.S. NIDA, 1991).

A number of clinical studies illustrate the scope of the problem. For instance, a study of 36 hospitals across the country conducted by the National Association for Perinatal Addictions Research and Education (NAPARE) in 1988 found that on average, 11% of pregnant women used heroin, methadone, amphetamines, PCP, marijuana, or cocaine (Chasnoff, Landress & Barrett, 1990). Another study reported that 17% of pregnant teenagers test positive for alcohol and other drugs by questionnaire, provider report or urine screen (Kokotailo, Adgar, Duggan, Repke & Joffe, 1992).

Based on an analysis of the 1988 National Hospital Discharge Survey, the U.S. General Accounting Office (GAO) identified approximately 14,000 infants with indications of maternal drug use during pregnancy. The report acknowledges that this figure substantially minimizes the problem because physicians and hospitals do not screen and test all women and their infants for drugs (Chasnoff et al., 1990; General Accounting Office [GAO], 1990).

PROFILE OF THE ADDICTED MOTHER

Studies show that the addicted pregnant woman in the scarce number of treatment slots available across the country is a 27- to 31-year-old high school dropout with three or four children, either living in a drug-abusing environment, or homeless. She has been using illegal substances for at least 10 years, and has grown up in a home with violence, sexual abuse, and substance-abusing relatives. This profile suggests the need for public health interventions that are augmented by clinical case management, child care, transportation, housing, and education (NIDA, 1994).

Unpublished data (NIDA, 1994) indicate that addicted pregnant women access drug treatment very late in their drug-taking careers. This is not surprising, considering that they face the very real risk of having a child taken away in many states. Because most primary care health care services and drug treatment services are not designed for needs of addicted mothers, child protective services and the court system become the gateway to drug treatment for most pregnant women in many communities. There are two problems with the child welfare and the family court systems as entry points for treatment. First, a mother must be seriously impaired to qualify, and secondly, adequate coordination between the family court system and the needed medical and social service systems rarely exists.

POOR MINORITY WOMEN ARE OVER-REPRESENTED

Although statistics characterize perinatal addiction as primarily affecting poor minorities, recent studies show these data not to be reliable. A clinical investigation conducted within Pinellas County, Florida, anonymously tested women entering private obstetric care and women entering public health clinics for prenatal care and found the overall incidence of drug use was similar in both groups (Chasnoff et al., 1990). A 1990 GAO report found that private hospitals serving primarily non-Medicaid patients screened infants for drug exposure less often than public hospitals. While some researchers have found a prevalence of substance abuse as low as 2%, other studies from inner city hospitals report that as many as half of all pregnant women test positive for illegal drugs.

According to public health experts, we lack complete information on the prevalence of addicted pregnant women and drug-exposed children partly because investigators have reviewed drug histories over the course of pregnancy in a representative sample of women at delivery, and partly due to methodological limitations to acquiring information through interview or biological assessment (Robbins & Mills, 1993).

STEP 2: IDENTIFY ALTERNATIVE POLICIES

There is an ongoing debate between public health professionals and policymakers about how best to address the problem of drug-dependent mothers and their families. Because public health professionals view perinatal substance abuse as a health care problem, their approach fosters expansion and coordination of community-based treatment programs. While the public health perspective accepts that some women will be unable to sustain total abstinence, they believe that the harm caused by drugs can be reduced with comprehensive treatment. On the other hand some policy makers who advocate criminal punishment as a deterrent to pregnant women, believe that punishment will stop women from using drugs. State laws reflect the variations in these very different perspectives. Within those states that have a strong public health perspective, the differences between each state law are incremental. But the contrast between the public health and the deterrent approach reflects major systematic distinctions.

Public Health Approach

Preventing Prenatal Drug Exposure and Its Consequences

To address the problem of drug-exposed children two broad categories of service needs must be addressed. The first is drug abuse treatment programs for biological parents of these children. The second is health and developmental services for the children. Presently, neither of these needs are being met.

The Need for Treatment Services

Approximately 280,000 pregnant women are estimated to need drug treatment annually. However, in the absence of scientific data, the actual numbers are not known (National Association of State Alcohol and Drug Abuse Directors [NASADAD], 1993).

A 1992 Rand study found that obstetricians in private institutions chose not to screen their patients for presence of illicit drugs because of limited treatment options and significant costs associated with screening. Private physicians also feared losing patients if it became known that they drug-screened their patients (Zellman, Jacobson, Du Plesis & DiMatteo, 1992).

A study conducted by the Southern Regional Project on Infant Mortality (1993) of 97 substance abuse treatment programs in Virginia, Oklahoma, Kentucky and Puerto Rico found that although 61% of the women interviewed qualified for Medicaid, only 14% were using Medicaid to pay for substance abuse treatment. A majority of the study programs were not eligible for reimbursement by Medicaid for services, even though federal law would allow it, since these services were not included in their state Medicaid plan.

It is difficult to estimate the need for treatment, given the barriers that exist. There is reason to believe, however, that the need is greater than estimated. In 1992 the designers of the Missouri State's Comprehensive Substance Abuse Treatment and Rehabilitation Program (CSTAR) planned for 2000 families annually. In 1994, 7,266 women and their children were treated . . . far greater than anyone had anticipated (Jordon, 1995). Chapter 12 describes how the CSTAR program was developed.

Prognosis for Drug-Exposed Infants

The lack of urgency over limited treatment services is sometimes based on the assumption that addicted pregnant women will not respond to treatment and that drug-exposed infants will have prolonged and chronic health problems regardless of what services are provided. This assumption, perpetuated by the media, has led the public to believe that these infants are "throwaway" kids. It is, however, largely unfounded. Most birth outcomes of substance abusing mothers are unremarkable. Chapters 2 and 3 provide the scientific evidence for this assertion.

The long-term impact of drug exposure on a child's physical, mental, and social well-being is as yet unknown. We do know that all children are not physically damaged as a result of maternal drug use. In fact, most effects of prenatal drug exposure are transient and responsive to treatment. A recent meta-analysis of followup studies of drug-exposed children found fewer statistically significant differences between children with and without in utero drug exposure later in life than there are at birth (Robbins & Mills, 1993). Children have a tremendous capacity to recuperate and accommodate if they grow up in an organized, nurturing environment (Olegard, 1992; Volpe, 1992; Werner, 1989).

IMPACT OF THE ENVIRONMENT

The environment plays a significant role in the development of prenatally drug-exposed children. For example, children living within the drug culture are susceptible to the toxic effects of cigarette smoke and secondary crack smoke within the environment. A recent review of nine U.S. studies in *The Lancet* showed that fathers who smoked cigarettes produced smaller babies and babies with higher rates of perinatal mortality. Babies of nonsmoking mothers whose fathers smoked more than 10 cigarettes a day had a greater frequency of severe malformations, independent of parental age and social class (Davis, 1991). Children have also developed neurologic symptoms such as seizures following passive inhalation of vaporized crack (Schwartz, 1989). Follow-up studies generally show that most differences observed at birth seem to disappear over time (Robbins & Mills,1993).

Many of the behaviors attributed to drug-exposed children are extremely common, especially in small or premature babies. A few adverse outcomes can be attributed to less effective mothering or to an unstable home environment rather than to a woman's use of drugs during pregnancy. The high rate of placement of these children away from the mother also suggests early childhood loss and separation (Robbins & Mills, 1993).

Some disabling effects of parental substance abuse are the consequence of broader social problems such as destitution, homelessness, and hunger. Many addicted mothers live with poverty, violence, abuse, neglect, prostitution, mental illness, and psychological and physical abandonment. Physical maltreatment by alcohol- or drug-involved mothers and fathers also has detrimental effects. Response to any one prenatal or postnatal environmental insult varies.

Cumulative multiple traumas such as drugs, poor nutrition, inadequate prenatal care, violence and neglect are predictive of poorer outcomes (Kronstadt, 1991; Werner, 1989; Zuckerman, 1991). In Werner's study, prenatal complications were consistently related to impairment of physical or psychological development only when they were combined with negative environmental factors such as family discord, parental mental illness, chronic poverty, or other consistently poor rearing conditions (Werner, 1989). If most children can recover from the trauma of prenatal drug exposure, what must the community provide in order to maximize the developmental potential of these children?

STEP 3: DETERMINE EVALUATION CRITERIA

Research shows that drug treatment for a pregnant women benefits the child by decreasing or eliminating the risk of drug exposure before birth, and improving the mother's ability to care for the child after birth. If drug-exposed children have an excellent chance for full and productive lives when they and their mothers receive treatment, what constitutes good treatment?

COMMUNITY-BASED CARE FOR FAMILIES WITH A DRUG-DEPENDENT MOTHER

For pregnant women, effective treatment requires an array of services connected by case management including basic services such as drug-free housing, child care, transportation, and language translation. While most of these services are available in urban communities, they seldom are coordinated in such a way that the needs of the whole family are addressed. Yet without this coordination, drug treatment loses its effectiveness.

To demonstrate what effective treatment is, we have created a graphic that displays the complex of services that constitutes comprehensive care. The model, developed by Haack and Darnell (Haack, Budetti, Darnell & Hudman, 1993), is based on information from key states and federal agencies concerned with substance abuse prevention and treatment. The sources included published research, conference proceedings, and special analyses derived from the Department of Health and Human Services, the New York State Division of Substance Abuse Services, and the National Association for Perinatal Addiction Research and Education (NAPARE).

The model is built on the assumption that infants have a sequence of developmental tasks to accomplish, each dependent on successful mastery of the earlier task, and that the mother has an indispensable role in this process. Therefore, services that improve an addicted mother's chances to live a drug-free existence also enhance the child's chances to grow and develop normally. Services that prevent or treat a child's developmental delays strengthen the potential for a healthy relationship between mother and child (Office for Substance Abuse Prevention [OSAP], 1992).

When community services are organized in a time sequence or according to the family's readiness for services, categories emerge as building blocks. The services within the model build on each other, and the strength or weakness of one service has the ability to weaken the effectiveness of other services. Interagency linkages and coordination and case management maximize the synergistic potential of the services. Transportation and child care improve access to and compliance with treatment.

Theoretical Framework

The guiding principles of Abraham Maslow's work (1954) were used as the theoretical framework for the model. Maslow's hierarchy of needs is built on two fundamental premises: (1) people's needs depend on what they have, and they are motivated only by needs not yet satisfied; (2) people's needs are arranged in a hierarchy of importance. Figure 1.1 demonstrates the application of Maslow's hierarchy to the Haack-Darnell Community Care model. As shown there are five need categories:

1. physiological needs;
2. safety and security needs;
3. affection and social activity needs;
4. esteem and status needs; and
5. self-realization needs.

Figure 1.2 displays the model components which are arranged according to Maslow's hierarchy of needs. Basic physiological needs begin at the left side of the figure and progress to higher needs, such as esteem and self-fulfillment, on the right. The basis for Maslow's theory is that lower needs must be satisfied before higher needs can be addressed. The effectiveness of the services on the right side of the model is therefore dependent on the strength of the services on the left. Column 1 lists sources through which addicted mothers may be identified.

Column 2: Survival Services

Housing, safety and food

If the family is homeless or without food, they will need services to address hunger and safety before they can respond to substance abuse treatment. Once the mother is detoxified and treated for substance abuse, she will need skills to help her live a drugfree life. She may need language and literacy skills, and communication assistance with providers or services. She may need education in parenting, life-skills, and employment skills as well as support and information concerning how to negotiate the numerous public and private systems that can provide assistance. She may need access to a telephone to call for appointments or to notify agencies of the family's place of residence.

Nonmedical services

Transportation, case management, child care, and community outreach are critical components of the service delivery model. These services are not typically provided as part of the traditional medical model.

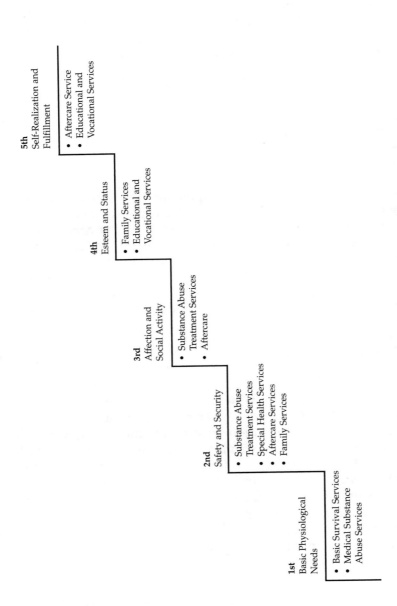

Figure 1.1 Maslow's Hierarchy of Needs Applied to the Model of Community-Based Care for Drug-Dependent Mothers and Their Children

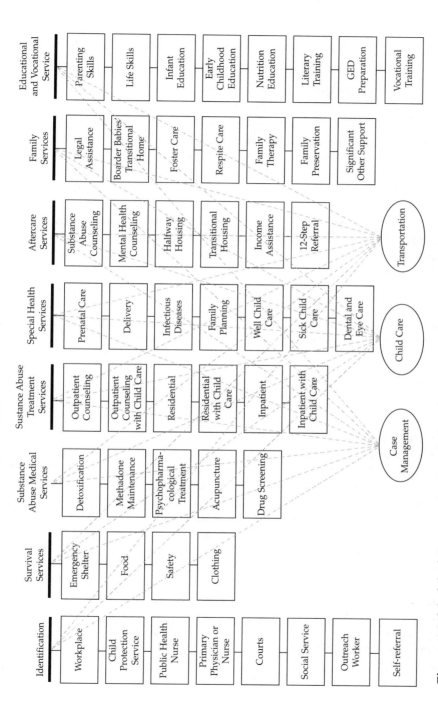

Figure 1.2 Model of Community-Based Care for Drug-Dependent Mothers and Their Children

Sources: Haack-Darnell Model of Community-Based Care for Drug-Dependent Mothers and Their Children, 1993. Used with permission.

However, without them, families are unable to access the most critical services.

Column 3: Medical Substance Abuse Services

While methadone maintenance is the standard of care in the U.S. for pregnant heroin addicts, not all experts agree. The practice of transferring heroin users to methadone in order to improve fetal growth and outcome is the subject of debate (Robbins & Mills, 1993); see Chapter 2 for a detailed discussion of the effects of heroin and methadone on the developing child. Indeed, other health care systems outside the United States do not subscribe to this practice. For example, the British National Health Service (NHS) would rather provide expensive in-hospital detoxification for an addicted mother than subject the child to the painful withdrawal associated with prenatal methadone maintenance (Joyce, 1995).

Detoxification

Although cocaine does not produce a classic withdrawal syndrome, a pronounced craving for the substance does occur upon cessation. The "crash" or postintoxication period gradually progresses from intense craving to symptoms of clinical depression. This period often produces increased risk for suicide. After the depressive phase of the crash, craving may return and be present for weeks or months (Mitchell, 1993).

The use of psychotropics to withdraw a pregnant mother must be considered on a case-by-case basis. Their effects on the mother and fetus must be taken into account, particularly with respect to the potential for teratogenic effects and to possible interactions with other drugs, such as methadone.

Behavioral management techniques are used to minimize the need for medication whenever possible. Although it is clear that cessation of the use of cocaine during pregnancy is best, the timing of withdrawal is important to the well-being of the mother and her child. Most experts believe withdrawal treatment in the second trimester is the most desirable, since the fetus can be monitored more effectively at that time. Although withdrawal treatment in the first or third trimester has been reported to cause the fetus to abort, motivated women have been withdrawn throughout pregnancy without complications (Robbins & Mills, 1993).

The pharmacological understanding of cocaine guides the treatment for intoxication and chronic abuse. For example the neurotransmitters, dopamine and norepinephrine, are directly affected by cocaine. The immediate intoxication and subsequent potential for psychotic or depressive responses can, in part, be explained by a dysregulation of these neurotransmitters in the brain. Antidepressants have been shown to be effective in preventing and treating these conditions. Unfortunately, antidepressant agents must be taken for at least 2 weeks to produce an effect. Therefore, the potential for relapse and need for behavioral intervention are great during this period. Acupuncture, an intervention that can be provided by a specially trained nurse, has also been useful for the amelioration of craving and other symptoms associated with cocaine use. Acupuncture is also safe as an adjunctive treatment for pregnant women (Mitchell, 1993).

Column 4: Substance Abuse Treatment Services

What constitutes appropriate treatment for addicted mothers goes well beyond the traditional Minnesota Model of 28-day treatment found so effective with White middle-class men or the Therapeutic Community Model of long-term residential treatment found so effective with male hard-core drug users. These models may be part of treatment, but to be effective, they must be provided in collaboration with other primary care and community services.

Column 5: Special Health Services

Prenatal care

According to the National Institute of Child Health and Human Development report to Congress (Robbins & Mills, 1993), the only scientific information now available concerning the prevention of adverse drug effects during pregnancy is the repeated observation that more prenatal care is associated with fewer adverse pregnancy and birth outcomes. The advantage of prenatal care may be explained by the differences between women who avail themselves of prenatal care and those who do not. Or it may be that prenatal care provides access to services that the woman needs to reduce or cease legal and illegal drug use, or to obtain treatment for infections, such as hepatitis, or sexually transmitted diseases (see chapter 5 for a complete discussion of health care needs). Pregnancy offers a critical opportunity, when addicted women may be more receptive to treatment that will benefit their babies. With rare exceptions, all mothers want to do what is best for their child. Despite this, very few prenatal services are designed to meet the needs of this population.

Pain during labor and delivery

Substance-abusing women often confuse the early signs of labor with signs of withdrawal, and medicate themselves with their drug of choice. If cocaine is used, labor may be stimulated. Therefore, it is important to ascertain an accurate recent drug history so that possible drug interactions during labor and delivery can be avoided. If self-medication has not occurred, analgesia and anesthesia administration during labor may include the same range of options available to all patients, with the following considerations: regional anesthesia may be the drug of choice; a higher dose of short-acting intramuscular narcotics may be required to compensate for tolerance to the drug, and methadone does not provide anesthesia (Mitchell, 1993).

Newborn withdrawal

Although "crack babies" have been erroneously described in the media as hopelessly addicted and suffering from withdrawal, experts believe it is inaccurate to use these terms (Zuckerman, 1991). The neurobehavioral functioning of the prenatally cocaine-exposed infant is not completely understood, because research findings are inconsistent.

Some cocaine-exposed infants can be poorly responsive and sleepy or irritable and hypersensitive to stimuli. However, it is not known whether these behaviors are due to a direct effect of cocaine, changes in the brain's neurotransmitters or withdrawal. Nevertheless, it is these behaviors that make the mother-child interaction less rewarding and more problematic.

Comorbid psychiatric problems

Although psychopharmacological treatment generally is contraindicated during pregnancy, it can be safely used to treat craving, depression, and anxiety after the infant is born. Many providers in the substance abuse treatment community, including members of the self-help community, object to the use of pharmacological treatment to assist in recovery (Institute of Medicine, 1990). This conflict is reflective of the lack of coordination between the substance abuse treatment system and the mental health treatment system.

Column 6: Aftercare Services

After the treatment of physical symptoms associated with substance dependence, women need ongoing counseling, drug-free living arrangements and the support of culturally sensitive self-help groups. In addition, they may need basic income assistance until they can function independently. These services may be needed for two years or longer.

Column 7: Family Services

Family preservation

Like so many interventions designed for intact middle-class families, traditional family therapy does not lend itself to the needs of addicted mothers and their children. A more practical approach is the family preservation model. The essential features of the family preservation model are: 24-hour, 7-day-a-week availability for families; small caseloads, usually not more than 2 families; services provided in the home; intervention focuses on family needs and strengths; short-term intensive services; and referral to support services and additional counseling.

From a policy perspective, family preservation interventions are timely. Congress has just enacted the Family Preservation and Family Support Act of 1993 (U.S. Congress. House. [1993]. Family Preservation and Family Support Act of 1993 contained in the Omnibus Budget Reconciliation Act of 1993. 1st sess. P.L. 103–66 103rd Cong. HR2264), which requires every state's highest court to examine why the family preservation tenets of the Adoption Assistance and Welfare Act of 1980 have not been fulfilled. The act directs courts to work with communities to develop strategies and programs that will serve families more comprehensively, while relieving overburdened court systems. Interdisciplinary teams help to develop practice models to accomplish the federal goals at the community level. In the very near future, all communities will be searching for reform strategies to conform to the law (U.S. Congress, 1993) (see Appendix B for Model Family Preservation Act Policy Statement).

Column 8: Educational and Vocational Services

Parenting skills

Drugs can disturb either side of the parent-child relationship by impairing the mother's ability to care for her child or by making the child irritable and difficult to care for. Prenatal drug abuse interferes with the normal regulation of the infant's prenatal physiologic processes; and postnatal drug abuse impairs the mother's ability to communicate and respond to the infant. Parent education can begin as soon as possible after the birth to promote effective caregiving and to prevent compounding the problems of the infant already at risk. It is important that a mother be told her infant's strengths as well as the weaknesses. The mother or caregiver can be taught to help the infant to relax by avoiding excessive handling and by protecting it from bright lights and noise.

Secondary prevention interventions have been designed to promote the attachment relationship, establish interactive reciprocity, and develop a communicative dialogue between mother and child. These techniques are critical to overcoming developmental delays. After the infant is stable at home, care should continue through a high-risk followup clinic, parent support groups, community liaison, and case management.

The preschool and school-aged child. As the delivery of primary health care becomes increasingly more available in school settings, health care providers and teachers can work together to provide the best educational strategies for drug-exposed children. Because many of these children come from poorly organized environments which lack nurturance and structure, it is important to view the child's behaviors as a deficit in learning, rather than as misconduct which requires special education.

Labeling a 3- or 4-year-old child as "drug-exposed" is the most detrimental thing society can do. In Chapter Ten, Lardner discusses this issue in depth. Even if a child was prenatally exposed to drugs, current physical or emotional problems may be due to other causes. It is more effective to focus on behaviors that signal risk for problems and school failure.

Teachers need to be aware of strategies that work with this population. For example, the traditional way to deal with children who appear to be disruptive is to isolate them from the group or give them "time out." The real danger of this practice is the negative self-image that it fosters within young children who have not learned to separate the deed from their own self-worth. Many of these children have experienced such inconsistent punishment that they do not know which behaviors are acceptable and which are not. Early childhood programs such as Head Start are an excellent place to begin teaching organizational skills while interjecting structure and predictability.

The successful programs that intervene with drug-exposed children and other vulnerable populations emphasize a strong relationship between program staff and each child and family. These programs provide a low adult-child ratio to promote the child's attachment and learning. They also establish a partnership with the mother or caregiver, both to role model respect and nurturance in interactions with the child and to provide support for the family.

Although some policymakers have made attempts to address the problem of perinatal addiction and drug-exposed children, little progress has been made in reaching a consensus on a national policy. Indeed, state and federal policies often collide in their effort to deter addictive behavior among parents in an effort to protect their children.

Criminal Punishment as a Deterrent

Because community services, as described above in Step 2, often are unavailable or inadequate to meet the needs of these families, informal support networks often erode, bringing deterioration and eventual child abuse and neglect charges against the parents. Many judges would like to order assistance that would strengthen these families, however, the courts have few tools to guide them in determining the safety of the home environment and the treatment needs of the family. Kelleher, Chaffin, Hollenberg & Fisher (1994) report that maltreating parents rarely receive a substance abuse evaluation, and that of those who are diagnosed, less that half are referred to substance abuse treatment.

Today over one million people are incarcerated in the U.S. This figure represents a doubling of the prison population, including a tripling of the female population, since 1980, an increase primarily due to non-violent drug-related offenses. Most of these women are mothers of small children (Kline, 1992).

In addition, due to the backlog in family courts, court-ordered treatment may be delayed for a year or longer. The inability of the courts to respond to these families in more efficient ways leads to punitive solutions, which often further traumatize the children. Today, half a million children live in foster homes—more than at any time in history. Neglect and caretaker absence account for the increase in these placements—eight out of ten involve parental drug problems (GAO, 1994).

Laws that punish addicted mothers are designed to deter drug use, but they also inhibit addicted women from seeking essential prenatal care, for fear of losing custody of their children. In prison, addicted pregnant women receive limited health care that often fails to meet their needs for prenatal care and drug treatment. The vast majority of addicted inmates lack access to drug treatment programs, and studies show that women continue to obtain drugs behind bars. In Washington, DC, recently, 10 Department of Corrections officers were charged with taking bribes (often consisting of sexual activity) from inmates at the DC jail in return for providing them with cocaine (York & Castaneda,

1993). Such conditions raise questions about the wisdom of incarcerating pregnant and drug-addicted women and the goal of protecting the unborn fetus.

To date, no national standards have been set in place for addressing the medical and drug treatment needs of female offenders, pregnant or otherwise, with or without HIV infection. Nor has there been any federal program targeting drug abuse research or treatment for women inmates, though there have been some initiatives in this direction. For example, the women's prison facility at Rikers Island in New York, has programs to address the comprehensive needs of its inmates. Of the 14,000 women in this facility, 25% suffer from syphilis; 25% have a current mental illness; 75% are drug abusers; 27% are HIV-positive; and 10% are pregnant. To address these health problems, the Rikers Health Service has expanded to provide health education and prevention programs as well as treatment. Although Rikers tries to connect the women with community services when they are discharged, the referral often fails because inmates lose eligibility for Medicaid benefits while in prison and have no way to pay for continued treatment (Ragghianti, 1994).

IMPACT ON CHILDREN

The children in families with addicted parents have been seriously affected by the policies which punish mothers, children placed in foster care experience serious disruptions in relationships and home environments. Children cared for in kinship arrangements with a grandmother or great-grandmother also may experience a strained and chaotic home environment (Howard, Beckwith, Rodning & Kropenske, 1989).

STEP 4: EVALUATE THE ALTERNATIVE POLICY

To evaluate the alternative policies, we will apply the following criteria: effectiveness, cost, equity and political viability. Below is a comparison of the criminal punishment as deterrent approach versus the public health harm reduction approach.

POLICY FAILURES

For the most part, policies have failed to make much of an overall difference in the problem of perinatal addiction. National antidrug efforts

TABLE 1.1 Comparison of Policy Alternatives

Evaluation criteria	Deterrence approaches	Harm reduction approaches
objectives	to use punishment in order to deter pregnant women fom using drugs	to assist pregnant women to make life-style changes that will reduce harm to their child
	to define prenatal drug use as child abuse or as a criminal offense	to promote prevention, treatment and educational interventions
effectiveness	**protecting babies from drug-exposure**	
	incarceration of mothers and foster care placement of children are the most common outcomes of deterrence approaches	research data indicate that mothers are very motivated to be drug-free while pregnant
	drugs are readily available in prison and there are no standards of care for pregnant women with drug problems	most babies are born without teratogenic effects if their mothers receive treatment
	foster care, which often involves multiple placement, compounds the stress on the child	children do overcome many developmental delays associated with maternal drug use with early intervention
cost	foster care per child averages $14,000 annually[1]	community-based primary care and substance abuse treatment for one child and mother cost $7,000[4]
	juvenile justice placements for older children can cost up to $70,000 annually[2]	therapeutic community residential drug treatment costs $50,000 for one mother and child[5]
	incarceration costs for one inmate per year averages $19,120[3]	

1. State of Maryland unpublished data, 1993.
2. State of New York unpublished data, 1993.
3. Criminal Justice Institute, *The Corrections Year Book*, 1993.
4. State of Missouri CSTAR program unpublished data, 1993.
5. Operation PAR St. Petersburg, Florida, unpublished data, 1993.

are fragmented and lack a strategy to combat the problem. The complexity and lack of coordinated government funding for health services hinder these families from obtaining the comprehensive care they need. While the U.S. conducts some of the most sophisticated drug research in the world, that research does not always translate into service delivery systems. Indeed, pregnant addicted women and their children have been historically a vulnerable population, mostly residing in medically underserved areas (Aday, 1993).

U.S. POLICIES DIFFER FROM THOSE OF OTHER WESTERN COUNTRIES

In countries where primary health care services are available to all citizens, it is more likely that addicted women will be treated earlier in their drug-taking careers. The U.S. is the only Western country that prosecutes addicted pregnant women for using drugs while pregnant. In most of Western Europe, pregnant addicted women not only have access to basic primary care for themselves and their children, but they also have access to drug treatment.

BARRIERS TO PRIMARY AND SECONDARY PREVENTION

While much is known about the prevention of the effects of perinatal drug use, many barriers exist to the provision of care for these families. The most effective way to prevent prenatal drug exposure is to help the mother to be drug free. As basic as this premise may seem, very few communities have adequate services to accomplish this end.

FEAR OF LEGAL LIABILITY

A survey of 78 drug treatment programs in New York City found that 54% denied treatment to pregnant women (GAO, 1990). One of the primary reasons cited for refusing treatment to pregnant women was the issue of legal liability.

INSURANCE COVERAGE

Medicaid will cover almost all hospital-based services. In the case of drug treatment, however, Medicaid usually covers detoxification up to 5 days, which is not adequate for detoxification of most drugs during pregnancy. Follow-up care in a residential treatment program is also rare. Darnell reviews funding resources in chapter 8.

MOST DRUG TREATMENT IS DESIGNED FOR MEN

Treatment needs of pregnant and parenting women are more complex than those of men. Many pregnant and parenting women with substance abuse problems have multiple diagnoses and require treatment for hepatitis, tuberculosis, and sexually transmitted diseases, which are difficult to accommodate within existing treatment programs. Providing ancillary services, such as dental care, is also problematic because of the high risk of AIDS among drug populations. The delay in obtaining Medicaid benefits also interferes with the procurement of family planning services such as Norplant and tubal ligations.

LACK OF PSYCHIATRIC SERVICES

The ability to address the mental health needs of addicted pregnant women requires specialized staff and services. Women using alcohol and other drugs during pregnancy often face the simultaneous stresses of poverty, addiction, and new motherhood without adequate support and social resources to assist them. As part of the problem that leads to and results from substance abuse, many women suffer from low self-esteem, anxiety, and depression. The lack of appropriate mental health treatment leads to relapse and treatment failure.

COMMUNITY RESISTANCE TO DRUG TREATMENT PROGRAMS

Establishing treatment centers for addicted pregnant women inevitably confronts the NIMBY ("not in my back yard") phenomenon. While the need for substance abuse treatment centers is great, people needing treatment are often seen as undesirable and dangerous. Moreover, communities are often fearful that the presence of substance abuse treatment centers will encourage and foster increased drug use or present dangers for children and other adults. This fear contributes to the maintenance of substance abuse treatment programs as satellites of mainstream medical and mental health services and ultimately encourages a climate of mistrust and lack of coordination between substance abuse treatment and mental health services.

STEP 5: SELECT THE PREFERRED POLICY

Those programs that successfully navigate the funding maze and overcome the punitive state policies to piece together exemplary programs do so with impressive ingenuity, sophistication, and financial and administrative resources. One such program is CSTAR (Comprehensive Substance Treatment and Rehabilitation), a Missouri State program. Figure 1.3 displays the services provided under CSTAR. The funding of CSTAR is unique to the communities it serves and is an example of creative use of available community resources.

THE CSTAR PROGRAM

CSTAR is a Missouri Alcohol and Drug Administration (ADA) approach to community-based, long-term drug abuse treatment for all addicted Missouri residents, including pregnant women and their children. One of the most innovative state substance abuse programs in the country, the program is designed to provide holistic treatment and support to anyone with a drug abuse problem in the state. Most of the substance abuse treatment is provided on an outpatient basis with supportive housing.

By shifting from a provider-driven to a client-driven treatment philosophy, the Missouri Department of Mental Health allowed CSTAR's services to be restructured to meet eligibility criteria for Medicaid reimbursement. A major restructuring of services and a seamless system of electronic processing enables all CSTAR providers to transmit data and invoices electronically to ADA. The system permits most services then to be reimbursed directly through Medicaid or other sources.

Clients and services ineligible for Medicaid are automatically identified and directed through the unique fiscal and billing system to the proper funding source. For example, child care and rental assistance are usually reimbursed through substance abuse block grants funded through the state. CSTAR is innovative not only in the comprehensive services it provides, but in its creative use of federal funding sources. The restructuring of services and the extra money from Medicaid made it possible to provide comprehensive treatment for pregnant women and their children. Between 1991 and 1994, CSTAR reported 522 babies born drugfree and 692 foster children returned to their families (Stuart, 1995). The program is an elegant example of how Medicaid and federal

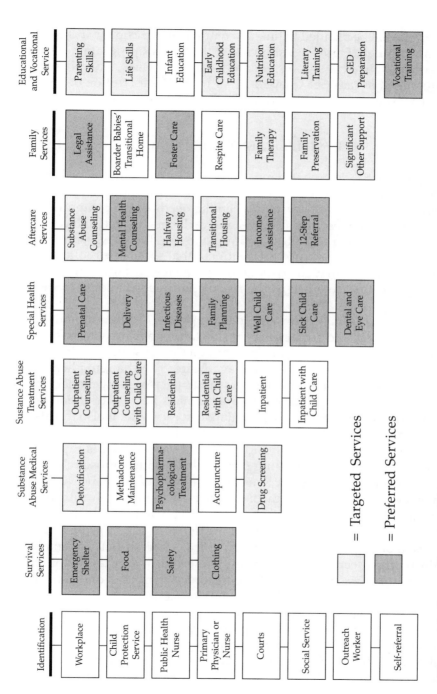

Figure 1.3 Comprehensive Substance Treatment and Rehabilitation Program (CSTAR), State of Missouri

Sources: Haack-Darnell Model of Community-Based Care for Drug-Dependent Mothers and Their Children, 1993. Used with permission.

block grants can be blended to finance comprehensive care for addicted pregnant women. Figure 1.3 shows that the CSTAR program nearly approximates the evaluation standard set by the Haack, Darnell and Budetti model of care. See Chapter 12 for Jordon's description of how the CSTAR program was created.

STEP 6: IMPLEMENT THE POLICY

Although the CSTAR program meets the standard of care set forth by our model, it is only one example of what can be accomplished within the public health delivery system when the needs of the community determine how the resources of the state can be maximized and coordinated. The funding of CSTAR is unique to the state of Missouri. It is presented not as an example of treatment that should be replicated throughout the country, since that may not be feasible, but rather as an example of creative use of the fiscal resources available to the state.

As states, cities, and communities grapple with the immediate financial, medical, and social needs of substance-abusing women and their children, policymakers and communities must struggle with the prospect of welfare reform and managed care. The changing health care delivery system provides an opportunity to create new models of care and new roles for public health practitioners in the prevention of the deleterious consequences of prenatal drug exposure. It also threatens to dismantle proven models such as CSTAR.

Before the advent of Medicaid managed care (which is rapidly becoming the source for funding perinatal substance-abuse related services), the case management and coordination of substance abuse treatment with other essential medical services was extremely difficult. Except in states like Missouri, which totally restructured their treatment system, most states have found the delivery of comprehensive services to be impossible. As a consequence, when addicted women sought prenatal care, rarely were they referred to substance abuse treatment. Likewise, substance abuse treatment personnel often failed to coordinate their services with prenatal services.

Within the changing health care environment, however, Medicaid managed care providers may be expected to deliver case management for necessary services even when they are not covered services. Unlike traditional Medicaid coverage, coverage through managed care enrollment creates a duty on the part of managed care plans to ensure access to covered services. Under waivers granted by the Secretary of HHS under Section 1115 of the Social Security Act, certain federal Medicaid payment restrictions have been lifted, thereby making coverage of substance abuse services more possible. See Chapter 8 for a full discussion of Medicaid. Moreover, the conceptual hallmark of managed care is prevention and early intervention to avert long-term health costs. Given the financial and health implications of perinatal substance abuse, managed care plans might be expected to promote access to services designed to ameliorate its effects. The full impact of Medicaid managed care cannot be predicted at this time.

CONCLUSIONS

If the public health system is to seize the opportunities presented by privatizing services through Medicaid managed care, public health workers will need to know how to negotiate contracts that maximize the potential for a comprehensive health care delivery system that accommodates the needs of pregnant addicted women and their children. With the shift to managed care comes the opportunity to create new treatment systems that can build on the lessons learned from the CSTAR program and from federally sponsored demonstration projects throughout the country.

The public policy and public health systems are critically involved in the development of effective solutions to the complex problem of drug-affected children and their families. It is clear that no one institution, agency, or discipline can provide a comprehensive model of care for addicted mothers and their children. Solutions must go beyond the eradication of a drug within a pregnant woman or the jailing of an addicted pregnant woman. The barriers to achieving these solutions reflect the weakest links of our social, medical and mental health service delivery service system. The ability to deliver comprehensive care to addicted mothers and their families requires contributions from every aspect of the public policy and public health care systems.

REFERENCES

Aday, L. (1993). *At risk in America: The health and health care needs of vulnerable populations in the United States.* San Francisco, CA: Jossey-Bass, Inc.

Centers for Disease Control and Prevention (1993). *HIV/AIDS Surveillance Report.* 5:3, 2–3.

Chasnoff, I. J., Landress, H. J., & Barrett, M. E. (1990). The prevalence of illicit drug and alcohol use during pregnancy and discrepancies in mandatory reporting in Pinellas County, Florida. *New England Journal of Medicine, 322,* 102–106.

Conners, S. (1992–1993). Medicaid Working Group. Data from patients with advanced-stage AIDS enrolled in Community Medical Alliance, Santa Barbara, California.

Davis, D. L. (1991). Parental smoking and fetal health. *The Lancet, 337*(12), 123.

Frank, D. A., Zukerman, B. S., Amaro, H., Aboagye, K., Bauchner, H., Cabral, H., Fried, L., Hingson, R., Kayne, H., & Levenson, S. M. (1988). Cocaine use during pregnancy: Prevalence and correlates. *Pediatrics, 82,* 888–895.

General Accounting Office (1990). *Prenatal care: Medicaid recipients and uninsured women obtain insufficient care* (GAO Publication No.HRD 87–137). Washington, DC: U.S. General Accounting Office.

Haack, M. R., Budetti, P., Darnell, J., & Hudman, J. (1993). *An analysis of resources to aid drug-exposed infants and their families.* Washington, DC: The George Washington University Center for Health Policy Research.

Howard, J., Beckwith, L., Rodning, C., & Kropenske, V. (1989). The development of young children of substance-abusing parents: Insights from seven years of intervention and research. *Zero to Three, 9*(5), 8–12.

Institute of Medicine. (1990). *Broadening the base of treatment for alcohol problems.* Washington, DC: National Academy Press.

Jordon, L. (1995, May). Personal Communication.

Joyce, E. (1995, June 23). Personal Communication.

Kelleher, K., Chaffin, M., Hollenberg, J., & Fisher, E. (1994). Alcohol and drug disorders among physically abusive and neglectful parents in a community-based sample. *American Journal of Public Health, 84,* 1586–1590.

Kline, S. (1992). A profile of female offenders in the Federal Bureau of Prisons. *Federal Prisons Journal, 3*(1), 33–35.

Kokotailo, P. K., Adgar, H., Duggan, A. K., Repke, J., & Joffe, A. (1992). Cigarette, alcohol, and other drug use by school-age, pregnant adolescents: Prevalence, detection, and associated risk factors. *Pediatrics, 90*(3), 328–334.

Kronstadt, D. (1991). Complex developmental issues of prenatal drug exposure. *The future of children, 1*(1), 36–49.

Maslow, A. H. (1954). *Motivation and personality.* New York: Harper and Row.

Mitchell J. L. (1993). *Pregnant, substance-using women: Treatment improvement protocol 2.* Rockville, MD: Center for Substance Abuse Treatment.

National Association for Perinatal Addiction Research and Education. (1988). A first: National hospital incidence survey. In: *Perinatal addiction research and education update.* Chicago, IL: National Association for Perinatal Addiction Research and Education.

National Association of State Alcohol and Drug Abuse Directors (1993). Unpublished statistical data. Washington, DC: Author.

National Institute on Drug Abuse (1991). *National Household Survey on Drug Abuse 1990.* Rockville, MD: Author.

National Institute on Drug Abuse (NIDA) (1994). Technical review conducted by the Perinatal 20 on a program of treatment research on drug-exposed women and their children. West Palm Beach, Florida.

Office for Substance Abuse Prevention. (1992). *Identifying the needs of drug-affected children* (OSAP Prevention Monograph 11). Rockville, MD: Author.

Olegard, R. (1992). Alcohol and Narcotics—Epidemiology and Pregnancy Risks. *International Journal of Technology Assessment in Health Care, 8(Supplement 1),* 101–105.

Patton, C. V., & Sawicki, D. S. (1993). *Basic methods of policy analysis and planning.* Englewood Cliffs, NJ: Prentice Hall, 2–5.

Racine, A., Joyce, T., & Anderson, R. (1993). The association between prenatal care and birth weight amond women exposed to cocaine in New York City. *Journal of the American Medical Association, 270,* 1581–1586.

Ragghianti, M. (1994, February 6). Save the innocent victims of prison. *Parade Magazine,* 14–15.

Robbins, L. N., & Mills, J. L. (1993). Effects of in utero exposure to street drugs. *American Journal of Public Health, 83*(supplement to vol.83), 3–32.

Shalala, Donna. (Secretary of the Department of Health and Human Services). (1996). *C-Span.* Washington, DC.

Schwartz, R. H. (1989). Passive inhalation of marijuana, phencyclidine, and free base cocaine ("crack") by infants. *American Journal of Diseases of Children, 143*(6), 644.

Southern Regional Project on Infant Mortality (1993). Study examines access to substance abuse treatment for women. *Special Delivery, 3*(1).

Stuart, E. (1995, May). Missouri says "yes" to drug-free births. *State Government News,* 25–27.

Suffett, F., & Brotman, R. A comprehensive care program for pregnant addicts: Obstetrical, neonatal and child development outcomes. *International Journal of Addictions, 19,* 199–219.

United Nations International Children's Educational Fund. (1992). *State of the world's children.* New York: Author, 23–24.

U.S. Department of Health and Human Services. (1992). *Healthy People 2000: National health promotion and disease prevention objectives.* Washington, DC: Author

U.S. Congress. House. (1993). *FP & FSA of 1993* contained in the OBRA of 1993. HR 2664. 103rd Congress, 1st session.

Volpe, J. J. (1992). Mechanisms of disease: Effect of cocaine use on the fetus.

New England Journal of Medicine, 327(6), 399–407.

Werner, E. E. (1989). Children of the garden island. *Scientific American, 260*(4), 106–111.

York, M. & Castaneda, R. (1993, Dec. 15). 12 on DC Force Arrested in Corruption Probe. *The Washington Post,* pp. A1, A19.

Zellman, G. L., Jacobson, P. D., DuPlesis, H., & DiMatteo, M. R. (1992). Health care system response to prenatal substance use: An exploratory analysis. *Rand Drug Policy Research Center.* Santa Monica, CA: Author.

Zuckerman, B. (1991). Drug-exposed infants: Understanding the medical risks. *The Future of Children, 1*(1), 26–34.

Zuckerman, B., Frank, D. A., Hingson, R., Levenson, S. M., Kayne, H., Parker, S., Amaro, H., Aboagye, K., Vinci, R., & Fried, L. (1989). Effects of maternal marijuana and cocaine use on fetal growth. *New England Journal of Medicine, 320*(12), 762–768.

PART I

Issues in Public Health

2

Teratogenic Effects of *In Utero* Exposure to Alcohol and Other Abusable Psychotropics

Ann Marie Pagliaro, R.N., and
Louis A. Pagliaro, Ph.D.

INTRODUCTION

This chapter focuses on the abusable psychotropics (Table 2.1) as human teratogens. The word "teratogen" is derived from the Greek words "terato," monster, and "genesis," origin or beginning. A teratogen is broadly defined as any factor (e.g., drug) associated with the production of physical or mental abnormalities in the developing embryo or fetus. It is estimated that some type of teratogenic effect can be found in 2 to 3% of all live births and that teratogenic effects, at least in part, account for 20% of the deaths that occur during the first 5 years of life. These effects, which can be acute and self-limiting or irreversible and long-term, may be displayed in a variety of ways among developing infants and children (Pagliaro & Pagliaro, 1995).

The type and degree of human teratogenic effects has been associated with many factors, including genetic, maternal/fetal environmental and unknown factors. The maternal/fetal environmental factors can be further categorized as concerned with radiation, disease, infections, and drugs. Although many prescribers and other health care providers are paying closer attention to the potential teratogenic effects associated with the use of selected drugs during pregnancy (see

31

TABLE 2.1   Major Abusable Psychotropics

Central Nervous System Depressants
> Opiates (e.g., codeine, heroin, meperidine, morphine,
>   pentazocine)
> Sedative-Hypnotics (e.g., alcohol [beer, wine, distilled
>   spirits]; barbiturates; benzodiazepines; miscellaneous)
> Volatile Solvents and Inhalants (e.g., gasoline; glue)

Central Nervous System Stimulants
> Amphetamines (e.g., dextroamphetamine)
> Caffeine (e.g., caffeinated soft drinks; coffee, tea)
> Cocaine (e.g., cocaine hydrochloride; crack cocaine)
> Nicotine (e.g., tobacco, cigarettes and cigars)

Psychedelics (partial list)
> Lysergic acid diethylamide (LSD)
> Mescaline (Peyote)
> Phencyclidine (PCP)
> Psilocybin (hallucinogenic mushrooms)
> Tetrahydrocannabinol (THC) (e.g., hashish; hashish oil;
>   marijuana)

Pagliaro & Pagliaro, 1995), their general knowledge and understanding of the possible teratogenic effects associated with the abusable psychotropics may be limited.

This chapter summarizes the results of published research and case reports examining the teratogenic effects associated with maternal abusable psychotropic use during pregnancy. Attention is given to human studies only because of the inherent difficulties associated with extrapolating data from animal studies to humans, including the determination of physiologic and genetic differences in teratogenic susceptibility and the establishment of comparable doses, stages of pregnancy, environmental conditions, ages, and health status (Hemminki & Vineis, 1985). A classic example of the problems associated with the extrapolation of the results of animal studies to humans is the thalidomide tragedy. When thalidomide was tested in several pregnant rodent species, no teratogenic effects were noted. However, when thalidomide was used by women during their first trimester of pregnancy to treat anxiety and insomnia, devastating teratogenic effects were produced (What Lessons, 1983).

PREVALENCE OF MATERNAL USE OF ABUSABLE PSYCHOTROPICS

Many adolescent girls and women use one or more of the abusable psychotropics some time during their pregnancies; the drug used is determined primarily by such factors as age, race, and socioeconomic status (Cornelius et al., 1993; Jorgensen, 1992; Wheeler, 1993). However, a reliable estimate of the nature and extent of abusable psychotropic use among this population group is not available. There are many reasons for this lack of data regarding maternal abusable psychotropic use. These include the fact that many abusable psychotropics (e.g., cocaine, heroin, marijuana) are illegal and, thus, their use is hidden or underreported. Although the moderate use of a particular abusable psychotropic may have limited harmful effects for the mother, it may be extremely toxic and pose high risk to the developing embryo or fetus as a result of differences in maternal and fetal metabolism, concentration, tissue sensitivity, and a variety of other factors that preclude a single direct cause-effect relationship (Griffith, Azuma, & Chasnoff, 1994).

Attention to the types of abusable psychotropics used and their patterns of use is important in order to retrospectively identify teratogenic risk to the developing embryo and fetus. Although there are limitations to this type of research, human teratogenic experiments cannot be ethically performed and the results of experiments involving animal models, as previously noted, cannot be relied upon to determine human teratogenic potential. In order to better identify the teratogenic risk associated with maternal abusable psychotropic use, attention must be given to the interaction of several factors including maternal factors (e.g., general health, maternal dose); placental factors; fetal factors (e.g., stage of fetal development); environmental factors; and specific abusable psychotropic factors (Cordier, Ha, Ayme, & Goujard, 1992; Pagliaro & Pagliaro, 1995; Van Allen, 1992) (Figure 2.1).

Maternal factors include uterine blood flow, concomitant medical conditions (e.g., diabetes, epilepsy, infections, thyroid disorders), and general health. Placental factors include the size and thickness of the placenta, placental blood flow, ability of the placenta to metabolize the abusable psychotropic to an inactive, active, or teratogenic metabolite, and placental age. Fetal factors include the stage of fetal development, the status of hepatic drug-metabolizing systems, the amount of hepatic blood flow through the ductus venosus, fetal blood pH, genetic predisposition, and concomitant exposure to other potential teratogens.

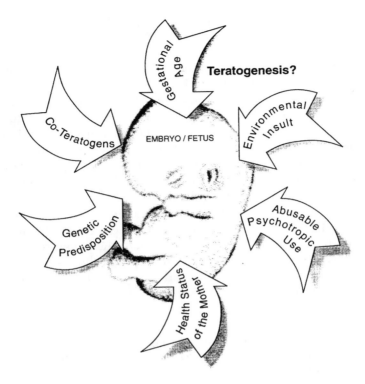

Figure 2.1 Various Factors Associated with Teratogenesis

Environmental factors include food additives (e.g., aspartame and nitrates), pesticides (e.g., chlordane), air and water pollutants, radiation, and toxins (e.g., mercury and organic solvents). Abusable psychotropic factors include the amount, frequency, and method of maternal use; distribution (concentration), metabolism and excretion; lipid solubility (partition coefficient); degree of ionization (pKa); molecular weight; concentration of free (nonprotein bound) drug; and the basic pharmacology (Gilbody, 1991; Pagliaro & Pagliaro, 1995).

However, of all the factors identified as being involved in producing a particular teratogenic effect, the most important factor is timing in regard to organogenesis (Figure 2.2). There is a critical period of greatest teratogenic susceptibility. Although this critical period of susceptibility varies slightly among different organ systems, teratogenic effects associated with major physical malformations are generally induced during the first trimester. It is important to note that teratogenic

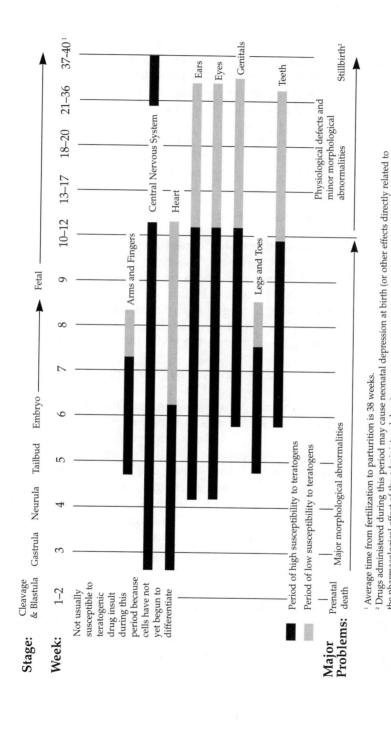

Figure 2.2   Critical Periods for Teratogenic Effect in Relation to Human Organogenesis

effects will not occur if exposure to a particular abusable psychotropic occurs after organogenesis is complete. For example, the maternal use of diazepam during pregnancy has been implicated in cleft palate anomaly. However, this teratogenic effect would not be observed if diazepam was used during pregnancy after fusion of the fetal palate. Thus, when evaluating the possible teratogenic potential of a particular abusable psychotropic, it is essential to identify if the abusable psychotropic, or another in the same class, has been implicated in producing a human teratogenic effect and the stage of embryo and fetal development at which time the exposure occurred.

TERATOGENIC EFFECTS OF ABUSABLE PSYCHOTROPICS

The potential teratogenic effects associated with alcohol and other abusable drugs are summarized below. The drugs discussed have been grouped in relation to their major psychotropic effects (i.e., CNS depressants, CNS stimulants, Psychedelics). Within each of these major sections, they have been further arranged in alphabetical order according to their nonproprietary United States Adopted Names. Commonly used brand names have been included in order to facilitate access to needed information.

The use of alcohol or other abusable psychotropics during pregnancy always involves some degree of risk to the developing embryo or fetus. Therefore, regardless of how safe an abusable psychotropic may appear to be, it should *not* be used during pregnancy unless it is clearly indicated and its benefits outweigh its potential risks. Adolescent girls and women who are pregnant or thinking about becoming pregnant should be encouraged to limit their use of the abusable psychotropics. Adolescent girls and women who display problematic patterns of abusable psychotropic use (e.g., abuse or compulsive use) should be referred to treatment programs aimed at promoting nonuse or, in the event that use has been discontinued, relapse prevention.

CENTRAL NERVOUS SYSTEM DEPRESSANTS

The central nervous system depressants discussed in this section include the opiates and sedative-hypnotics. Although the central nervous system depressants have been associated with various levels of teratogenic risk, data accumulated over the last several decades only support a particularly strong relationship for the sedative-hypnotic, alcohol. For this reason, a more comprehensive discussion of alcohol has been included. No reports of cases involving maternal solvent and inhalant use (e.g., gasoline, glue) were found. However, as with the other abusable psychotropics, the associated pharmacologic effects would be expected to occur in the neonate if solvents and inhalants were used by the mother near term.

OPIATES

Several cases have been reported implicating teratogenic insult with maternal opiate use during pregnancy. However, a review of this literature provides only weak support for teratogenic effects involving codeine, heroin, meperidine (Demerol®), methadone, morphine, and pentazocine (Talwin®).

Heroin

Maternal heroin use during pregnancy has been associated with many problems for the fetus and newborn; however, teratogenesis does not appear to be one of them. Although intrauterine growth retardation is common among infants born to heroin-addicted mothers, this effect has not been consistently reported. Neonates exposed to heroin near term commonly experience the heroin withdrawal syndrome. A 13.5% first-year mortality rate also has been reported for these neonates, as has an increased incidence of the Sudden Infant Death Syndrome (SIDS). However, these data are confounded because mothers who use heroin during pregnancy frequently use alcohol, cocaine, nicotine, and other abusable psychotropics (see below under "Alcohol and Nicotine"). Whereas intrauterine growth retardation has been attributed by some researchers to a decreased cell number, this finding also can be related to such confounding variables as poor maternal nutrition and the use of other abusable psychotropics.

Methadone (Dolophine®)

The maternal use of methadone during pregnancy has not been associated with physical abnormalities among neonates. However, these infants may be small for their gestational ages, an effect that has not been consistently reported and which a more recent study has attributed to confounding variables, such as poor maternal nutrition and concurrent alcohol and nicotine use. About 80% of infants born to mothers who have used methadone during their pregnancies experience the methadone withdrawal syndrome. Convulsions during unmedicated withdrawal occur more frequently among these neonates than among those neonates exposed *in utero* to heroin. Although data are conflicting, the Sudden Infant Death Syndrome (SIDS) also has been associated with methadone exposure *in utero*, which may be explained by a decreased ventilatory response to carbon dioxide among these infants. However, as with other effects, the interpretation of SIDS data is complicated by maternal alcohol and nicotine use during pregnancy, particularly because there has been a reported relationship between tobacco smoke and SIDS.

Whenever possible, adolescent girls and women who use methadone, including adolescent girls and women enrolled in methadone maintenance programs, should undergo detoxification before becoming pregnant. If methadone detoxification is to be used, it should be attempted between the 14th and 28th week of gestation with a slow tapering of the dosage. Methadone detoxification during the first trimester has been associated with an increased incidence of spontaneous abortions. When attempted during the third trimester, methadone detoxification has been associated with fetal distress.

ALCOHOL

Alcohol (ethanol; ethyl alcohol) is a known human teratogen. As such, it has the potential to affect all fetuses of mothers who consume it during their pregnancies (Day & Richardson, 1991; Larroque, 1992). Once ingested and absorbed into the bloodstream, alcohol crosses readily from the maternal circulation to the fetal circulation (Pagliaro & Pagliaro, 1995). It is also found in significant levels in the amniotic fluid even after the ingestion of a single moderate dose. Alcohol is "eliminated from the amniotic fluid at one-half the elimination rate from the maternal blood." Thus, alcohol remains in the amniotic fluid and fetal circulation after "there is none present in the maternal blood stream" (Tranmer, 1985, pp. 489–490).

Unfortunately, many adolescent girls and women drink quantities of alcohol that are known to be harmful to their unborn babies (Cornelius et al., 1994; Leonard, Boettcher, & Brust, 1991; Substance abuse, 1994). In fact, the National Institute on Alcohol Abuse and Alcoholism (1987) has estimated this number to be approximately 16% or one out of six women of childbearing age. Based upon a comprehensive and extensive review of the literature, this figure could be conservatively increased by 50 to 100% to approximately 1 out of 3 to 4 adolescent girls and women of childbearing age. However, even if there is a lack of agreement regarding the exact percentage of fetuses at risk, there is consensus that the Fetal Alcohol Syndrome (FAS) is currently the leading cause of mental retardation and is totally preventable (Pagliaro & Pagliaro, 1995).

Fetal Alcohol Syndrome

The teratogenic effects associated with the use of alcohol during pregnancy have been long known. However, the specific physical, mental, and developmental characteristics associated with the FAS were not formally identified until the early 1970s (Jones, Smith, Ulleland, & Streussguth, 1973) (Table 2.2). Subsequently, clinicians and scientists have used this list of physical characteristics, particularly the associated craniofacial features (Figure 2.3), to assist them with the identification of affected infants and children. Although the characteristic features of the FAS vary among affected children and can present difficulties in clinical identification (Edwards, 1981; Little, Snell, & Rosenfeld, 1990), the consistent use of these general criteria has been found to be generally reliable for identifying the FAS (Abel, Martier, Kruger, Ager, & Sokol, 1993).

In addition to the use of these characteristics, a consensus case definition for the FAS was established by the Fetal Alcohol Study Group of the Research Society on Alcoholism (Sokol & Clarren, 1989). This consensus case definition includes the following three major criteria:

1. Prenatal and/or postnatal growth retardation (weight and/or length or height below the 10th percentile when corrected for gestational age);
2. Central nervous system involvement (including neurological abnormality, developmental delay, behavioral dysfunction or deficit, intellectual impairment and/or structural abnormalities, such as microcephaly [head circumference below the third percentile] or brain malformations found on imaging studies or autopsy); and
3. A characteristic face, currently qualitatively described as including short palpebral fissures, an elongated mid-face, a long and flattened philtrum, thin upper lip, and flattened maxilla. (p. 598)

The reported incidence of FAS (Table 2.3) has varied widely for a number of reasons including: unreliability of self-reports of maternal drinking (i.e., consistently biased underreporting) (Ernhart, Morrow-

TABLE 2.2 Abnormalities Associated with FAS*

Category	Abnormality	Percentage occurrence
Growth	Prenatal Growth Deficiency	100
Craniofacies	Short Palpebral Fissures	100
	Microcephaly	91
	Maxillary Hypoplasia	64
	Epicanthic Folds	36
	Micrognathia	27
	Cleft Palate	18
Development	Developmental Delay	100
	Postnatal Growth Deficiency	100
Limbs	Altered Palmar Crease Pattern	73
	Joint Anomalies	73
Heart	Cardiac Anomalies	70
Other	Fine-Motor Dysfunction	80
	Anomalous External Genitalia	36
	Capillary Hemangiomata	36

* This list is based on Jones et al. (1973) and has been expanded by several authors (e.g., Committee on Substance Abuse and Committee on Children with Disabilities, 1993; Pagliaro & Pagliaro, 1995) in order to account for additional features (e.g., asymmetrical or low-set ears; flat or absent philtrum; hypoplastic, flat midface; short nose; and thin vermilion of the upper lip) commonly noted by other researchers (e.g., Carones, Brancato, Venturi, Bianchi, & Magni, 1992; Clarren & Smith, 1978; Froster & Baird, 1992; Haddad & Messer, 1994; Lewis, 1983).

Tlucak, Sokol, & Martier, 1988); qualitative and quasiexperimental methods of data collection (e.g., case report, retrospective studies) (Abel & Sokol, 1987); and possible confusion, or overlap, with Fetal Alcohol Effects (FAE) (Remkes, 1993; Wallace, 1991). The incidence of the FAS in North America varies among cultural, ethnic, and social groups, with the highest incidence reported among Blacks and native Americans (Abel & Sokol, 1987, 1991; Burd & Moffatt, 1994; Gordis & Alexander, 1992).

FAE and FAS

"Fetal alcohol effects" is a term that is used to identify neonates and children who exhibit fewer of the characteristics deemed necessary, by definition or convention, for the establishment of a proper diagnosis of the FAS (Barbour, 1990; Burns, 1990; Caruso & Bensel, 1993; Ginsberg,

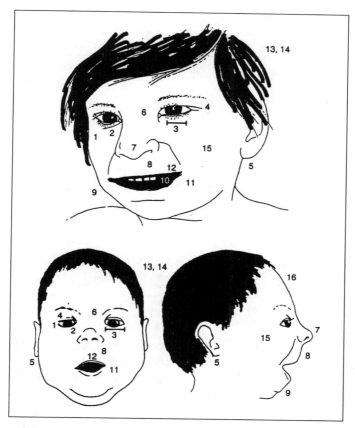

Figure 2.3

Eyes

1. ptosis (drooping lid)
2. strabismus (squint)
3. shortened palpebral
   fissure (opening between
   eyelids)
4. epicanthal fold

Ears

5. smaller or larger than
   normal, malformed,
   or low-set

Nose

6. low nasal bridge
7. short with high or upturned
   nasal tip

Mouth

8. philtrum (groove in upper lip):
   underdeveloped or absent
9. micrognathia (small jaw) or
   retrognathia (posteriorly
   displaced jaw)
10. teeth: absent enamel,
    malformed, or maloccluded
11. wide mouth
12. thin vermilion border of
    upper lip

Head

13. microcephaly (small head size)
14. abnormally shaped cranium
15. mid-face hypoplasia (broad,
    flat face)
16. narrow receding forehead

TABLE 2.3 Reported Incidence of FAS

Incidence*	Country (group)	Reference
1:8	Canada (Native Americans)	Robinson, Conry, and Conry, 1987
1:250	U.S.A. (Native Americans)	Duimstra et al., 1993
1:333–500	Europe (mixed)	Hill, Hegemier, & Tennyson, 1989
1:500	Worldwide (mixed)	Abel & Sokol, 1987
1:500–1000	Western Hemisphere (mixed)	Clarren & Smith, 1978
1:700	U.S.A. (mixed)	Bertucci & Krafchik, 1994
1:1000	U.S.A. (mixed)	Rosett et al., 1983
1:1500–3000	Western Hemisphere (mixed)	Abel & Sokol, 1991
1:3000	U.S.A. (mixed)	Shoemaker, 1993

* per live births.

Blacker, Abel, & Sokol, 1991; Smitherman, 1994). Other terminologies also have been suggested and have been used in the clinical literature (e.g., alcohol-related birth defects [ARBD] [Harris, Osborn, Weinberg, Loock, & Junaid, 1993; Jacobson et al., 1993; Sokol & Clarren, 1989).

We strongly disagree with the use of these terminologies and argue that the infants and children who display fewer of the classic characteristics of the FAS be diagnosed more appropriately as having a less severe form of FAS and not a different syndrome. We argue that this approach to diagnosing the FAS would:

1. more accurately reflect the anticipated normal distribution of the effects of the FAS among affected infants and children in the general population or its subsets;
2. indicate more completely the extent of the FAS in the general population;
3. represent more fully the nature of the FAS;
4. clearly identify that even "modest social drinking" during pregnancy places the exposed fetus at significant risk for the FAS;
5. reflect the fact that the severity of teratogenic effects is not only related to alcohol, but also to other factors (see Figure 2.1); and
6. allow and encourage the development of more rational and

comprehensive prevention and treatment strategies (Pagliaro & Pagliaro, 1995).

Long-term sequelae of the FAS

While significant attention has been given to the diagnosis of FAS among neonates, the long-term sequelae associated with such a diagnosis generally have not received adequate attention. A comprehensive review and analysis of the published literature indicates that the long-term sequelae of the FAS can be divided into four general areas: (1) growth retardation; (2) developmental deficits in cognitive skills; (3) developmental deficits in motor skills; and (4) mental disorders (Table 2.4). As noted in Table 2.4, the long-term sequelae appear to be quite stable. Thus, the effects associated with the FAS do not end in infancy, but persist into childhood, adolescence, and, unfortunately, throughout adulthood (Smitherman, 1994; Spohr, Willms, & Steinhausen, 1993). The lifelong effects of the FAS on human growth and development, although troubling, should not be ignored. In this regard, we concur with Streissguth, Randels, and Smith (1992) that, for infants and children affected with the FAS and their parents and caregivers, "more realistic expectations for performance during childhood and adolescence may result in the availability of more appropriate services, less frustration, and improved behavioral outcome in later adolescence and adulthood" (p. 564).

Alcohol is a known human teratogen that can cause significant, lifelong deficits in relation to growth, cognitive function, psychomotor skills, and psychological health. Although some authors (e.g., Knupfer, 1991; Walpole, Zubrick, Pontré, & Lawrence, 1991) disagree, we concur with the recommendation made by the National Institute of Child Health and Human Development, the American Academy of Pediatrics, and the U.S. Surgeon General (American Academy of Pediatrics, 1993; Johnson, Reeves, & Jackson, 1983; Schydlower & Perrin, 1993), and others (e.g., Caruso & Bensel, 1993; Casiro, 1991; Leonard et al., 1991; Olson, 1994; Streissguth, Sampson, & Olson et al., 1994), that adolescent girls and women who are pregnant or planning to become pregnant totally *abstain* from alcohol consumption. This recommendation is based on the observations that, first, no safe level of alcohol use has been demonstrated and, second, there is no known cure for the FAS. In this regard, it is essential that prevention and treatment programs be developed to assist adolescent girls and women with this recommendation, particularly those mothers for whom abstinence may be difficult (i.e., adolescent girls and women who use alcohol compulsively).

TABLE 2.4 Long-Term Sequelae of FAS

Age	Number of cases (sample size)	Sequelae	Comments	Reference
Birth	20	**growth retardation**	Exposure to alcohol *in utero* throughout the mother's entire pregnancy resulted in prenatal growth retardation affecting body length, weight, and head circumference.	Autti-Rämö et al., 1992
0, 8, 18, & 36 mo.	595		Smaller physical size noted among alcohol-exposed neonates, which did *not* demonstrate a postnatal "catch-up" by 3 years of age (i.e., the relative smaller size noted at birth was maintained).	Geva, Gold-schmidt, Stoffer, & Day, 1993
5 mo. to 15 yr.	6		"All were small at birth, though their mothers were not underweight, and none has shown any catch-up in growth despite being offered adequate nutrition by their caring foster families." (p. 607)	Collins & Turner, 1978
6.5 and 13 mo.	412		Postnatal growth retardation was strongly correlated with maternal drinking during the second and third trimesters, but not with drinking at conception. Maternal nutritional intake during pregnancy did *not* appear to significantly influence postpartum check-up growth. The findings support the contention "that symmetrical intrauterine	Jacobson, Jacobson, & Sokol, 1994

TABLE 2.4 continued

			growth retardation is most likely to be associated with persistently smaller size later in life." (p. 321)	
18 mo.	505		"Prenatal alcohol exposure during the second and third trimesters was related to growth deficits (weight, height, and head circumference) in the offspring at 18 months of age." (p. 914)	Day et al., 1991
5 y.o.	2		Twin girls with FAS were followed since birth. Growth retardation was noted at birth and by 5 years of age they were still "both small for their ages." (p. 615)	Harris et al., 1993
6 y.o.	152		Alcohol consumption during pregnancy was associated with "shorter mean height and smaller mean head circumference in children at age six." (p. 991)	Russell, Czarnecki, Cowan, McPherson, & Mudar, 1991
6 y.o.	668		"At 6 years of age, children who were prenatally exposed to alcohol were significantly smaller in weight, height, head circumference, and palpebral fissure width." (p. 786)	Day, Richardson, Geva, & Robles, 1994
10 y.o.	60		"We found that the characteristic craniofacial malformations of FAS diminish with time, but *microcephaly* and, to a lesser degree, *short stature* and underweight (in boys) persist; in female adolescents body weight normalises." (p. 907)	Spohr et al. 1993

continued

TABLE 2.4 *continued*

Age	Number of cases (sample size)	Sequelae	Comments	Reference
12 to 40 y.o.	61		"Short stature and microcephaly appeared to be the most prominent growth deficiencies as the children got older . . . although their weight was somewhat closer to the mean." (pp. 1961, 1966)	Streissguth et al., 1991
13 mo.	382	developmental deficits in cognitive skills	Significant deficits noted in infants whose mothers drank heavily. "Effects of second and third trimester drinking were as strong or stronger than those of drinking at the time of conception." (p. 174)	Jacobson et al., 1993
27 mo. (mean)	60		Number of children with cognitive impairment (i.e., mental or verbal performance 2 standard deviations below normal) increased in relation to the duration of intrauterine alcohol exposure (i.e., exposure during all three trimesters was related to significantly increased numbers of children with cognitive impairment in comparison to exposure during only the first or first and second trimesters).	Autti-Rämö et al., 1992
5 y.o.	2		Stanford-Binet IQs of 71 and 72 were determined at 5 years of age for twin sisters born with FAS. Note that an IQ range of 20 to 95 (with a mode of ~70) has been reported for children	Harris et al., 1993

TABLE 2.4 continued

			with FAS (Carney & Chermak, 1991; Robinson et al., 1987; Streissguth et al., 1991).	
6 y.o.	175		Verbal IQ, as measured by the Wechsler Preschool and Primary Scale of Intelligence, and linguistic ability, as measured by the Token Test for Children, was significantly lower among children born to women who drank alcohol during pregnancy.	Russell et al., 1991
6 to 12 y.o.	27		"The results of the present study are consistent with previous reports of expressive and receptive language deficits among FAS children." (p. 132)	Carney & Chermak, 1991
10 y.o.	60		"Persistent mental retardation is the major sequela of intrauterine alcohol exposure in many cases, and environmental and educational factors do not have strong compensatory effects on the intellectual development of affected children". (p. 907)	Spoh et al., 1993
Children of "various ages"			Most children displayed some degree of cognitive deficit with a large percentage classified as mentally. retarded. The cognitive deficits and IQ bands appeared to be longitudinally stable (i.e., intelligence generally did not improve with age over time).	Stein- hausen, Willms, & Spohr, 1993
14 y.o.	464		"Earlier reports of prenatal, alcohol-related neurobehavioral deficits in childhood have now been extended into	Streissguth, Barr et al., 1994

continued

TABLE 2.4 continued

Age	Number of cases (sample size)	Sequelae	Comments	Reference
			adolescence." The neurobehavioral deficits were related to "the acquisition of reading and arithmetic skills." (pp. 248, 252)	
14 y.o.	462		"The 14-year attention/ memory deficits observed in the present study appear to be the adolescent sequelae of deficits observed earlier in development." (p. 202)	Streissguth, Sampson, Olson, Bookstein, Barr et al., 1994
12 to 40 y.o.	61		"The developmental and cognitive handicaps persist as long in life as these patients have been studied... the average IQ was 68." (pp. 1961, 1966)	Streissguth et al., 1991
12 mo.	80	develop- mental deficits in psycho- motor skills	Significant retardation of gross motor development was noted in all groups of infants exposed to alcohol *in utero*. However, it was more severe if alcohol consumption was continued toward the end of pregnancy.	Autti-Rämö & Granström, 1991
13 mo.	382		Significant deficits were noted among children whose mothers drank heavily. "Effects of second and third trimester drinking were as strong or stronger than those of drinking at the time of conception." (p. 174)	Jacobson et al., 1993

TABLE 2.4 continued

18 mo.	5		Psychomotor skills, as determined by Bayley Psychomotor Development Index, showed some variability over time, but ended being 1 to 3 standard deviations below normal for 60% of the infants studied who had FAS.	Harris et al., 1993
5 y.o.	2		In terms of overall motor performance, twin girls with FAS were found to perform at 60% to 65% of their age level; "percentile scores . . . were all at either the 1st or 2nd percentile, indicating that 98% to 99% of age-mates were performing at higher levels." (p. 165)	Harris et al., 1993
7.5 y.o.	486	**mental disorders**	". . . the learning problems evidenced by these children are the school-age sequelae of CNS dysfunction originating from in utero alcohol exposure." (p. 668)	Streissguth, Barr, & Sampson, 1990
children of "various ages"	158		An "excess of psychopathology" was noted among children diagnosed with FAS. These mental disorders, particularly attention-deficit hyperactivity disorder and various affective and sleep disorders, were noted in almost 66% of the children and tended to persist over time. (p. 990)	Steinhausen, Willms, & Spohr, 1993
children 3 to 17 y.o.	46		Among the 46 children, 18 (39%) were diagnosed with attention-deficit hyperactivity disorder.	Caruso & Bensel, 1993

OTHER SEDATIVE-HYPNOTICS

The other sedative-hypnotics include barbiturates, benzodiazepines, and miscellaneous sedative hypnotics. A more comprehensive discussion of alcohol was included because of the increased accumulation of evidence regarding its teratogenic effects and their sequelae among affected infants, children, and adolescents.

BARBITURATES

The barbiturates include mephobarbital, pentobarbital, phenobarbital, and secobarbital. Although the use of the barbiturates has decreased as a result of the synthesis of the benzodiazepines, they are still generally available and are used therapeutically for the treatment of seizure disorders unresponsive to other anticonvulsant therapy. The use of the barbiturates during pregnancy has generally been associated with a number of teratogenic effects. However, confounding variables, particularly maternal epilepsy, have not yet been completely ruled out as principal or coteratogenic factors.

Mephobarbital (Mebaral®)

A statistically significant increase in fetal malformations was noted in a Japanese study (Nakane, Okuma, Takahashi et al., 1980) that examined the use of mephobarbital during pregnancy. Other studies (e.g., Hill, Verniaud, Horning et al., 1974; Speidel & Meadow, 1972) have linked such teratogenic effects as anencephaly; heart anomalies (e.g., atrial septal defect, ventricular septal defect, patent ductus arteriosus, and others); cleft lip and palate; congenital hip dislocation; craniofacial anomalies (e.g., large fontanelles, broad alveolar ridge, broad nasal ridge, low hairline); developmental delay; digital thumb; inguinal hernia; nail hypoplasia; strabismus; and talipes equinus with mephobarbital use during pregnancy (see also *Phenobarbital*, a major metabolite of mephobarbital).

Pentobarbital (Nembutal®)

Although one early study (Fealy, 1958) indicated that pentobarbital was safe for the fetus when used during labor, its known pharmacology and reports associating other barbiturates with teratogenic effects during pregnancy and labor suggest that pentobarbital be used with caution. Neonatal respiratory depression and the barbiturate withdrawal syndrome can be expected when pentobarbital is used near term. More data are needed.

Phenobarbital

Phenobarbital appears to present a significant risk for human teratogenesis. Once the preferred anticonvulsant for use during pregnancy because only one case of teratogenesis was reported, it is no longer generally recommended. Phenobarbital has been associated with several cases of teratogenesis involving various fetal malformations. The teratogenic effects of phenobarbital were substantiated in the report of the Collaborative Study Group in Japan. These effects include anencephaly, cardiac defects (various), cleft lip and palate, congenital dislocated hip, developmental delay, hydrocephalus, hypoplastic phalanges, hypospadias, microcephaly, myelomeningocele, neonatal phenobarbital withdrawal syndrome, ocular agenesis, pre- and postnatal growth retardation, psychomotor retardation, short nose with a low-set nasal bridge, talipes equinovarus, and wide fontanelle. However, confounding variables, such as the mother's seizure disorder, may contribute to the observed teratogenic effects.

BENZODIAZEPINES

The benzodiazepines include chlordiazepoxide, diazepam, lorazepam, nitrazepam, and oxazepam. The use of these abusable psychotropics during pregnancy has been associated with various degrees of teratogenic effects, particularly cleft lip and palate. However, data are conflicting and the use of benzodiazepines during pregnancy appears to have a low teratogenic risk.

Chlordiazepoxide (Librium®; Solium®)

The use of chlordiazepoxide during pregnancy was previously thought to be clearly associated with teratogenic risk. Initial data provided evidence that fetal exposure to chlordiazepoxide during the first 42 days after conception resulted in a 4 1/2-fold greater risk of severe congenital abnormalities. An increased fetal death rate also was observed with chlordiazepoxide use during pregnancy. However, subsequent studies (e.g., Hartz, Heinonen, Shapiro, Siskind, & Slone, 1975; Milkovich & Van den Berg, 1974) failed to support these findings and some researchers have concluded that because of the diversity of the anomalies reported in the earlier studies, it is doubtful that chlordiazepoxide was responsible. Regardless of these conflicting findings, babies born to mothers who receive chlordiazepoxide therapy during the antenatal period may manifest various CNS symptoms, including convulsions, depression, hyperexcitability, respiratory depression, somnolence, and a chlordiazepoxide withdrawal syndrome. Generally, the chlordiazepoxide withdrawal syndrome, manifested by crying, insomnia, irritability, and poor feeding, abates over several days with complete recovery.

Diazepam *(Valium®)*

Earlier reports implicated diazepam with cleft lip and palate and limb and digit malformations. However, more recent data indicate that it is unlikely that therapeutic doses of diazepam are teratogenic. The report of the cleft lip and palate malformations was associated with an acute overdose (580 mg) during the first trimester. Diazepam has been related to neonatal hypothermia, hypotonia, low Apgar scores, poor feeding, and a diazepam withdrawal syndrome when used during the third trimester near term. The effects are generally fully reversible with proper recognition and care (see also *Oxazepam*, a major metabolite of diazepam).

Lorazepam *(Ativan®)*

Maternal use of lorazepam near term has been associated with lethargy, poor muscle tone, and respiratory depression in the neonate. These effects are generally fully reversible with proper recognition and appropriate care. Physical malformations have not been reported. More data are needed.

Nitrazepam (Mogadon®)

Nitrazepam appears to present a low risk for human teratogenesis. However, the use of nitrazepam during pregnancy has been associated with neonatal CNS depression, a nitrazepam withdrawal syndrome, and cleft lip and palate. More data are needed.

Oxazepam (Serax®)

Oxazepam appears to present a low risk for human teratogenesis. In one study, the use of oxazepam during pregnancy was associated with cleft lip and palate. More data are needed.

CENTRAL NERVOUS SYSTEM STIMULANTS

The central nervous system stimulants include caffeine, cocaine, dextroamphetamine, methylphenidate, and nicotine. Results are mixed in regard to the teratogenic effects associated with this group of abusable psychotropics.

Caffeine

Caffeine, in the form of coffee, tea, and other beverages (e.g., caffeinated soft drinks), is probably consumed to a greater extent by pregnant adolescent girls and women than any other abusable psychotropic, including alcohol. Although research has not been as prolific as that for alcohol, some studies have associated caffeine consumption with birth defects. The consumption of eight or more cups of coffee per day was related to fetal limb defects in three case reports, but more recent studies have shown that the only teratogenic effect associated with caffeine is reduced birth weight. This effect was associated with the consumption of 3 or more cups of coffee per day. However, a significant correlation between increased caffeine consumption during pregnancy and fetal loss also has been reported. Although these data would generally support the relative safety of caffeine use during pregnancy, pregnant adolescent girls and women should be encouraged to minimize their caffeine use, particularly if they smoke tobacco cigarettes. Tobacco smoking, which is significantly correlated with coffee consumption, is an obvious confounding factor in the interpretation of data supporting the possible teratogenic effects of caffeine.

Cocaine

Cocaine use during pregnancy increased significantly during the 1980s and remains the most commonly used *illicit* abusable psychotropic among pregnant adolescent girls and women, particularly in North American inner cities. Cocaine use during pregnancy has been associated with intrauterine death (including spontaneous abortions), low birth weight, preterm delivery, neonatal seizures, neonatal tachycardia, intrauterine growth retardation, and a variety of fetal physical anomalies, particularly affecting the ophthalmic and urogenital systems. Autopsies of fetuses exposed to cocaine *in utero* often reveal cerebral hemorrhages. However, some researchers have attributed these effects to confounding factors associated with maternal cocaine use (e.g., poor nutrition; inadequate prenatal care). When used by the mother near term, the neonate may experience CNS excitation. There also appears to be a significantly higher incidence of behavioral and learning disorders (e.g., attention deficit hyperactivity disorder) among preschoolers and school-age children exposed to cocaine *in utero*.

The teratogenic effects associated with maternal use of cocaine during pregnancy remain inconclusive because of the difficulties associated with interpreting and evaluating research data. For example, the retrospective case report methodology that is generally used has several inherent limitations, including inaccuracy of reported information. These limitations make definitive conclusions highly speculative. In addition, adolescent girls and women who use cocaine commonly use alcohol, a known teratogen, to "come down" from a cocaine high, thus further confounding interpretation of data. A general consensus appears to be forming that cocaine use at high dosages, as is commonly associated with injectable use or the use of smokable crack or rock forms of cocaine, probably has a significant, but low, potential for inducing teratogenic effects. More data are needed.

Dextroamphetamine (Dexedrine®)

Although data are contradictory regarding the teratogenic effects of dextroamphetamine exposure *in utero*, it appears that there is a moderate risk for human teratogenesis. Maternal use of dextroamphetamine during the first trimester has been associated with congenital heart disease, biliary atresia, cleft lip and palate, prematurity, and small size for gestational age. However, a prospective study found no increase in fetal malformations. More data are needed.

Methylphenidate (Ritalin®)

Methylphenidate is a CNS stimulant that is closely related to the amphetamines. It is widely used for the treatment of attention deficit hyperactivity disorder among school-age children and adolescents and, more recently, adults. A study of 11 neonates exposed to methylphenidate *in utero* found no significant increase in malformations. More data are needed.

Nicotine: Tobacco Smoking

Tobacco smoking during pregnancy is teratogenic to the fetus. There is an inverse relationship between the number of cigarettes smoked per day and the birth weight of neonates born to adolescent girls and women who smoke; neonates born to mothers who smoke are an average of 200 g (100–400 g) smaller and have a shorter body length than do neonates born to mothers who do not smoke. Fortunately, a period of accelerated growth occurs during the first year of life and, generally, no differences in body weight or length are observed among infants at

1 year of age born to mothers who smoke and those who do not. Adolescent girls and women who cease smoking during the first trimester have infants of normal size.

Adolescent girls and women who smoke have higher rates of spontaneous abortions, abruptio placentae, placenta previa, and higher perinatal mortality rates than do mothers who do not smoke. Mothers who smoke also may have a higher fetal malformation rate, but data are inconclusive. The risk of the sudden infant death syndrome (SIDS) is up to 4.4 times higher for infants born to mothers who smoked during pregnancy than for infants born to mothers who did not smoke during pregnancy. Adolescent girls and women should be advised not to smoke during pregnancy. As with other abusable psychotropics, the teratogenic effects of heavy tobacco smoking are confounded by alcohol use, another known human teratogen.

PSYCHEDELICS

The psychedelics comprise a variety of drugs and substances that generally are used for their hallucinatory effects and to expand consciousness. No studies were found that reported teratogenic effects associated with the maternal use of psilocybin (magic mushrooms) or peyote (mescaline) during pregnancy. However, several studies, which are discussed in this section, were found for lysergic acid diethylamide (LSD), phencyclidine (PCP), and tetrahydrocannabinol in its various forms of cannabis (i.e., hashish; hash oil; marijuana).

Lysergic Acid Diethylamide (LSD)

LSD use during pregnancy was previously associated with a number of reports of fetal anomalies including bladder exstrophy; chromosomal breakage; eye, CNS, and limb defects; and inguinal hernias. However, more recent studies have found no association between LSD exposure *in utero* and fetal malformations, even though LSD has been widely used by adolescent girls and women of childbearing age for several decades. Although one study linked LSD use to an increased incidence of spontaneous abortions, available data suggest that LSD does not appear to present a significant risk for human teratogenesis. More data are needed.

Phencyclidine (PCP)

Phencyclidine is reportedly used by 0.8% of the population during pregnancy, often in combination with other abusable psychotropics.

However, PCP does not appear to present a significant risk for human teratogenesis. Only one case was reported associating PCP use during pregnancy with the birth of a malformed infant. Phencyclidine use during pregnancy also has been associated with a withdrawal phenomenon among neonates (i.e., abnormal suck, irritability, jitteriness). More data are needed.

Tetrahydrocannabinol (THC): Cannabis Smoking

Cannabis (including hashish, hash oil, and marijuana) smoking during pregnancy has not been clearly associated with teratogenic effects. Thus, tetrahydrocannabinol (THC), the principal active psychedelic ingredient in cannabis does not appear to present a significant risk for human teratogenesis. Although there are scattered case reports of fetal defects and neurobehavioral problems among infants born to mothers who reportedly smoked cannabis, these effects appear to be dependent upon pre- and postnatal environmental factors and are limited to low birth weight and minor temporary neurologic symptoms (e.g., tremors). Given the widespread use of cannabis by adolescent girls and women and the relative paucity of reported teratogenic effects, the teratogenic potential of cannabis, if it does exist, appears to be low.

CONCLUSIONS

Teratogenesis is a complex process that is influenced by many factors including maternal, placental, fetal, environmental, and abusable psychotropic factors. To minimize the risk for and incidence of abusable psychotropic-induced teratogenesis, it is necessary to recognize that any abusable psychotropic has the potential to cause teratogenic effects. Adolescent girls and women should be encouraged to abstain from, or to minimize, their use of the abusable psychotropics during pregnancy. In particular, they should be advised to avoid alcohol use, in that strong evidence has been provided associating the use of this abusable psychotropic with significant teratogenic effects (i.e., FAS). The effects of FAS are not limited to the neonatal period or first year of life, but persist throughout life, affecting growth and development in many significant ways. Whenever possible, health care providers should avoid prescribing abusable psychotropics (e.g., opiates, sedative-hypnotics) to adolescent girls and women of childbearing age unless the perceived benefit outweighs the potential risk. When abusable psychotropics are used during the antenatal period, their respective withdrawal syndromes can be expected to be observed among neonates and require appropriate care. In addition, most abusable psychotropics used near term can cause expected pharmacologic effects and toxicities in the neonate. Fortunately, these effects are generally reversible with proper recognition and care.

Public health and other health care providers should be aware of the teratogenic effects associated with the abusable psychotropics. Further research examining the relationship between abusable psychotropic use by pregnant adolescent girls and women and the developing child also is needed. There is extensive documentation indicating that maternal alcohol drinking and tobacco smoking result in serious risk for teratogenic effects. However, a large percentage of pregnant adolescent girls and women continue to unnecessarily expose themselves and their unborn babies to these abusable psychotropics. Health care providers must be alert to the likelihood of teratogenic effects associated with abusable psychotropic use and advise adolescent girls and women regarding the possible harmful effects to their unborn babies when used during pregnancy, including the possible long-term effects of alcohol use (i.e., FAS).

The available information regarding the teratogenic effects of the abusable psychotropics presented in this chapter can be used to plan public policy and to advise adolescent girls and women in an effort to decrease the incidence of preventable abusable psychotropic-induced teratogenic effects. When teratogenic effects have occurred as a result of abusable psychotropic exposure *in utero,* it is essential that long-range plans be developed in order to optimize the development and potential of these children.

REFERENCES

Abel, E. L., Martier, S., Kruger, M., Ager, J., & Sokol, R. J. (1993). Ratings of fetal alcohol syndrome facial features by medical providers and biomedical scientists. *Alcoholism: Clinical and Experimental Research, 17,* 717–721.

Abel, E. L., & Sokol, R. J. (1987). Incidence of fetal alcohol syndrome and economic impact of FAS-related anomalies. *Drug and Alcohol Dependence, 19,* 51–70.

Abel, E. L., & Sokol, R. J. (1991). A revised conservative estimate of the incidence of FAS and economic impact. *Alcoholism: Clinical and Experimental Research, 15,* 514–524.

Autti-Rämö, I., & Granström, M.-L. (1991). The psychomotor development during the first year of life of infants exposed to intrauterine alcohol of various duration: Fetal alcohol exposure and development. *Neuropediatrics, 22,* 59–64.

Autti-Rämö, I., Korkman, M., Hilakivi-Clarke, L., Lehtonen, M., Halmesmäki, & Granström, M.-L. (1992). Mental development of 2-year-old children exposed to alcohol in utero. *The Journal of Pediatrics, 120,* 740–746.

Barbour, B. G. (1990). Alcohol and pregnancy. *Journal of Nurse-Midwifery, 35*(2), 78–85.

Bertucci, V., & Krafchik, B. R. (1994). Diagnosis: Fetal alcohol syndrome. *Pediatric Dermatology, 11,* 180.

Burd, L., & Moffat, M. E. K. (1994). Epidemiology of fetal alcohol syndrome in American Indians, Alaskan Natives, and Canadian Aboriginal Peoples: A review of the literature. *Public Health Reports, 109,* 688–693.

Burns, E. M. (1990). The effects of stress during the brain growth spurt. In J. J. Fitzpatrick, R. L. Taunton, & J. Q. Benoliel (Eds.), *Annual review of nursing research* (pp. 57–82). New York: Springer Publishing.

Carney, L. J., & Chermak, G. D. (1991). Performance of American Indian children with fetal alcohol syndrome on the test of language development. *Journal of Communicative Disorders, 24,* 123–134.

Carones, F., Brancato, R., Venturi, E., Bianchi, S., & Magni, R. (1992). Corneal endothelial anomalies in the fetal alcohol syndrome. *Archives of Ophthalmology, 110,* 1128–1131.

Caruso, K., & Bensel, R. (1993). Fetal alcohol syndrome and fetal alcohol effects: The University of Minnesota experience. *Minnesota Medicine, 76,* 25–29.

Casiro, O. G. (1991). Drinking and pregnancy. *Canadian Medical Association Journal, 145,* 1552, 1554.

Clarren, S. K., & Smith, D. W. (1978). Medical progress: The fetal alcohol syndrome. *The New England Journal of Medicine, 298,* 1063–1067.

Coffey, T. G. (1966). Beer Street: Gin Lane. Some views of 18th-century drinking. *Quarterly Journal of Studies on Alcohol, 27,* 669–692.

Collins, E., & Turner, G. (1978). Six children affected by maternal alcoholism. *The Medical Journal of Australia, 2,* 606–608.

Committee on Substance Abuse and Committee on Children with Disabilities. (1993). Fetal alcohol syndrome and fetal alcohol effects. *Pediatrics, 91,* 1004–1006.

Cordier, S., Ha, M.-C., Ayme, S., & Goujard, J. (1992). Maternal occupational exposure and congenital malformations. *Scandinavian Journal of Work Environment Health, 18,* 11–17.

Cornelius, M. D., Day, N. L., Cornelius, J. R., Geva, D., Taylor, P. M., &

Richardson, G. A. (1993). Drinking patterns and correlates of drinking among pregnant teenagers. *Alcoholism: Clinical and Experimental Research, 17,* 290–294.

Cornelius, M. D., Richardson, G. A., Day, N. L., Cornelius, J. R., Geva, D., & Taylor, P. M. (1994). A comparison of prenatal drinking in two recent samples of adolescents and adults. *Journal of Studies on Alcohol, 55,* 412–419.

Day, N. L., Goldschmidt, L., Robles, N., Richardson, G., Cornelius, M., Taylor, P., Geva, D., & Stoffer, D. (1991). Prenatal alcohol exposure and offspring growth at 18 months of age: The predictive validity of two measures of drinking. *Alcoholism: Clinical and Experimental Research, 15,* 914–918.

Day, N. L., & Richardson, G. A. (1991). Prenatal alcohol exposure: A continuum of effects. *Seminars in Perinatology, 15,* 271–279.

Day, N. L., Richardson, G. A., Geva, D., & Robles, N. (1994). Alcohol, marijuana, and tobacco: Effects of prenatal exposure on offspring growth and morphology at age six. *Alcoholism: Clinical and Experimental Research, 18*(4), 786–794.

Duimstra, C., Johnson, D., Kutsch, C., Wang, B., Zentner, M., Kellerman, S., & Welty, T. (1993). A fetal alcohol syndrome surveillance pilot project in American Indian communities in the Northern Plains. *Public Health Reports, 108,* 225–229.

Edwards, M. S. (1981). Fetal alcohol syndrome. *The Journal of Nursing Care, 11,* 6–14.

Ernhart, C. B., Morrow-Tlucak, M., Sokol, R. J., & Martier, S. (1988). Underreporting of alcohol use in pregnancy. *Alcoholism: Clinical and Experimental Research, 12,* 506–511.

Fealy, J. (1958). Placental transmission of pentobarbital sodium. *Obstetrics and Gynecology, 11,* 342–349.

Froster, U. G., & Baird, P. A. (1992). Congenital defects of the limbs and alcohol exposure in pregnancy: Data from a population based study. *American Journal of Medical Genetics, 44,* 782–785.

Geva, D., Goldschmidt, L., Stoffer, D., & Day, N. L. (1993). A longitudinal analysis of the effect of prenatal alcohol exposure on growth. *Alcoholism: Clinical and Experimental Research, 17,* 1124–1129.

Gilbody, J. S. (1991). Effects of maternal drug addiction on the fetus. *Adverse Drug Reactions and Acute Toxicology Reviews, 10,* 77–88.

Ginsberg, K. A., Blacker, C. M., Abel, E. L., & Sokol, R. J. (1991). Fetal alcohol exposure and adverse pregnancy outcomes. *Contributions to Gynecology and Obstetrics, 18,* 115–129.

Gordis, E., & Alexander, D. (1992). From the National Institutes of Health: Progress toward preventing and understanding alcohol-induced fetal injury. *Journal of the American Medical Association, 268,* 3183.

Griffith, D. R., Azuma, S. D., & Chasnoff, I. J. (1994). Three-year outcome of children exposed prenatally to drugs. *Journal of American Child and Adolescent Psychiatry, 33,* 20–27.

Haddad, J., & Messer, J. (1994). Fetal alcohol syndrome: Report of three siblings. *Neopediatrics, 25,* 109–111.

Harris, S. R., Osborn, J. A., Weinberg, J., Loock, C., & Junaid, K. (1993). Effects of prenatal alcohol exposure on neuromotor and cognitive development during early childhood: A series of case reports. *Physical Therapy, 73,* 608–617.

Hartz, S. C., Heinonen, O. P., Shapiro, S., Siskind, V., & Slone, D. (1975). Antenatal exposure to meprobamate and chlordiazepoxide in relation to malformations, mental development, and childhood mortality. *New England Journal of Medicine, 292,* 726–728.

Hemminki, K., & Vineis, P. (1985). Extrapolation of the evidence on teratogenicity of chemicals between humans and experimental animals: Chemicals other than drugs. *Teratogenesis, Carcinogenesis, and Muta-genesis, 5,* 251–318.

Hill, R. M., Hegemier, S., & Tennyson, L. M. (1989). The fetal alcohol syndrome: A multihandicapped child. *Neurotoxicology, 10,* 585–596.

Hill, R. M., Verniaud, W. M., Horning, M. G., McCulley, L. B., & Morgan, N. F. (1974). Infants exposed in utero to antiepileptic drugs. *American Journal of Diseases of Children, 127,* 645–653.

Jacobson, J. L., Jacobson, S. W., Sokol, R. J., Martier, S. S., Ager, J. W., & Kaplan-Estrin, M. G. (1993). Teratogenic effects of alcohol on infant development. *Alcoholism: Clinical and Experimental Research,* 174–183.

Johnson, C. D., Reeves, K. O., & Jackson, D. (1983). Alcohol and sex. *Heart and Lung, 12,* 93–97.

Jones, K. L., Smith, D. W., Ulleland, C. N., & Streussguth, P. (1973). Pattern of malformation of offspring of chronic alcoholic mothers. *Lancet, 1,* 1267–1271.

Jorgensen, K. M. (1992). The drug-exposed infant. *Critical Care Nursing Clinics of North America, 4,* 481–485.

Knupfer, G. (1991). Abstaining for foetal health: The fiction that even light drinking is dangerous. *British Journal of Addiction, 86,* 1063–1073.

Larroque, B. (1992). Alcohol and the fetus. *International Journal of Epidemiology, 21*(Suppl. 1), S8–S16.

Leonard, B. J., Boettcher, L. M., & Brust, J. D. (1991). Alcohol-related birth defects. *Minnesota Medicine, 74,* 23–25.

Lewis, D. D. (1983). Alcohol & pregnancy outcome. *Midwives Chronicle & Nursing Notes, 12,* 420–422.

Little, B. B., Snell, L. M., & Rosenfeld, C. R. (1990). Failure to recognize fetal alcohol syndrome in newborn infants. *American Journal of Diseases of Children, 144,* 1142–1146.

Milkovich, L., & Van den Berg, G. J. (1974). Effects of prenatal meprobamate and chlordiazepoxide hydrochloride on human embryonic and fetal development. *New England Journal of Medicine, 291,* 1268–1271.

Nakane, Y., Okuma, T., Takahashi, R., Sato, Y., Wade, T., Sato, T., Fukushima, Y., Kumashiro, H., Ono, T., Takahashi, T., Aoki, Y., Kazamatsuri, H., Inami, M., Komai, S., Seino, M., Miyakoshi, M., Tanimura, T., Hazama, H., Kawahara, R., Otsuki, S., Hosokawa, K., Inanaga, K., Nakazawa, Y., & Yamamoto, K. (1980). Multi-institutional study on the teratogenicity and fetal toxicity of antiepileptic drugs: A report of a collaborative study group in Japan. *Epilepsia, 21,* 663–680.

National Institute on Alcohol Abuse and Alcoholism. (1987). *Program strategies for preventing fetal alcohol syndrome and alcohol-related birth defects* (DHHS Publication No. ADM 87–1482). Washington, DC: U.S. Government Printing Office.

Olson, C. H. (1994). The effects of prenatal alcohol exposure on child development. *Infants and Young Children, 6,* 10–25.

Pagliaro, L. A., & Pagliaro, A. M. (1995). Drugs as human teratogens. In L. A. Pagliaro & A. M. Pagliaro (Eds.), *Problems in pediatric drug therapy* (3rd ed., pp. 105–243). Hamilton, IL: Drug Intelligence.

Remkes, T. (1993, June). Saying no - Completely. *The Canadian Nurse,* 25–28.

Robinson, G. C., Conry, J. L., & Conry, R. F. (1987). Clinical profile and prevalence of fetal alcohol syndrome in an isolated community in British Columbia. *CMAJ, 137,* 203–207.

Rosett, H. L., Weiner, L., Lee, A., Zuckerman, B., Dooling, E., & Oppenheimer, E. (1983). Patterns of alcohol consumption and fetal development. *Journal of the American College of Obstetricians and Gynecologists, 61,* 539–546.

Russell, M., Czarnecki, D. M., Cowan, R., McPherson, E., & Mudar, P. J. (1991). Measures of maternal alcohol use as predictors of development in early childhood. *Alcoholism: Clinical and Experimental Research, 15,* 991–1000.

Schydlower, M., & Perrin, J. (1993). Prevention of fetal alcohol syndrome [Letter to the editor]. *Pediatrics, 92,* 739.

Shoemaker, F. W. (1993). Prevention of fetal alcohol syndrome [Letter to the editor]. *Pediatrics, 92,* 738–739.

Smitherman, C. H. (1994). The lasting impact of fetal alcohol syndrome and fetal alcohol effect on children and adolescents. *Journal of Pediatric Health Care, 8,* 121–126.

Sokol, R. J., & Clarren, S. K. (1989). Guidelines for use of terminology describing the impact of prenatal alcohol on the offspring. *Alcoholism: Clinical and Experimental Research, 13,* 597–598.

Speidel, B. D., & Meadow, S. R. (1972). Maternal epilepsy and abnormalities of the fetus and newborn. *Lancet, 2*, 839–843.

Spohr, H. L., Willms, J., & Steinhausen, H. C. (1993). Prenatal alcohol exposure and long-term developmental consequences. *The Lancet, 34*(8850), 907–910.

Steinhausen, H.-C., Willms, J., & Spohr, H.-L. (1993). Long-term psychopathological and cognitive outcome of children with fetal alcohol syndrome. *Journal of the American Academy of Child and Adolescent Psychiatry, 32*, 990–994.

Streissguth, A. P., Aase, J. M., Clarren, S. K., Randels, S. P., LaDue, R. A., & Smith, D. F. (1991). *Journal of the American Medical Association, 265*, 1961–1967.

Streissguth, A. P., Barr, H. M., Olson, H. C., Sampson, P. D., Bookstein, F. L., & Burgess, D. M. (1994). Drinking during pregnancy decreases word attack and arithmetic scores on standardized tests: Adolescent data from a population-based prospective study. *Alcoholism: Clinical and Experimental Research, 18*, 248–254.

Streissguth, A. P., Barr, H. M., & Sampson, P. D. (1990). Moderate prenatal alcohol exposure: Effects on child IQ and learning problems at age $7^1/_2$ years. *Alcoholism: Clinical and Experimental Research, 14*, 662–669.

Streissguth, A. P., Randels, S. P., & Smith, D. F. (1992). Fetal alcohol syndrome [letter to the editor]. *Journal of the American Academy of Child and Adolescent Psychiatry, 31*, 563–564.

Streissguth, A. P., Sampson, P. D., Barr, H. M., Bookstein, F. L., & Olson, H. C. (1994). The effects of prenatal exposure to alcohol and tobacco: Contributions from the Seattle longitudinal prospective study and implications for public policy. In H. L. Needleman & D. Bellinger (Eds.), *Prenatal exposure to toxicants: Developmental consequences* (pp. 148–183). Baltimore, MD: John Hopkins University.

Streissguth, A. P., Sampson, P. D., Olson, H. C., Bookstein, F. L., Barr, H. M., Scott, M., Feldman, J., & Mirsky, A. F. (1994). Maternal drinking during pregnancy: Attention and short-term memory in 14-year-old offspring: A longitudinal prospective study. *Alcoholism: Clinical and Experimental Research, 18*, 202–218.

Substance abuse: Frequent alcohol consumption among women of childbearing age. (1994). *Weekly Epidemiological Record, 69*, 180–182.

Tranmer, J. E. (1985). Disposition of ethanol in maternal venous blood and the amniotic fluid. *Journal of Obstetric, Gynecologic, and Neonatal Nursing, 14*(6), 484–490.

Ulleland, C. N. (1972). The offspring of alcoholic mothers. *Annals of the New York Academy of Sciences, 197*, 167–169.

Van Allen, M. I. (1992). Structural anomalies resulting from vascular disruption.

Pediatric Clinics of North America, 39, 255–277.

Wallace, P. (1991). Prevalence of fetal alcohol syndrome largely unknown. *Iowa Medicine, 81,* 381.

Walpole, I., Zubrick, S., Pontré, J., & Lawrence, C. (1991). Low to moderate maternal alcohol use before and during pregnancy, and neurobehavioural outcome in the newborn infant. *Developmental Medicine and Child Neurology, 33,* 875–883.

What lessons did thalidomide teach us? (1983). *Pharmaceutical Journal, 233,* 438–439.

Wheeler, S. F. (1993). Substance abuse during pregnancy. *Primary Care, 20,* 191–207.

3

Developmental Outcomes Associated with *In Utero* Exposure to Alcohol and Other Drugs

Judith J. Carta, Ph.D., Scott R. McConnell, Ph.D.,
Mary A. McEvoy, Ph.D., Charles R. Greenwood, Ph.D.,
Jane B. Atwater, Ph.D., Kathleen Baggett,
and Rosanne Williams, Ph.D

O ver the past two decades, researchers from a variety of disciplines have explored the effects of prenatal exposure to a variety of licit and illicit drugs on the neurological and behavioral development of young children. Initially, this research focused primarily on simple effects models, examining direct effects of one suspected substance (or, in limited instances, a small class of substances) on specific aspects of child outcome. Based on both the results of this early research *and* a critical and ongoing appraisal of its core assumptions, methodological approach, and implications, research on prenatal drug exposure has recently entered its "second generation" (Lester & Tronick, 1994). In this contemporary phase, researchers interested in outcomes associated with prenatal exposure to drugs in humans are expanding their attention to polydrug exposure, larger and more diverse study samples, assessment and analysis of correlates and comorbidity factors, and more direct and careful assessment of postnatal environmental and contextual factors.

This chapter will describe the earlier work on this problem, identify some of its shortcomings, and then present a model for conducting studies in this area using a new research paradigm. The chapter will highlight some preliminary findings of the Early Childhood Research Institute on Substance Abuse, a consortium of researchers from the Universities of Kansas, Minnesota, and South Dakota. This group has been conducting a longitudinal study examining environmental factors influencing risk and resilience in children prenatally exposed to alcohol and other drugs. This work is describing the developmental outcomes as well as the interactions that take place between these children and their caregivers within natural contexts. This research is leading to an understanding of the interactional processes within the home and school that affect early school success and failure for these and similar children who come from environments with multiple challenges.

FIRST GENERATION OF RESEARCH

The first generation of research identified children prenatally exposed to alcohol, cocaine, and other illicit substances as a high-risk group for developmental problems. Investigators began to identify a wide variety of medical risks associated with substance exposure during the prenatal and perinatal periods, including prematurity, lower birthweight, and decreased head circumference, impaired neurological function, neuromotor problems, intraventricular hemorrhage, strokes, and congenital malformations (e.g., Chasnoff, 1988a; Chasnoff, Burns, & Burns, 1987; Zuckerman, Amaro, Bauchner, & Cabral, 1989). This early set of studies identified biological and behavioral characteristics, common in infants who were exposed prenatally to drugs and alcohol, that make the care of these children more difficult. Documented effects include protracted high-pitched cries, tremors, inconsolability, irritability, inability to organize normal sleep-wake cycles, and hyperactivity when exposed to multiple stimuli (Finnegan, 1986; Griffith & Freier, 1992; Oro & Dixon, 1987). In addition, some of these infants were reported to avoid eye contact and become overexcited when they were exposed to multiple stimuli, such as being talked to and rocked at the same time (Griffith & Freier, 1992). Researchers who identified these characteristics pointed out that while these factors are sometimes associated with poor outcomes in and of themselves, they may also occasion the development of child-caregiver interaction patterns that jeopardize later development (Chasnoff et al., 1987; Freier, 1994; Lester & Tronick, 1994).

The first generation of research also contributed some limited information about children exposed to illicit drugs after the initial period of infancy. A small set of studies pointed out, for example, that some of these children had significant cognitive impairments, language delays, and hyperactivity (e.g., Chasnoff, Griffith, & Azuma, 1992; Fried & Watkinson, 1990; Wilson, McCreary, Kean, & Baxter, 1979). In a comprehensive review of early experimental studies of children with a history of prenatal drug exposure, the greatest *proportion* of adverse outcomes for these children was identified in the social and cognitive domains (Carta et al., 1994).

The first generation of research has not revealed the long-term effects of children's prenatal exposure to illicit drugs on their developmental outcomes (Griffith, 1992). Very few of these studies have examined these children's outcomes beyond the first few years of life (Carta et al., 1994; Singer, Arendt, & Minnes, 1993). Some studies taken as a whole reveal a slight trend toward increased adverse outcomes as children enter the preschool years. Some researchers have explained this increasing trend by pointing out that prenatal exposure to drugs may affect subtle areas of children's functioning that are difficult to assess in early infancy. These more subtle effects, they note, may not be measurable until children reach preschool or school age (Allen, Palormares, DeForest, Sprinkle, & Reynolds, 1991; Dixon & Bejar, 1989). For example, in one longitudinal study, children prenatally exposed to marijuana did not show adverse outcomes during the first 2 years of life, but did exhibit cognitive and language delays at 3 years (Fried, 1989). Similarly, a group of children prenatally exposed to cocaine and other substances and followed since birth by Chasnoff performed no differently than a nonexposed comparison group on cognitive and motor measures through age 2 (Chasnoff, Griffith, Freier, & Murray, 1992). At 3 years, however, the children with a history of prenatal exposure scored lower on verbal and reasoning tasks and were more likely to be rated by their mothers as having behavior problems (Chasnoff, Griffith, & Azuma, 1992). While numerous hypotheses have been offered to explain these "sleeper" effects, a better understanding of the operating mechanisms awaits the next generation of research.

SHORTCOMINGS OF THE FIRST GENERATION OF RESEARCH

Recently, researchers have begun to evaluate critically the status and significance of this earlier research. Critiques have included summaries and analyses of findings to date (Carta et al., 1994; Coles, Platzman, Smith, Jones, & Falek, 1992; Lutiger, Graham, Einarson, & Koren, 1991); reviews and restatements of underlying conceptual models for this research (Beeghly & Tronick, 1994; Lester & Tronick, 1994; Zuckerman, 1993), critical appraisals and recommendations for new and expanded methodology (Freier, 1994), and major restatement and rethinking of the overall consequences of prenatal exposure and its role as a causal variable in child development outcomes (Carta et al., 1994; Lester & Tronick, 1994; Mayes, Granger, Bornstein, & Zuckerman, 1992). While the defining characteristics of this "second generation" of research are still being developed, several strong themes have emerged. These themes include (a) larger and more diverse study samples; (b) more direct and careful modeling of polydrug exposure; (c) repeated assessment across infancy, preschool, and middle childhood to capture subtle, transient, and emergent effects; (d) multiple measures of development to capture these effects; and (e) more direct assessment and analysis of distal and proximal environmental factors that may mediate outcome.

SAMPLE CHARACTERISTICS

Early research on the effects of prenatal exposure to licit and illicit drugs, particularly cocaine, was frequently based on small- to medium-size convenience samples drawn from clinical settings (e.g., Chasnoff, Griffith, Freier, & Murray, 1992; Rodning, Beckwith, & Howard, 1989). These samples tended to include large proportions of minority-culture and low-socioeconomic-status children. While there is evidence that prenatal substance exposure does occur at moderate levels in minority and low-income communities, there is also evidence that the condition is not restricted to these communities (Chasnoff, Landress, & Barrett, 1990). Additionally, many of the samples in these early studies were originally quite small, and (if followed longitudinally) suffered tremendous attrition (Carta et al., 1994), leaving too few participants for sophisticated parametric analyses at the conclusion of data collection. The new generation of research on the developmental effects of prenatal exposure must recruit more ethnically and economically diverse samples, both to provide variance on process and outcome measures *and* to expand the generalizability of this work.

POLYDRUG EXPOSURE

Early research on prenatal exposure in human populations built fairly simple models, often examining the effects of single substances (e.g., cocaine—Chasnoff, Griffith, Freier, & Murray, 1992; heroin—Chasnoff et al., 1987; alcohol—Landesman-Dwyer, Ragozin, & Little, 1981; nicotine—Nieburg, Marks, McLaren, & Remington, 1985). However, there is much evidence t o suggest that polydrug use may be more prevalent or typical, and that exposure to these multiple substances may be an important factor in subsequent child development (e.g., Amaro, Zuckerman, & Cabral, 1989; Chasnoff, 1988b; Lester & Tronick, 1994). While simple-effects models of the consequences of exposure to single substances can be achieved, these models rarely occur naturally in human populations. Thus, the second generation of research on pre-natal exposure must account for and analyze the effects of polydrug use during pregnancy, and begin to describe the unique and combined effects of prenatal exposure to various substances.

REPEATED ASSESSMENTS

Early research on the developmental consequences of prenatal expo-sure, particularly to cocaine, was characterized by particular attention to assessment during the first days and months of infancy and initial findings that occasionally failed to replicate (Carta et al., 1994). Recent reviews of conceptual foundations and methodological practices in research on prenatal exposure have suggested, however, that effects in various domains (e.g., neurological, neurobehavioral, behavioral, and developmental) may either be very subtle (e.g., Tronick, Frank, Cabral, & Zuckerman, 1994), may not be apparent until children reach more advanced ages (e.g., Lester & Tronick, 1994), or may be interactional (Freier, 1994). To characterize more subtle, emergent effects on the behavior, development, and interaction of young children exposed prenatally to drugs and alcohol, longitudinal prospective studies with repeated measures collected over extended periods of time are needed.

Additionally, thorough assessment and analysis of the develop-mental and other consequences of prenatal substance exposure requires multiple measures across domains. As noted earlier, many of the effects identified to date appear either transient, subtle, or some-what unreliable (cf. Zuckerman, 1993). Several recent methodological and substantive reviews of this research have suggested that more detailed assessment, across more domains of child performance and interaction, are essential to capture and describe more completely the effects of prenatal exposure and its pre-, peri-, and postnatal correlates (Lester & Tronick, 1994).

ASSESSMENT OF ENVIRONMENTAL FACTORS

Perhaps the greatest single change to characterize the "second generation" of research on the developmental consequences of prenatal substance exposure is increased attention to, and expanded methods for, describing, assessing, and analyzing environmental and contextual factors in the lives of children and families. The need to consider *postnatal environmental* factors more completely was a persistent theme of a recent special issue of the *Infant Mental Health Journal* (Summer, 1994). In this issue, Lester and Tronick (1994) presented a "systems approach" model for the study of cocaine exposure in which child outcomes are mediated by a number of factors, including drug exposure and prenatal environment; the lifestyle, behavior, and personality of the child's mother and other caregivers; and the interactions (or "mutual regulation") between the child and caregiver(s). Lester and Tronick argued that "drugs have a direct acute effect [during the perinatal period] and an indirect long-term effect. . . . The longer term drug effect is indirect, mediated by environmental factors" (1994, p. 112). This theme was reiterated and expanded in the same issue by Beeghly and Tronick (1994) and Freier (1994), who each argue for increased attention to interactions between drug-exposed children and their social and physical environment with specific attention to mutual regulation functions and their effect on subsequent development. The second generation of research must include an expanded methodology for describing, assessing, and analyzing environmental and contextual factors in the lives of children and families. This is especially true in view of the many environmental factors that may jeopardize children growing up in a lifestyle affected by substances.

SECOND GENERATION OF RESEARCH

Children exposed prenatally to alcohol and other drugs are raised in varied environments, often characterized by the presence of multiple factors of substantial risk and few protections or curative influences. These factors must be considered in understanding their developmental outcomes. Some examples of those environmental risks are described below.

FAMILY VARIABLES

Poverty often is a factor affecting the development of children with a history of prenatal substance exposure. Mothers who abuse drugs and/or alcohol must often cope with a multitude of financial and social difficulties, including poor housing, inadequate income, and single parenthood (Regan, Ehrlich, & Finnegan, 1987). Ultimately, because poverty strains caregivers' economic, social, and educational resources, it can profoundly affect caregivers' abilities to provide a consistent nurturing environment (McLoyd, 1990; Zigler & Hall, 1989).

Another difficulty often faced by children prenatally drug exposed or living with a drug-using lifestyle is the *inconsistency of their family and home environment.* Women who continue to abuse substances after the birth of their child often lose custody of their child within 1 year of their child's birth (Tittle & St. Clair, 1989). In some areas of the country, as many as 60% of drug-exposed infants are placed in foster care (Select Committee on Children, Youth, and Families, 1989) and are growing faster than any other population in the foster care system (McCullough, 1991). These children are often shifted from one home to another and separated from their siblings due to the shortage of foster parents willing to care for their special needs. These children are more likely to remain in foster care longer than other children, due to the barriers to adoption and the uncertainty about the appropriateness of adoption for drug-exposed children. It is not uncommon for children who face the continuous trauma of being placed and becoming attached, being shifted and separated, and dealing with loss and grief over and over again to experience emotional and behavioral problems during their childhood years (Griffith, 1992).

EXPOSURE TO VIOLENCE

This is another environmental risk factor faced by children living in a substance-using lifestyle that may occur both in their homes and in their communities (Gropper, 1985). If a child's mother is using drugs, she and the child have a greater likelihood of being surrounded by many other family members and friends who abuse substances (Zuckerman, 1991). Women in these environments are at risk for becoming victims of violence even during pregnancy (Amaro, Fried, Cabral, & Zuckerman, 1990). Children within these environments are more likely to witness violent acts in their homes and in their neighborhoods. A growing body of evidence indicates that witnessing violence can have a profound effect on children's social and emotional outcomes (Garbarino, Kostelny, & Dubrow, 1991; Hughes, 1988). Underscoring this point, some researchers have concluded that children growing up in violent neighborhoods have begun to display the symptoms of post-traumatic stress disorder, including depressed interest in activities, guilt, violent outbursts and rage, difficulty concentrating, and a decline in cognitive performance (Hyman, Zelikoff, & Clarke, 1988; Pynoos & Eth, 1985).

CAREGIVER CHARACTERISTICS

For children who do not go into foster care, continued abuse of alcohol or illicit drugs can significantly affect their parents' abilities to be effective parents (Howard, Beckwith, Rodning, & Kropenske, 1989). Leif (1985) reported that children of women who continue to abuse drugs often experience inconsistent parenting, with mothers behaving one way when under the influence of substances and another way when they are straight. Similarly, women who are taking methadone to control their addictions may neglect to feed or care for their children, or if they are withdrawing, they may be abusive and irritable (Regan, Ehrlich, & Finnegan, 1987). Thus, the quality of caregiving of parents who continue to abuse substances can be seriously undermined.

One of the most prominent risk characteristics of women who abuse drugs and alcohol is the high rate at which these women report past *histories of incest and rape* (Schaefer & Evans, 1989). Estimates of the prevalence of childhood sexual abuse among women in substance abuse treatment centers approach 90% (Amaro et al., 1990). In addition, these women are at increased risk for being physically or sexually assaulted as adults. Many aspects of their lifestyles may predispose women to violence. For example, women in substance-impaired states who are estranged from their families of origin, homeless, or who exchange sex for illicit substances are at higher risk for becoming victims of violence (Covington & Cohen, 1984; Inciardi, 1989; Rieker & Mills, 1984; Rolfs, Goldberg, & Sharran, 1990). Children in these situations may be neglected because the victimized parent is not able to focus on the child's needs.

Considering the lifelong histories of abuse frequently associated with substance abuse, it is not surprising that these women are also at increased risk for adjustment and emotional disorders. Limited psychological resources and impairments in psychological functioning among substance abusing women are widely reported in the literature (Burns, Melamed, & Burns, 1985; Hesselbrock, Meyer, & Kumes, 1985; Miller & Resnick, 1993). A recent prevalence study by the National Institute of Mental Health estimated that individuals with a history of alcohol or drug abuse are seven times more likely to suffer from *mental disorders* than individuals in the general population (Reiger, Farmer, & Roe, 1990).

Specific patterns of risk for psychological disorders have been reported for women substance abusers. Women tend to be at elevated risk for mood disorder (Ross, Glaser, & Stiansy, 1988). Several studies have noted that more than 50% of women in inpatient substance abuse treatment centers present with major *depression* (Hesselbrock et al., 1985). The rate of clinical depression has been reported to be even higher when women in this group are pregnant. In a sample of pregnant women in a methadone treatment program, 75% presented with major depression (Burns et al., 1985). Maternal characteristics such as depression and anxiety have been reported to affect the interactions that caregivers have with their infants (Cohn, Campbell, Matias, & Hopkins, 1990; Crnic, Greenberg, Ragozin, Robinson, & Basham, 1983; Field, Healy, Goldstein, & Guthertz, 1990).

Limited social resources and *impairments in social functioning* long have been recognized as issues of concern for women within the substance-abusing lifestyle. Women who abuse substances often lack basic skills for surviving in today's society, such as availing themselves of community resources, managing finances, finding adequate child care, and pursuing educational and vocational activities (Leif, 1985). Not only do these women often tend to be disconnected from their families, which predisposes them to more unstable living conditions (Shinn, Knickman, & Weitzman, 1991), but they are also likely to experience difficulties in establishing and maintaining interpersonal relationships (Burns et al., 1985; Fiks, Johnson, & Rosen, 1985; Tucker, 1979). Substance-abusing women have been reported to be living in more isolated conditions during pregnancy than nonabusing women (Fiks et al., 1985; Kelley, Walsh, & Thompson, 1991) or to be engaged in ambivalent or negative relationships (Fiks et. al, 1985).

All of the caregiver characteristics described above are likely to affect caregivers' abilities to understand their own children. A commonly expressed clinical concern among professionals providing services to this population is caregivers' *lack of understanding of child development* and behavior (Burns, Chetnik, Burns, & Clark, 1991; Chasnoff & Griffith, 1991; Griffith, 1988). Their limited education in general and their lack of continuing well-child pediatric follow-up result in fewer opportunities for caregivers to gain knowledge of child development (Dawson, Doorninick, William, & Robinson, 1989; Smith, Spiers, & Freese, 1987). Sometimes this lack of understanding leads to unrealistic behavioral expectations of their children. These unrealistic expectations can result in authoritarian and excessively negative approaches to parenting (Bauman & Levine, 1986; Wolfe, 1985).

In summary, consideration of the caregiver characteristics of prenatally drug-exposed children, which frequently include histories of physical and sexual abuse, emotional disorders such as anxiety and depression, lack of social support systems and social skills, and a limited knowledge of child development, is critical to understanding additional risk factors in the postnatal environment. Each of these characteristics has implications for caregiver and child interactions.

INTERACTIONAL RISK FACTORS

A final category of risk that can potentially affect children's long-term development is related to the child's interactions with objects and with persons in their environment. The most obvious environmental risk interaction in a home with ongoing substance abuse is the child's *exposure to the abused substances* themselves. Children have been known to ingest illicit drugs and are often the passive recipients of their smoke.

Another set of interactional risk factors relates to the way in which the child and caregiver interact. Factors associated with a caregiver's drug dependence may seriously affect the *caregiver-child interactions* in a variety of ways. At one extreme, a caregiver under the influence of drugs may not feed children, may neglect to keep infants clean and dry, or, if in a state of withdrawal may be irritable or abusive. At a lesser extreme, caregivers may not be responsive or engage their children in quality exchanges (patterns known to facilitate children's development). In summary, children growing up within environments of ongoing substance use face an abundance of risks within the context of their families, their environments, and the interactions they have with their caregivers. This myriad of factors must be considered in the second generation of research as we attempt to determine the outcomes of children prenatally exposed to substances.

ADVANCES IN ASSESSING CAREGIVING RISK
AND PROTECTIVE FACTORS

Attention to contextual variables, and to transactional models of risk and development that include frequent assessment of multiple aspects of children's environments, has long been a cornerstone in the study of other aspects of child development. Patterson and his colleagues (e.g., Patterson, 1982) have developed a complex, causal model for the development of antisocial behavior that relies substantially on the direct, *in vivo* assessment of interactions between children and family members (or peers) over extended periods of time. Patterson's model of coercive social processes accounts for the development of antisocial behavior through assessment and analysis of a host of environmental factors, including interactional components (e.g., coercive interactions); more molar aspects of child rearing (e.g., parental monitoring); stable characteristics of the child and caregivers (e.g., maternal depression); and cultural, demographic, or socioeconomic variables.

Environmental models also have been used to expand the descriptions of the developmental course of other children at risk, including premature or low birthweight children and children with disabilities. For instance, Bradley et al. (1994) demonstrated validity of a cumulative risk model, in which environmental factors affect developmental outcome in combination rather than through separate, distinct mechanisms. Additionally, Bradley and colleagues adapted earlier research on resilience in children to develop a composite measure of outcome. In this protocol, children were assessed across multiple domains, and outcome was defined as a shared function of performance on all behavioral and developmental measures. Finally, Bradley and colleagues demonstrated that several classes of environmental variables function as "protective factors," and that the accumulation of these factors above a particular threshold increased the likelihood that individual children would achieve desired developmental outcomes.

Although the studies described above did not focus specifically on prenatal exposure to alcohol or other drugs, the methods in these studies hold particular promise for the problem at hand. In particular, these models illustrate various approaches to assessing and analyzing distal and proximal variables that affect children's developmental outcomes. While many of these studies rely on methodological practices not routinely applied in research on prenatal exposure (i.e., longitudinal, *in vivo* and interactional assessment), the principles and methods employed appear to hold special merit for this "second generation" of research on prenatal drug exposure.

Thus, a more complete description of the developmental outcomes of children exposed prenatally to drugs and alcohol, *and* a more complete analysis of the multiple factors associated with these outcomes, requires a more careful and thorough assessment and analysis of the caregiving environments of these children, and changes in these environments both in isolation *and* in interaction with child behavior over time.

A CONCEPTUAL MODEL TO SUPPORT THE
SECOND GENERATION OF RESEARCH

One of the major limitations in addressing the role of environment has been the gap between theory and assessment, resulting in an inadequate measurement and analysis of environmental factors. Thus, while many authors (e.g., Brazelton, Koslowski, & Main, 1974; Tronick, 1989) agree that proximal social factors, such as quality of caregiving, may be more critical in determining child outcomes than larger distal factors, such as SES (socioeconomic status), seldom have direct observational instruments been used to measure such influences.

The work of the Early Childhood Research Institute on Substance Abuse (ECRISA) is based on the view that the development of new interventions and adaptation of existing interventions, those that address the unique needs of drug- and alcohol-exposed children, will be enhanced if guided and informed by longitudinal and experimental data describing the behavioral development of these children as they interact with caregivers and peers in natural settings. This approach, termed *ecobehavioral assessment and analysis* (Greenwood, Carta, & Atwater, 1991), is a transactional ecological-developmental framework that enables us to describe behavioral process within environmental process and to understand the effects of qualitatively different interactions that children experience over time and situations.

Ecobehavioral analysis is an approach to measuring environments concerned with the ecology (its topographical features and the persons within it) and the interactions that occur between the ecology and the behavior of caregivers and children (Carta & Greenwood, 1985; Greenwood & Carta, 1987). A vortex illustrating interaction and transaction within the ecological context is an appropriate metaphor for this set of dynamic relations (see Figure 3.1). One of the goals of ecobehavioral analysis is to determine child behaviors that are most clearly related to negative as well as promising outcomes, such as reduced developmental gain or improved levels of social competence.

Once these critical "decelerating" or "accelerating" behaviors are determined, a second goal of ecobehavioral analysis is to determine the arrangements of ecological variables, including caregiver behavior, that set the occasion for and that establish accelerator behaviors (Greenwood, Delquadri, Stanley, Terry, & Hall, 1985). These accelerator behaviors and their associated ecological (functional situational) factors can then become targets for interventions aimed at improving outcomes.

The ecobehavioral framework supports both proximal and distal analyses of environmental effects. Proximal effects are defined in terms of momentary interactions between children and caregivers and the physical environment (e.g., Sameroff & Fiese, 1990). Distal effects (see Figure 3.1) are defined in terms of the effects of molar environmental factors that affect infant-caregiver by Bronfenbrenner as leveled ecological systems (1989); Thurman & Widerstrom (1990) as ecological system/individual linkage; and by Wahler (1980) as setting events that affect interactions at the proximal level (Greenwood et al., 1992). The ecobehavioral approach provides a useful theoretical basis for forming, operationalizing, and testing multivariate hypotheses concerning environmental effects on child development, including an accounting of natural as well as intervention/services over time. Based on this approach, we have developed and validated and continue to identify and validate new interventions. Findings from our longitudinal studies are providing information on caregiver-child interactions that are most predictive of successful as opposed to high-risk developmental outcomes. These interactions will be the keystones for developing new interventions for drug- and alcohol-exposed children.

PRELIMINARY FINDINGS OF THE EARLY CHILDHOOD RESEARCH INSTITUTE

The ECRISA builds on the tradition of using multiple measures of the child within an environmental context for predicting long-term outcomes. As part of a larger project funded by the Office of Special Education Programs within the Department of Education, the ECRISA is currently carrying out a longitudinal study of children prenatally exposed to illicit drugs and alcohol between birth and 5 years of age. The goal of this study is to describe children's development and significant features of their caregiving environments, and children's interactions with caregivers and teachers within those environments.

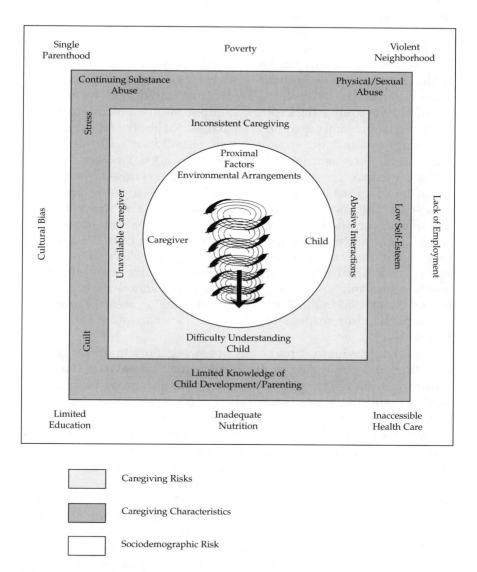

Figure 3.1 Multiple Levels of Risk Affecting Caregiver-Child Interaction in Drug-Using Lifestyle

This descriptive information is being used to identify targets of educational interventions that are being validated in other projects of the Institute.

The descriptive study employs a sequential cohort design with three cohorts defined by the age at which we begin following a child: birth, 18 months, and 36 months. Thus, we are obtaining data on 5 years of development within a 2-year time frame. Cohorts are composed of two groups: the exposed group, composed of children with documented prenatal exposure to illicit drugs or alcohol (60 per cohort); and a nonexposed group, composed of children with no known exposure to illicit drugs or alcohol (30 per cohort), who are matched on race, birthweight, and SES. Children in the exposed group have fallen into two subgroups equal in number: (a) a group primarily exposed to alcohol (but not cocaine) and (b) a group primarily exposed to cocaine (which might or might not be accompanied by alcohol). These children have been recruited from over 125 agencies serving children and families in the geographic vicinity of our three research sites. Participants are distributed equally across the three Institute sites and have been recruited from: (a) inner-city and suburban neighborhood in the Kansas City metropolitan area, (b) inner-city and suburban Minneapolis-St. Paul, and (c) urban and rural areas of South Dakota.

In keeping with the philosophy of assessing multiple areas of risk over time and employing multiple measures, we have used a fairly broad spectrum of assessments to examine family and home variables, mothers' substance use history during pregnancy and during the course of the study, child developmental variables (both general and domain-specific), play skills, and behavior problems (see Table 3.1). Ecobehavioral assessment is used to evaluate children's interactions with their caregivers in their homes, and when applicable, in their child care or preschool settings. Most of these measures are administered repeatedly to all children during their 2-year participation in the project. With few exceptions, all assessments, observations, and interviews have been carried out in children's home environments.

A total of 270 children and their families has been recruited into the study since initiation of the study in February of 1993. Since that time, our annual rate of attrition has been only 2.1%. We consider this a major achievement in light of the fact that some of our families have moved as often as three times within a 4-month period and many of them have no phone service. We have instituted several procedures to retain participants in the study. First is the use of an ethnically diverse professional staff of family liaisons responsible for contact, rapport, and maintenance of family participants. This staff makes monthly visits for this purpose. We contact families and routinely verify information on addresses, and phone numbers for themselves and other members of their social network (Hans, 1991). We also compensate families for their time involved in the study (Capaldi & Patterson, 1987). Additionally, we make strong efforts to encourage a low staff turnover (Hart & Risley, 1989). Our use of a professional staff of observers and assessors, who administer tests and conduct observations in the home, allows children and family members to experience a sense of continuity with the project. Finally, we realize and act on our ethical obligation of assisting families in getting the help they need for their children and for the broad range of problems they may experience (Hans, 1991).

STUDY RESULTS

A preliminary analysis of some of the first data collected on the first set of children taking part in our longitudinal study yields the following preliminary findings.

First, as is true in most studies of prenatal substance use, children in the exposed group have been exposed to more than one substance, and this was especially true for children exposed to cocaine. For example, 43 of the 52 children prenatally exposed to cocaine (83%) were also exposed to one or more illicit drugs such as marijuana, amphetamines, barbiturates or psychedelics, or substantial amounts of alcohol. Of the 84 children included in the exposed group because of their prenatal exposure to alcohol, only 17 (or 20%) were exposed to one or more illicit drugs.

Second, drug-exposed children as a group scored within normal limits on standard IQ tests. For example, children from our exposed and nonexposed groups are performing at approximately the same levels on the Bayley Scales of Infant Development at 20 months (mean MDI for exposed = 96, for nonexposed = 101 and on the Stanford-Binet mean IQs for the exposed group = 96, for the nonexposed group = 95). What we have noted, however, is an increasing tendency for children in each of the older cohorts (i.e., at 21 and 39 months) in both the exposed and nonexposed groups to score lower at each successive age on both the cognitive and communication subscales on the Battelle Developmental Inventory (BDI). Mean deviation quotients on the cog-

TABLE 3.1 ECRISA Assessment Protocol

Assessment domains	Instruments
Prenatal and early childhood medical history	Substance Use Questionnaire
Family	Family Profile, Family Support Scale
Neonatal behavior	Neonatal Behavioral Assessment Scale
Language	Sequenced Inventory of Child Development, Test of Language Development
Play skills	Object Play Observation System
Behavior problems	Achenbach Child Behavior Checklist
Home environment	Home Observation for Measurement of the Environment
Caregiving ecology and interactions	Code for the Interactive Recording of Children's Learning Environment (CIRCLE)
Behavior in child care and preschool	CIRCLE, Student Behavior Rating Scale

nitive subscale for the exposed group at 3, 21, and 39 mos. were 97, 90, and 84; the mean deviation quotients for the nonexposed group at the same age levels were 98, 94, and 84. This same decreasing pattern for the older groups at 3, 21, and 39-month testing was apparent on the communication subscale, with mean deviation quotients of 96, 90, 97, 94, and 80. The mean deviation quotients for both the cognitive and communication subscales for both exposed and nonexposed group at 39 months are more than 1 standard deviation below the mean deviation quotient of 100 for this assessment. This decline in the second year of life, sometimes called the "2-year slump" has been frequently reported for infants from low SES backgrounds (Escalona, 1982; Golden & Birns, 1976). We hypothesize that the developmental trajectories of children from low SES backgrounds in the present study will show a similar decline that will be mediated by environmental risk and protective factors.

Many differences between the exposed and nonexposed group were identified on measures of physical and social aspects of the home environment through the use of the Infant-Toddler (IT-HOME) and Early Childhood (EC-HOME) tests administered every 6 months. Even though exposed and nonexposed groups were matched on SES, we have identified differences on the IT-HOME at 6 and 24 months on all but one subscale, indicating a large discrepancy between the groups in the quantity and quality of support and stimulation provided to the child in the home environment. The subscales on which differences between exposed and nonexposed were most likely to be found on the IT-HOME were the level of caregiver involvement and the caregiver's acceptance of child behavior. The subscale on which greatest differences were found between the groups on the EC-HOME was the variety of stimulation provided in the home. All three of the indicators of caregiving quality have been identified as factors that discriminate between resilient and nonresilient children (see Bradley et al., 1994). It may be hypothesized that these HOME factors may be moderated by family risk factors (such as continued drug use) or child factors related to exposure status.

The study also examined the relationship of other more distal environmental risk factors to children's overall development level as measured by the BDI. Using a cumulative risk approach similar to Sameroff and his colleagues (Sameroff, Seifer, Barocas, Zax, & Greenspan, 1987), we identified a set of risk factors based on evidence in the literature documenting their negative effect on developmental outcomes. For this preliminary analysis, we identified them as: annual income less than $10,000, membership outside of the dominant culture, a primary caregiver who did not complete high school, a single caregiver who did not have the support of other adults, and a child who had experienced out-of-home placement at least once. Similar to the findings of others (Rutter, 1980; Sameroff, Seifer, Barocas, Zax, & Greenspan, 1987), we found a strong relationship between the number of cumulative risk factors (and not necessarily the specific type of factors) and children's developmental outcomes. Children in the exposed group who experienced fewer than two environmental risk factors had a mean deviation quotient (DQ) of 96 (see Figure 3.2). When children in the exposed group experienced two or more risk factors, their DQs were significantly lower and decreased with each additional risk.

Children with five risk factors obtained a mean DQ of 83, significantly lower than those with 0 or 1 risk factor ($p < .015$). Thus far, no similar relationship between the number of risk factors and developmental outcomes for children in the nonexposed group has been identified. In future analyses, proximal caregiving variables will be included in the analyses of risk factors. We expect them to provide similar findings.

We have begun some analyses of patterns of interaction between caregivers and their children as measured by the Code for Interactive Recording of Children's Learning Environments (CIRCLE) (Atwater, Montagna, Creighton, Williams, & Hou, 1993), an ecobehavioral observation system used to assess children in their home environments. Preliminary analyses have shown some significant differences of caregiver and child behaviors between the exposed and nonexposed groups. For example, observations taken when children were 18 months indicated that the primary caregivers of the exposed group spent much less time talking with their child and eliciting child language through verbal prompts or expansions. One of the largest differences we have identified in the behaviors of the children has been in their play with objects. Children in the exposed group at both 18 and 36 months spent much less time playing with toys appropriately or engaged in pretend play. These preliminary findings lend support to our hypothesis that children with a history of substance exposure will experience a greater range of risks in their caregiving environments.

We also have identified differences in ecobehavioral observations of caregiver-child interactions as a function of children's level of environmental risks using the cumulative risk index described above. Using the same list of factors shown to be related to performance on the Battelle Developmental Inventory, children were classified as "high environmental risk" (exposed to two or more factors) or "low environmental risk" (zero or one factor). When groups were divided in this way, many more differences in home environment variables as well as caregiver and child behavior variables were identified between groups. For example, caregivers in the high environmental risk group were less likely to engage in positive vocal responding to their child, to be closely involved with their child and talk to or attempt to elicit language from their child than were caregivers in the low environmental risk group. Children in the high environmental risk group were also much more likely to be observed with no materials in their vicinity with which to play or explore. These data provide preliminary

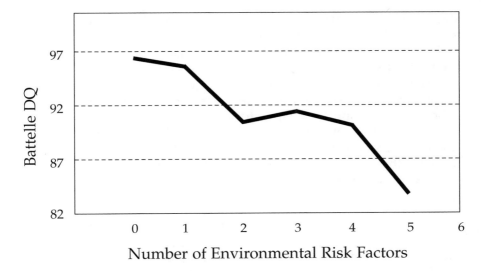

Figure 3.2 Relationship between Cumulative Environmental Risk and Developmental Outcome for High-Exposure Group

support for the hypothesis that children with a history of substance exposure who experience the effects of cumulative risk factors will demonstrate greater developmental delays than children with fewer risk factors and that these effects will be moderated by their ongoing patterns of interactions within the caregiving environments.

SUMMARY AND FUTURE DIRECTIONS

Our preliminary data show few differences thus far on standardized assessments—a finding we share with many other researchers working with drug-exposed children. Many researchers report, however, that standardized tests given in structured one-on-one assessment situations tend to minimize difficulties these children have in less structured classroom situations. Our observational data tend to confirm this, showing a much greater discrepancy in rates of language behavior between the low- and high-risk groups. Our observations of the caregiving context also direct us to some explanations for the lower language performance of the children in the high-risk group. Though these data are still very preliminary, they reveal how observational data can help amplify the picture of development provided by standardized assessments. Used in conjunction with information about the family and home environment, and gathering these data across several points in time, provides a more comprehensive explanation of outcomes for these children than was offered by the first generation of research. In the future, we will concentrate our efforts in identifying the protective factors that may help our understanding of children who succeed in spite of their history of prenatal exposure and other risk factors. This information will eventually lead us to information about successful patterns of caregiving that will form the basis of interventions that can be used by other parents and child care providers of infants affected by drug exposure and other environmental risks.

REFERENCES

Allen, L. F., Palomares, R. S., DeForest, P., Sprinkle, B., & Reynolds, C. R. (1991). The effects of intrauterine cocaine exposure: Transient or teratogenic? *Archives of Clinical Neuropsychology, 6,* 133–146.

Amaro, H., Fried, L. E., Cabral, H. , & Zuckerman, B. (1990). Violence during pregnancy and substance use. *American Journal of Public Health, 80,* 575– 583.

Amaro, H., Zuckerman, B., & Cabral, H. (1989). Drug use among adolescent mothers: Profile of risk. *Pediatrics, 84,* 144–151.

Atwater, J., Montagna, D., Creighton, M., Williams, R., & Hou, S. (1993). *CIRCLE-2: Code for Interactive Recording of Caregiving and Learning Environments-Infancy through early childhood.* Kansas City, KS: Early Childhood Research Institute on Substance Abuse.

Bauman, P., & Levine, S. (1986). The development of children of drug addicts. *The International Journal of the Addictions, 21,* 849–863.

Beeghly, M., & Tronick, E. Z. (1994). Effects of prenatal cocaine exposure in early infancy: Toxic effects on the process of mutual regulation. *Infant Mental Health Journal, 15,* 158–175.

Bradley, R. H., Whiteside, L., Mundfrom, D., Casey, P., Kelleher, K., & Pope, S. (1994). Early indications of resilience and their relation to experiences in the home environments of low birthweight, premature children living in poverty. *Child Development, 65,* 346–360.

Brazelton, T. B., Koslowski, B., & Main, M. (1974). The origins of reciprocity: The early mother-infant interaction. In M. Lewis & L. A. Rosenblum (Eds.) *The effect of the infant on its caregiver* (pp. 45–76). New York: Wiley.

Bronfenbrenner, U. (1989). Ecological system theories. *Annals of Child Development, 6,* 187–249.

Burns, K., Chethik, L., Burns, W. J., & Clark, R. (1991). Dyadic disturbances in cocaine-abusing mothers and their infants. *Journal of Clinical Psychology, 47,* 316–319.

Burns, K., Melamed, J., & Burns, W. (1985). Chemical dependence and clinical depression in pregnancy. *Journal of Clinical Psychology, 41,* 851–854.

Capaldi, D. M., & Patterson, G. R. (1987). An approach to the problem of recruitment and retention rates for longitudinal research. *Behavioral Assessment, 9,* 169–177.

Carta, J. J., & Greenwood, C. R. (1985). Ecobehavioral assessment: A methodology for expanding the evaluation of early intervention programs. *Topics in Early Childhood Special Education, 5,* 88–104.

Carta, J. J., Sideridis, G., Rinkle, P., Guimaraes, S., Greenwood, C., Bagget, K., Peterson, P., Atwater, J., McEvoy, M., & McConnell, S. (1994). Behavioral outcomes of infants and young children prenatally exposed to illicit drugs. *Topics in Early Childhood Special Education, 13,* 243–254.

Chasnoff, I. J. (1988a). Cocaine: Effects on pregnancy and the neonate. In I. J. Chasnoff (Ed.), *Drugs, alcohol, pregnancy and parenting.* (pp. 9–38). Hingham, MA: Kluwer Academic Publishers.

Chasnoff, I. J. (1988b). Drug use in pregnancy: Parameters of risk. *Pediatric Clinics of North America, 35,* 1403.

Chasnoff, I. J., Burns, K. A., & Burns, W. J. (1987). Cocaine use in pregnancy: Perinatal morbidity and mortality. *Neurotoxicology and Teratology, 9,* 291–293.

Chasnoff, I. J., & Griffith, D. (1991). Maternal cocaine use: Neonatal outcomes. In H. E. Fitzgerald, M. Lester, & M. W. Yogman (Eds.), *Theory and research in behavioral pediatrics* (pp. 1–17). New York: Plenum Press.

Chasnoff, I. J., Griffith, D. R., & Azuma, S. (1992). Intrauterine cocaine/polydrug exposure: Three-year outcome. *Pediatric Research, 31,* 9.

Chasnoff, I. J., Griffith, D. R., Freier, C., & Murray, J. (1992). Cocaine/polydrug use in pregnancy: Two-year follow-up. *Pediatrics, 89,* 284–289.

Chasnoff, I. J., Landress, G. D., & Barrett, R. (1990). The prevalence of illicit-drug or alcohol use during pregnancy and discrepancies in mandatory reporting in Pinellas County, Florida. *The New England Journal of Medicine, 322,* 1202–1206.

Cohn, J. F., Campbell, S. B., Matias, R., & Hopkins, J. (1990). Face-to-face interactions of postpartum depressed and non-depressed mother-infant pairs at 2 months. *Developmental Psychology, 26,* 15–23.

Coles, C. C., Platzman, K. A., Smith, I., James, M. E., & Falek, A. (1992). Effects of cocaine and alcohol use in pregnancy on neonatal growth and neurobehavioral status. *Neurotoxicology and Teratology, 14,* 23–33.

Covington, S., & Cohen, J. (1984). Women, alcohol, and sexuality. *Advances in Alcohol Substance Abuse, 4,* 41–56.

Crnic, K. A., Greenberg, M. T., Ragozin, A. S., Robinson, N. M., & Basham, R. B. B. (1983). Effects of stress and social support on mothers and premature and full-term infants. *Child Development, 54,* 209–217.

Dawson, P., Doorninick, V., William, J., & Robinson, J. L. (1989). Effects of home-based informal social support on child health. *Journal of Developmental and Behavioral Pediatrics, 10,* 63–67.

Dixon, S., & Bejar, R. (1989). Echoencephalographic findings in neonates associated with maternal cocaine and methamphetamine use: Incidence and clinical correlates. *The Journal of Pediatrics, 115,* 770–778.

Escalona, S. K. (1982). Babies at double hazard: Early development of infants at biologic and social risk. *Pediatrics, 70,* 670–676.

Field, T. M., Healy, B., Goldstein, S., & Guthertz, M. (1990). Behavior-state matching and synchrony in mother-infant interactions of non-depressed versus depressed dyads. *Developmental Psychology, 26,* 7–14.

Fiks, K. B., Johnson, H. L., & Rosen, R. S. (1985). Methadone maintained mothers: Three-year follow-up of parental functioning. *The International Journal of the Addictions, 20,* 651–660.

Finnegan, L. P. (1986). Neonatal abstinence syndrome: Assessment and pharmocotherapy. In F. F. Rubaltelli & B. Granati (Eds.), *Neonatal therapy update* (pp. 122–146). New York: Excerpta Medica.

Freier, K. (1994). In utero drug exposure and maternal-infant interaction: The complexities of the dyad and their enviroment. *Infant Mental Health Journal, 15,* 176–188.

Fried, P. A. (1989). Cigarettes and marijuana: Are there measurable long-term neurobehavioral teratogenic effects? *Neurotoxicology, 10,* 577–584.

Fried, P. A., & Watkinson, B. (1990). 36- and 48-month neurobehavioral follow-up of children prenatally exposed to marijuana, cigarettes, and alcohol. *Developmental and Behavioral Pediatrics, 11,* 49–58.

Garbarino, J., Kostelny, K., & Dubrow, N. (1991). What children can tell us about living in danger. *American Psychologist, 46,* 376–383.

Golden, M., & Birns, B. (1976). Social class and infant intelligence. In M. Lewis (Ed.), *Origins of intelligence: Infancy and early childhood* (pp. 73–95). New York: Plenum Press.

Greenwood, C. R., & Carta, J. J. (1987). An ecobehavioral analysis of instruction within special education. *Focus on Exceptional Children, 19,* 1–12.

Greenwood, C. R., Carta, J. J., & Atwater, J. J. (1991). Ecobehavioral analysis in the classroom: Review and implications. *Journal of Behavioral Education, 1,* 59–77.

Greenwood, C. R., Carta, J. J., Hart, B., Kamps, D., Terry, B., Arreaga-Mayer, C., Atwater, J., Walker, D., Risley, T., & Delquadri, J. (1992). Out of the laboratory and into the community: 26 years of applied behavior analysis at the Juniper Gardens Children's Project. *American Psychologist, 47,* 1464–1474.

Greenwood, C. R., Delquadri, J., Stanley, S. O., Terry, B., & Hall, R. V. (1985). Assessment of eco-behavioral interaction in school settings. *Behavioral Assessment, 7,* 331–347.

Griffith, D. R. (1988). The effects of perinatal cocaine exposure on infant neurobehavior and early maternal-infant interactions. In I. J. Chasnoff (Ed.), *Drugs, alcohol, and pregnancy* (pp. 105–114). Boston, MA: Kuwer Academic Publishers.

Griffith, D. R. (1992, September). Prenatal exposure to cocaine and other drugs: Developmental and educational prognosis. *Phi Delta Kappan, 30–34.*

Griffith, D. R., & Freier, C. (1992). Methodological issues in the assessment of the mother-child interactions of substance-abusing women and their children. *NIDA Research Monographs, 117,* 228–247.

Gropper, B. (1985). Probing the links between drugs and crime. *National Institute of Justice Research in Brief.* Washington, DC: U. S. Department of Justice.

Hans, S. L. (1991). Following drug-exposed infants into middle childhood: Challenges to researchers. *NIDA Research Monographs, 114,* 310–322.

Hart, B., & Risley, T. R. (1989). The longitudinal study of interactive systems. *Education and Treatment of Children, 12,* 347–358.

Hesselbrock, M. N., Meyer, R. E., & Kumes, J. J. (1985). Psychopathology in hospitalized alcoholics. *Archives of General Psychiatry, 42,* 1050–1055.

Howard, J., Beckwith, L., Rodning, C., & Kropenske, V. (1989). The development of young children of substance-abusing parents: Insights from seven years of intervention and research. *Zero to Three, 9,* 5–8.

Hughes, H. M. (1988). Psychological and behavioral correlates of family violence in child witness and victims. *American Journal of Orthopsychiatry, 58,* 77–90.

Hyman, I. A., Zelikoff, W., & Clarke, J. (1988). Psychological and physical abuse in the schools: A paradigm for understanding post-traumatic stress disorder in children and youth. *Journal of Traumatic Stress, 2,* 243–267.

Inciardi, J. A. (1989). Trading sex for crack among juvenile drug users: A research note. *Contemporary Drug Problems, 16,* 689–700.

Kelley, S. J., Walsh, J. H., & Thompson, K. (1991). Birth outcomes, health problems, and neglect with prenatal exposure to cocaine. *Pediatric Nursing, 17,* 130–135.

Leif, N. (1985). The drug user as parent. *The International Journal of Addiction, 201,* 63–97.

Landesman-Dwyer, S., Ragozin, A. S., & Little, R. (1981). Behavioral correlates of prenatal alcohol exposure: A four-year follow-up study. *Neurobehavioral*

Toxicology and Teratology, 3, 187–193.

Lester, B. M. & Tronick, E. Z. (1994). The effects of cocaine exposure and child outcome. *Infant Mental Health Journal, 15,* 107–120.

Lutiger, B., Graham, K., Einarson, T. R., & Koren, G. (1991). Relationship between gestational cocaine use and pregnancy outcome: A meta-analysis. *Teratology, 44,* 405–414.

Mayes, L. C., Granger, R. H., Bornstein, M. H., & Zuckerman, B. (1992). The problem of prenatal cocaine use: A rush to judgment. *Journal of the American Medical Association, 267,* 406–408.

McCullough, C. B. (1991). The child welfare response. *In The Future of Children, 1,* 61–71.

McLoyd, V. C. (1990). The impact of economic hardship on black families and children: Psychological distress, parenting, and socioemotional development. *Child Development, 61,* 311–346.

Miller, W. H., & Resnick, M. P. (1993). Comorbidity in pregnant patients in a psychiatric inpatient setting. *American Journal of Drug and Alcohol Abuse, 19,* 177–185.

Nieburg, P., Marks, J. S., McLaren, N. M., & Remington, P. L. (1985). The fetal tobacco syndrome. *Journal of the American Medical Association, 253,* 2998–2999.

Oro, A. S., & Dixon, S. D. (1987). Perinatal cocaine and methamphetamine exposure: Maternal and neonatal correlates. *The Journal of Pediatrics,* 571–577.

Patterson, G. R. (1982). *Coercive family process.* Eugene, OR: Castalia.

Pynoos, R., & Eth, S. (1985). Children traumatized by witnessing acts of personal violence: Homicide, rape, and suicide behavior. In S. Eth & R. Pynoos (Eds.), *Post-traumatic stress disorder in children* (pp. 17–22). Washington, DC: American Psychiatric Press.

Regan, D., Ehrlich, S., & Finnegan, L. (1987). Infants of drug addicts: At risk for child abuse, neglect, and placement in foster care. *Neurotoxicology and Teratology, 9,* 315–319.

Reiger, D. A., Farmer, M. E., & Roe, D. S. (1990). Comorbidity of mental disorders with alcohol and other drug abuse. *Journal of the American Medical Association, 264,* 2511–2518.

Rieker, C. E. & Mills, T. (1984). Victims of violence and psychiatric illness. *American Journal of Psychiatry, 141,* 378–383.

Rodning, C., Beckwith, L., & Howard, J. (1989). Characteristics of attachment organization and play organization in prenatally drug-exposed toddlers. *Development and Psychopathology, 1,* 277–289.

Rolfs, R. T., Goldberg, M., & Sharran, R. G. (1990). Risk factors for syphilis: Cocaine use and prostitution. *American Journal of Public Health, 80,* 853–857.

Ross, H. E., Glaser, F. B., & Stiansy, S. (1988). Sex differences in the prevalence of psychiatric disorders in patients with drug and alcohol abuse. *British Journal of Addictions, 83,* 1179–1192.

Rutter, M. (1980). *Changing youth in a changing society: Patterns of adolescent development and disorder.* Cambridge, MA: Harvard University Press.

Sameroff, A. J., & Fiese, B. H. (1990). Transactional regulation and early intervention. In S. J., Meisels & J. Shonkoff (Eds.), *Handbook of early childhood intervention* (pp. 119–149). New York: Cambridge University Press.

Sameroff, A., Seifer, R., Barocas, B., Zax, M., & Greenspan, S. (1987). IQ scores of four-year-old children: Social-environmental risk factors. *Pediatrics, 79,* 343–350.

Schaefer, S., & Evans, S. (1987). Women, sexuality, and the process of recovery. *Journal of Chemical Dependency Treatment, 1,* 91–120.

Select Committee on Children, Youth and Families, U. S. House of Representatives, 101st Congress, First Session. (1989). *Born hooked: Confronting the impact of perinatal substance abuse.* Washington, DC: U. S. Government Printing Office.

Shinn, M., Knickman, J. R., & Weitzman, B. B. (1991). Social relationships and vulnerability to becoming homeless among poor families. *American Psychologist, 46,* 1180–1187.

Singer, L., Arendt, R., & Minnes, S. (1993). Neurodevelopmental effects of cocaine. *Clinics in Perinatology, 20,* 245–262.

Smith, K. E., Spiers, M. V., & Freese, M. P. (1987). Adolescent mothers' successful participation in well-baby care programs. *Journal of Adolescent Health Care, 8,* 193–197.

Thurman, S. K., & Widerstrom, A. H. (1990). *Infants and young children with special needs: A developmental and ecological approach* (2nd ed.). Baltimore: Paul H. Brookes.

Tittle, B., & St. Clair, N. (1989). Promoting the health and development of drug-exposed infants through a comprehensive clinic model. *Zero to Three, 9,* 18–20.

Tronick, E. Z. (1989). Emotions and emotional communication in infants. *American Psychologist, 44,* 112–119.

Tronick, E. Z., Frank, D. A., Cabral, H., & Zuckerman, B. (1994). A dose response effect of in utero cocaine exposure on infant neurobehavioral functioning. *Pediatric Research, 35,* (#4), Pt. 2 Abs. #152, 28A.

Tucker, M. B., (1979). A descriptive and comparative analysis of the social support structure of heroine-addicted women. In *Addicted women: Family dynamics, self perceptions, and support systems* (pp. 254–268). NIDA Services, Research Monograph Series. Rockville, MD: Department of Health, Education, and Welfare.

Wahler, R. G. (1980). The insular mother: Her problems in parent-child treatment. *Journal of Applied Behavior Analysis, 13,* 207–219.

Wilson, G. S., McCreary, R., Kean, J., & Baxter, C. (1979). The development of preschool children of heroin-addicted mothers: A controlled study. *Pediatrics, 63,* 135–141.

Wolfe, D. A. (1985). Child abusive parents: An empirical review and analysis. *Psychological Bulletin, 97,* 462–482.

Zigler, E., & Hall, N. (1989). Physical child abuse in America: Past, present, and future. In D. Cicchetti & V. Carlson (Eds.), *Child maltreatment: Theory and research on the causes and consequences of child abuse and neglect* (pp. 38–75). New York: Cambridge University Press.

Zuckerman, B. (1991). Selected methodologic issues in investigations of prenatal effects of cocaine: Lessons from the past. In M. Kibey & K. Asghar (Eds.), *Methodological issues in controlled studies of effects of prenatal exposure to drug abuse.* (pp. 45–54) (NIDA Research Monograph No. 114). Rockville, MD: National Institute on Drug Abuse.

Zuckerman, B. (1993, July). *Behaviors of drug-exposed offspring.* Presentation made at the NIDA Technical Review Meeting on "Behaviors of Drug-Exposed Offspring: Research Update." Washington, DC.

Zuckerman, B., Amaro, H., Bauchner, H., & Cabral, H. (1989). Depressive symptoms during pregnancy: Relationship to poor health behaviors. *American Journal of Obstetrics and Gynecology, 160,* 1107–1111.

4

Criminalization of Drug Use During Pregnancy: A Case Study*

Philip H. Jos, Ph.D., Mary Faith Marshall, Ph.D., and Martin Perlmutter, Ph.D.[†]

T he conflict between pregnant women freely using cocaine and the well-being of fetuses presents a difficult social problem. Since 1985, at least 200 women in 30 states have been criminally prosecuted for using illicit drugs or alcohol during pregnancy. Such policies enjoy considerable public and political support. Nonetheless, treatment programs that include referral to law enforcement officials raise serious ethical and legal issues for hospitals and health care providers. In this paper, we assess the development of one medical university's controversial treatment program for pregnant women addicted to cocaine.

In October 1989, the Medical University of South Carolina (MUSC) instituted a new program, called the Interagency Policy on Management of Substance Abuse During Pregnancy (Medical University of South Carolina, 1989), designed "to ensure appropriate management of patients abusing illegal drugs during pregnancy." This program required some pregnant women to seek drug counseling and prenatal care under the threat of criminal sanctions. This bold manner of dealing

* Previously published as "The Charleston Policy on Cocaine Use During Pregnancy: A Cautionary Tale," by P. H. Jos, M. F. Marshall, and M. Perlmutter, *Journal of Law, Medicine & Ethics*, 23(2) (1995): 120–28. Reprinted with the permission of the American Society of Law, Medicine & Ethics.
† Acknowledgments:
We are indebted to David J. Annibale, M.D., Arthur L. Caplan, Ph.D., Wendy Chavkin, M.D., M.P.H., James F. Childress, Ph.D., B. Natalie Demers, M.H.A., John C. Fletcher, Ph.D., Franklin G. Miller, Ph.D., Lawrence J. Nelson, Ph.D., J.D., John A. Robertson, J.D., Robert M. Sade, M.D., and Donna Taylor, J.D., for their comments on earlier drafts of the manuscript.

with the problem attracted national attention. Five years later, on September 1, 1994, MUSC agreed to discontinue the policy, which, by that time, had resulted in the arrest of 42 pregnant women who had tested positive for cocaine but did not follow up on recommended treatment for chemical dependency. The academic medical center, located in Charleston, South Carolina, made the change in a settlement with the Civil Rights Division of the Department of Health and Human Services (DHHS). After the policy was discontinued, the federal Office of Protection from Research Risks (OPRR) determined that the program constituted human experimentation conducted without requisite Internal Review Board (IRB) scrutiny and approval, and deferred renewal of MUSC's Multiple Project Assurance for at least 1 year, pending sufficient corrective action by MUSC (Memorandum, Oct. 5, 1993). MUSC still faces a multimillion dollar class action lawsuit brought on behalf of several women who were jailed under the policy (*Ferguson and Roe et al., v. City of Charleston et al.,* 1993).

The evolution of the Interagency Policy is not a simple story, but a complex tale involving diverse professional interests addressing a seemingly intractable social problem. We describe the policy, and consider the way in which it was developed, adopted, and came to incorporate both detection of drug use and referral for criminal prosecution. After reviewing some legal and ethical issues associated with cocaine abuse by pregnant women, we explain how a sense of crisis, the nature of the target population, and clinical medicine's way of conceptualizing problems each contributed to an overly narrow definition of the problem. The result was a treatment program with wide appeal but of dubious effectiveness. We conclude by reflecting on the role of medicine in addressing complex social problems, and by briefly assessing the proposed successor policy, which does not include criminal sanctions.

THE INTERAGENCY POLICY

The Interagency Policy applied to patients attending the obstetrics clinic at MUSC, which primarily serves patients who are indigent or on Medicaid. It did not apply to private obstetrical patients. The policy required patient education about the harmful effects of substance abuse during pregnancy, either on the patient's first visit to the clinic or during her initial hospitalization. Patients watched a video presentation of the harmful effects of substance abuse during pregnancy and were given a written statement, from the obstetrics service, which both reviewed complications of street drug abuse during pregnancy and offered patients assistance in obtaining treatment for substance abuse. The statement also warned patients that protection of unborn and newborn children from the harms of illegal drug abuse could involve the Charleston police, the Solicitor of the Ninth Judicial Court, and the Protective Services Division of the Department of Social Services (DSS). Patients were required to sign a document stating the following: "I have seen a video on substance abuse and have been advised of the risks to myself and my baby. I understand that the MUSC Medical Center staff is willing to assist me in obtaining assistance for drug abuse treatment." The patient's signature, Social Security Number, the date, and the signature of a witness were recorded on the document (Medical University of South Carolina, 1989, p. 5).

The policy required that women who met certain criteria undergo urine screening for illegal drugs. Screening criteria included the absence of prenatal care, late prenatal care after 24 weeks of gestation, incomplete prenatal care, abruptio placentae, intrauterine fetal death, preterm labor of no obvious cause, intrauterine growth retardation of no obvious cause, previous known drug or alcohol abuse, and unexplained congenital abnormalities. The policy defined illegal drugs as "heroin, crack/cocaine, amphetamines and any other drug illegally ingested by the patient that medical authorities deem a threat to the life and safety of the unborn child." Once obtained, the urine samples entered a legal chain of custody.

When a patient's urine screen was positive for illegal drugs, the high-risk obstetrical case manager was notified by the resident physician. If the patient had not seen the educational video, she was shown the video and was required to sign the statement indicating the dangers and consequences of continued drug use. An appointment was made with the substance abuse clinic, a follow-up appointment was made with the obstetrics clinic, and appointment letters were given to the patient. Patients who screened positive also were given a letter, from the Solicitor of the Ninth Judicial Circuit, stating that the patient had tested positive for drugs, was being afforded an opportunity for rehabilitation, and warning that "if you fail to attend Substance Abuse and Pre-Natal care you will be arrested by Charleston City Police and prosecuted by the Office of Solicitor" (Medical University of South Carolina, 1989)."

Operational guidelines of the Charleston police department stated that a criminal report would be made and an arrest warrant issued for patients who tested positive for drugs and failed to keep scheduled appointments for substance abuse therapy or for prenatal care. Those who tested positive for illegal drugs a second time would be taken into immediate custody on their medical release, even if time did not permit the securing of an arrest warrant. "[Aggravated] circumstances and/or refusal by the patient to agree to voluntary assistance may justify arrest at the first report of drug abuse." Any patient who delivered a child who tested positive for illegal drugs would be arrested immediately after her medical release, and the newborn child would be taken into protective custody by the DSS. If the gestation was 27 weeks or less, the patient was charged with possession of an illegal substance. If the gestation was 28 weeks or more, the patient was charged with possession and distribution of an illegal substance to persons under eighteen. If, during delivery, the patient or her child tested positive for illegal drugs, the mother was charged with unlawful neglect of a child (Medical University of South Carolina, 1989, p. 6).

THE ORIGINS OF THE INTERAGENCY POLICY

In 1988, a physician in MUSC's Department of Obstetrics and Gynecology and that department's high-risk case manager became concerned about an apparent increase in cocaine use among pregnant women. They were alarmed by reports that 10% or more of all infants are exposed to cocaine *in utero*, and they saw a sharp rise in positive urine drug tests in their own clinic. Drug screening, which began in October 1988, found only two to four positive tests per month during the initial months, but showed more than twenty positive test results in August 1989. In the first year of screening, 119 expectant mothers had tested positive, so data suggested a growing sense of an urgent problem (Medical University of South Carolina, 1989). Newborn Nursery and Neonatal Intensive Care Unit (NICU) staff witnessed an increasing number of newborns presenting with effects of maternal cocaine use, such as withdrawal, irritability, lethargy, stiff muscle tone, problems eating and sleeping, cardiovascular dysfunction, and aversion to loud sounds or handling (Medical University of South Carolina, 1989, p. 7).

This genuine concern for the health of babies born to drug-abusing mothers was heightened by the apparent inability of existing clinical protocols to change the pattern of drug abuse. Of the 119 women who tested positive for cocaine before the policy was established, 104 delivered their infants before a second drug screening occurred. Each of the remaining 15 patients tested positive when she returned in preterm labor, even though each had received counseling by a hospital nurse and a social worker regarding the risks of cocaine use while pregnant. Moreover, follow up care at the Charleston County Substance Abuse Clinic had been arranged in every case, but not one of the mothers kept her appointment. It was clear that existing treatment strategies were failing and that complacency would have been irresponsible.

By August 1989, concern had grown that something had to be done to "add some teeth to our counseling efforts" (Medical University of South Carolina, 1989). MUSC personnel approached the Ninth Circuit solicitor and the City of Charleston Police Department. This initial contact set the tone for the discussions that followed. The solicitor enthusiastically embraced the development of a revised policy, and took the position that hospital officials had no choice but to report positive drug tests to the police. "There's no patient-doctor privilege on this. If you don't report it, it's a crime." A task force was assembled by the solicitor's office, consisting of representatives from MUSC, the police department, the solicitor's office, the DSS, and the Charleston County Substance Abuse Commission. The group met in September and October, and drafted the Interagency Policy that was implemented in mid-October 1989. The policy was developed and implemented very quickly, in less than 2 months. The policy was never submitted for review either to MUSC's IRB, its Medical Center Ethics Committee, or to any outside evaluators. Early misgivings on the part of agencies whose goals were more rehabilitative than punitive eased when they were assured that criminal sanctions would apply only after initial efforts at treatment had failed (Memorandum, Oct. 5, 1993). During the first months of the policy's operation, several hospital employees, including the nursing manager and the medical director of the NICU, pointed out perceived flaws in the policy, such as "thinly veiled discrimination against . . . poor black women," and the lack of sufficient treatment facilities in Charleston. Such concerns were otherwise rarely expressed.

This swift pace of policy development stemmed from a sense of urgency surrounding the problem of cocaine abuse by pregnant women. The threat to fetal well-being posed by cocaine abuse is emotionally charged in ways that other, more common but legal behaviors that endanger fetal health, such as alcohol use, tobacco use, poor prenatal care, and inadequate diet, are not. In internal documents and press

interviews, the policy's formulators repeatedly referred to the enor-
mity of the problem. Within the obstetrics clinic, both genuine concern
for fetal well-being and outrage at the behavior of the pregnant women
were expressed. During the period when the policy was developed,
the specter of an epidemic of drug use was sufficiently well established
to trigger the appointment of a drug czar in Washington to emphasize
the severity of the drug crisis. A surge of media attention in 1988 and
1989, which focused on an "epidemic" of "pregnant addicts" and "coke
babies," also fueled the sense of crisis. Some of these stories (and, to
some extent, the development of the policy) were triggered by a study
based on a survey of 36 hospitals, 34 of which were urban, that estimated that 11% of pregnant women had used an illegal drug during
pregnancy (Chasnoff, 1989).

In this context, a more deliberative Interagency Policy planning
process involving affected groups never evolved. The clinicians sought
outside help for a seemingly intractable problem, but law enforcement
officials quickly framed the problem narrowly: How do we get women
to attend treatment sessions? The adequacy of existing treatment facilities was not seriously addressed, nor were the controversial legal and
ethical issues attending punitive sanctions.

Internal review was limited to MUSC's attorney, whose primary
concern was with the institution's vulnerability to breach of confidentiality complaints. The routine path of administrative approval was
followed, but neither MUSC's Medical Center Ethics Committee nor
its IRB were included in this process.

DISCUSSION

LEGAL AND ETHICAL CONFLICTS

Legal controversies surrounding maternal rights and the status of the
fetus are enormously complex. Informed in large part by the controversies surrounding the constitutionality of antiabortion statutes, the
courts have ruled repeatedly in recent years on the rights of the pregnant woman, the compelling state interests surrounding pregnancy,
and the legal standing of the fetus. The weight of judicial rulings continues to favor maternal rights even though some lower courts have
been willing to overrule maternal autonomy to prevent harm to the
fetus (Nelson & Milliken, 1988; Blank, 1993; Merrick, 1993).

Although inconsistency arises between jurisdictions, the unmistakable trend is toward greater acknowledgment of fetal rights in tort law (Blank, 1993). And even though no state has specifically criminalized substance abuse during pregnancy, some states have criminalized fetal homicide and manslaughter. Others, such as Minnesota, have non-punitive reporting statutes that include the use of controlled substances by pregnant women for nonmedical purposes as prenatal neglect. However, these have not been interpreted by the courts in ways that support judicial intervention on behalf of the fetus (Nelson & Milliken, 1988).

Moreover, standing Supreme Court decisions have rejected claims that maternal rights can be overwhelmed by fetal rights. The future status of the *Roe v. Wade* (1973) decision is uncertain, but the Court has refused to accept that a compelling state interest in protecting viable fetuses allows or sanctions compulsory treatment of the mother. In *Colautti v. Franklin* (1979) the Court struck down a statute because it failed to guarantee that a woman's health must always prevail over the fetus's life and health. A subsequent ruling confirmed this view and rejected statutes that require a tradeoff between maternal health and fetal survival. Nelson and Milliken (1988) conclude that "when the health interests of a woman and her fetus conflict, the state appears to be constitutionally bound to place the woman's interests above the fetus."

Nonetheless, prosecutors in 30 states, lacking both established precedent and clear statutory authority, have taken legal action against pregnant substance abusers on other grounds, such as child abuse, delivery of a controlled substance, and manslaughter. While some district courts have upheld such convictions, no criminal conviction involving *in utero* transmission of a controlled substance has been upheld by higher courts. The Florida Supreme Court rejected lower court rulings and unanimously overturned the conviction of Jennifer Johnson on child abuse and controlled substance charges (*Florida v. Johnson*, 1989). A divided Ohio Supreme Court reached similar conclusions (*State v. Gray*, 1990). In a 1992 South Carolina case, post-conviction relief for the charge of child abuse and neglect was granted to Rosena Tolliver, who used cocaine while pregnant, "on the grounds that the act she allegedly committed did not constitute a violation of the code section" (*Tolliver v. South Carolina*, 1992). In finding against the state, the court ruled that extending the meaning of the word "child" to include "fetus" in the South Carolina Code of Laws is illegitimate, because it violates the word's plain and ordinary meaning, and clearly was not the intention of the legislature (*Bryant v. City of Charleston*, 1988).

The 1993 lawsuit against MUSC, brought by three of the women incarcerated by the Interagency Policy, seeks compensatory and punitive damages and does not focus on the legal status of the fetus. Instead, the suit claims violations of the former patients' constitutional rights to privacy and liberty, and particularly violations of the patients' right to privacy in medical information, their right to refuse medical treatment, and their right to procreate. It also claims that the policy is "an unconstitutional experiment on African-American women," thereby violating the patients' constitutional right to equal protection under the law. Finally, the suit claims a violation of the right to confidentiality guaranteed to patients of substance abuse treatment programs under Federal and South Carolina law (*Ferguson and Roe*, 1993).

Many of these legal concerns are reflected in widely-held presumptive ethical standards for clinical care. Respect for a patient's privacy imposes a duty on health care clinicians to maintain patient confidentiality, which supports a fiduciary relationship between clinician and patient. Clinicians must protect patients' right to control information that pertains to them and that may affect their lives. Both patients and clinicians are negatively affected by the loss of this protected relationship. Moreover, consultation with a physician or a health care facility for a specific purpose does not provide an open-ended consent for investigation of unrelated medical conditions, even if the search is physically noninvasive, as with a urine test (*Skinner v. Railway Labor Executives Assn.* 1989).

The patient's right to informed consent and its corollary, the right to refuse treatment, are also well-established American legal doctrines and bioethical standards. Clinicians must adhere to the informed consent process, involving disclosure, understanding, and voluntariness; and they must respect the patient's right to refuse treatment. Treatment refusals can be overridden only when patients are incapable decision makers or pose a danger to themselves or to others. Trust within the therapeutic relationship depends on the patient's confidence that the clinician is concerned with her well-being. Breaches of confidentiality, medical coercion, and participation in the punitive incarceration of a patient undermine that trust, and so are *prima facie* objectionable (Nelson & Milliken, 1988). Professional associations are especially sensitive to the ways in which punitive policies may undermine the clinician's single-minded commitment to the well-being of the patient. Thus, in addition to their skepticism regarding the efficacy of punitive treatment, most public health organizations, including the American Medical Association, the American Academy of Pediatrics, the American

College of Obstetrics and Gynecology, the American Society of Addiction Medicine, and the American Nurses Association, reject the imposition of criminal sanctions as inappropriate to the caregiver's role. (See Appendix A.)

Of course, none of this takes into account the moral claims that might be made on behalf of the fetus (Robertson, 1983). Protecting the fetus from harm is seen by some as a preeminent duty that overrides other considerations. For the fashioners of the policy, the *prima facie* reasons against the policy conflicted with the belief that cocaine use on the part of the woman posed a direct and overwhelming threat to the health of the fetus, and that the fetus was therefore entitled to extraordinary measures of societal protection. They held that the yet-to-be-born are entitled to some of the same protections that abused children enjoy, and that both child abuse and abuse of the yet-to-be-born provide exceptions to norms of health care delivery, such as confidentiality, the right to refuse treatment, and the involvement of physicians in law enforcement efforts. A prominent university official publicly defended the policy with this comparison: "If you walked in on a woman that was beating her little toddler with a stick, is it illegal to grab that stick and say don't you do that anymore . . . I'm gonna call the police?" (60 Minutes News Magazine, Nov. 20, 1994).

So, the conflict was between well-established professional norms of health care delivery and the well-being of the yet-to-be-born child, whose health was being compromised by the illegal behavior of its mother. Ordinary therapeutic norms that inform the clinical relationship were seen to interfere with the protection of the fetus. The mother's refusal to take advantage of opportunities for therapy, informed by these norms, is what occasioned the involvement of the solicitor's office. The hope was that the threat of punishment would motivate the mother to therapy after the encouragement of nurses and social workers had failed.

Outcomes: Symbolic Divisiveness

The fact that conventional standards of health care were so quickly overridden needs further explanation. Concern for the well-being of the fetus, while significant, is not enough to account for the policy or for the swiftness of its execution. Fetal well-being would have led to a broader conception of the problem. First, it would have included testing and treatment protocols for all obstetrical patients, not just clinic patients. Second, the Interagency Policy would have included consideration of tobacco, alcohol, or other impediments to a healthy pregnancy; it would not have been restricted to illegal substances. The solicitor was well aware that the scope of the policy enhanced its political and public appeal. As he explained, "[t]here's not enough political will to move after pregnant women who use alcohol or cigarettes. There is, though, a political basis for this Interagency Program" (Siegel, 1994).

One result of the policy's narrow scope was that a particular population—poor, mostly African-American women—was disproportionately affected by the policy, a consequence that is at the heart of the still pending lawsuit and the sanctions levied by the Civil Rights Office of the DHHS. Had alcohol been chosen or had private obstetrical patients been included, the policy would have been less susceptible to the charge of targeting a poor, largely African-American population for punitive treatment.

The political basis of the policy is not solely due to the gender, race, and social class of the targeted population. Ingesting illegal drugs while pregnant is a potent symbol of selfishness and irresponsibility. Compromising the health of one's yet-to-be-born child to satisfy physical desires is anathema to the common expectation that mothers should protect their children. Harming an innocent and defenseless child-to-be is perceived as beyond the pale. It represents not merely a lapse of judgment, but also a serious moral failing: behavior that is both unnatural and illegal. This perspective helps explain why crack babies become a powerful symbol, an occasion for reaffirming a commitment to basic human values in a disturbed public order. The importance of a moral norm as basic as providing care and protection for innocent children helps explain the shift to a more punitive treatment model. Addicted mothers are seen as victimizers of innocent human babies, and consequently as deserving of retribution.

Indeed, the task force's decisions reflect a larger public belief that if women do not take care of their babies, they deserve to be punished and their children must be protected from their influence (Daniels, 1993). On this account, once mothers refuse their chance to mend their ways, they forfeit their rights to conventional therapy. Punishment replaces therapy as a model, a substitution that is legitimate because the offending behavior is, in fact, illegal.

By attaching sanctions to individual behaviors that society deems abhorrent, punitive social policies provide a powerful reminder of the importance of taking personal responsibility for one's actions. Precisely because such behavior violates deep-seated moral norms, questions of the rights of the mother, of racial discrimination, of patient confidentiality, and of the efficacy of coercion in altering the behavior of pregnant addicts fade from view in the face of what appears to be a fundamental decline in social order (Daniels, 1993). Even the effectiveness of the policy as therapy for the mother, or as helping the yet-to-be-born child, is less important than the moral outrage that the policy directs at the pregnant woman. The severity of the problem of crack addiction is only part of the larger collective anxieties that it symbolizes (Daniels, 1993).

During the policy's development, the nature of the target population and the numerous obstacles to effective treatment confined discourse to a discussion of personal habits and behavior. The problem came to be narrowly defined in such a way that criminal sanctions appeared to be the only solution to an otherwise insoluble problem, a last-ditch effort to coerce intransigent women into drug therapy. This preempted serious consideration of underlying social and cultural dimensions of the problem, and in turn facilitated stigmatizing patients as deserving of criminal sanctions.

This phenomenon is not unique to Charleston. The social construction of target populations as deviant, for example, gays and drug addicts, often results in punitive policies (Daniels, 1993). Public officials need fear little electoral retaliation from such groups, and the general public is likely to approve of treating them harshly (Sherman, 1991). As a result, strong incentives exist to treat such groups punitively, whether or not such treatment will effectively change their behavior (Daniels, 1993) or deal with the problems that occasioned the treatment. The case for incarceration rests on the idea that women must be held personally accountable for the choice of ingesting illegal substances that harm innocent yet-to-be-born children.

Paradoxically, the ability to make informed choices is precisely what cocaine so often destroys. At times, society legitimately takes action against those whose cognitive abilities are severely impaired or underdeveloped; court officers are appointed to act on behalf of children, the mentally imbalanced are removed from society, the old and infirm are sometimes committed to institutions. But this is a last resort—something done only after attempts to restore the individual's ability to make his or her own choices have failed. What is striking about the Charleston experience is how a consensus formed that everything had, in fact, been done to help these women restore a sense of personal responsibility and that the referral for criminal prosecution *was* a last resort, despite the lack of support (such as transportation, child care, and the like) that might have made rehabilitation visits possible, and the lack of adequate long-term residential treatment centers with child care capabilities and women-only services (Chavkin, 1991; Chavkin et al., 1993). A women-only residential treatment center for substance abusing pregnant women did not exist in Charleston or anywhere else in the State of South Carolina at the time the Interagency Policy was adopted.

OUTCOMES: EMPIRICAL UNCERTAINTY

One of the most serious consequences of the haste with which the policy was developed has been the inability to assess the tangible outcomes of MUSC's treatment program. No scientifically sound evaluative mechanism was built into this new and controversial approach to treatment. A more deliberative approach with broader consultation might have resulted in a policy design allowing for accurate assessment of treatment outcomes.

Proponents of the Interagency Policy reasoned that the threat of arrest would provide an incentive for participation in treatment programs, and that enhanced participation in such programs would produce healthier babies and healthier mothers to care for them. The principal designers of the policy published an article, in October 1990, that not only reported a dramatic decrease in positive drug tests at the clinic but also attributed at least some of the decrease to the Interagency Policy. More direct claims of a causal relationship between the policy and decreased crack cocaine use by clinic patients were made by two of the authors on numerous television talk shows. However, it is difficult to know how much, if any, of the decrease in positive drug tests was due to the Interagency Policy. The authors acknowledged that "other systems may be similarly responsible," including media efforts at public education and stepped-up efforts by law enforcement officials at reducing the availability of cocaine. Moreover, the authors were not able to establish the extent of illegal drug use among the MUSC obstetrical population because not all patients were screened, nor could they account for the impact of other regional obstetrical care programs on the clinic's population. In addition, they were not able to determine whether declining numbers of positive drugs tests were caused by women avoiding treatment at MUSC because they feared incarceration. Evidence indicates that shame and fear of losing one's children are major factors that deter drug-addicted mothers from seeking treatments, and both factors are inherent in the policy.

After the policy had been in operation for 4 years, other researchers at MUSC attempted to conduct a more rigorous and comprehensive study to address still-unanswered questions regarding the effects of the policy on patterns of health care usage. However, the inability to measure the overall incidence of drug positivity before and after the policy and to rule out alternative variables proved insurmountable. Additional confounding variables which might have altered the clinic population were identified, including a state program fostering private obstetric care of Medicaid-funded patients, improved public funding of obstetrics services to Medicaid patients, and the availability of long-acting contraception.

The Interagency Policy, therefore, produced little additional evidence regarding the efficacy of punitive intervention or its effects on mothers or the children removed from their influence. As a result, the debate about such policies is increasingly polarized and political. The empirical outcomes for patients are unclear to this day, to be settled by litigation instead of by scientific evaluation.

CONCLUSION: MEDICINE AND SOCIAL PROBLEMS

The Charleston case represents a comprehensive collaboration between health professionals and law enforcement officials. Health care and criminal justice are, in many ways, strange bedfellows. Health care is defined by the clinical encounter, which is personal, private, based on trust, voluntary, and therapeutic. Criminal justice is impersonal, public, based on rules, coercive, and retributive. But they can join forces if the deviant behavior that the clinician is treating is against the law. In the Charleston case, law enforcement became a natural and welcome ally in inducing women to attend drug therapy.

The alliance between health care and criminal justice is conceptual as well. Clinical medicine often displays a particular method of conceptualizing problems, one that endeavors to observe and quantify individual deviations from statistical normality (Stone, 1993). Once measured, such individual characteristics are taken as fixed, stable properties of individuals, rather than as products of the interaction between individuals and the social environment. The crack addiction of individual women became the problem that was susceptible to medical treatment. Individualizing the problem in this way has an important effect on treatment strategies. When crack addiction is identified as the problem, the pregnant woman becomes the patient;

substance use is the disease; substance abuse counselors are the appropriate caregivers; counseling is the appropriate therapy; and success is the elimination of the drug use, at least during the pregnancy. Because counseling is a treatment into which patients typically enter only reluctantly, the criminal justice system with its threat of sanctions becomes a natural ally of the health care professional. The patient's reluctance to enter therapy precludes successful treatment and must be overcome by coercion if not by persuasion. In this way, both medicine and law enforcement officials oversimplified a complex social problem.

This kind of clinical reasoning ignores behaviors such as inadequate diet, addiction to alcohol or tobacco, and absence of prenatal care, all of which adversely affect the health of the pregnant woman and her fetus. More important, clinical reason highlights individual behavior, but tends to ignore larger structural and relational issues, which lead to crack addiction and which separately compromise the health of the mother and her fetus. Thus, crack addiction emerges in communities that are alienated from health care institutions—communities characterized by poverty, lack of education, absence of opportunity, and domestic violence. Health care providers, of course, are in no position to solve such fundamental problems, but the Interagency Policy failed to take them into account in any serious way. No provisions were made for transportation to the therapy, no child care was available, and no residential facilities were available. A serious commitment would at least address these difficulties to make therapy accessible. The crafters of the Charleston policy explicitly rejected such efforts. The solicitor decried such a use of resources as "blaming society" for individual irresponsibility. "These women want day care and free transportation, but who's taking care of their kids when they're on coke?" (Siegel, 1994).

Two additional consequences of conceptualizing crack addiction as an individual clinical problem and of isolating it from the larger collection of factors compromise the health of the addict. First, it is more difficult to determine the extent of harm suffered by drug users. Poor nutrition and polydrug use compound the effects of cocaine use in ways that make it difficult to distinguish the effects of cocaine from other negative influences on childbearing that are associated with poverty (Halpern, 1993). Thus, it is unclear how much decreased birth weight, smaller head circumference, and neurobehavioral dysfunction are due specifically to cocaine use, as opposed to poor nutrition or other factors. Some evidence suggests that long-term effects of cocaine use may not be as serious as initial research reports suggested (Frank,

1988; Zuckerman, 1989). Chasnoff compares infants born to drug users with a control group, and reports extremely small differences in mental development. One interpretation of these findings is that environmental factors associated with poverty are equally damaging for infants born to nondrug users.

Second, isolating crack addiction as a specific, individual medical problem also carries with it a predisposition toward a legalistic, rights-based approach to the issue. This framing of the issue encourages attempts to weigh the interests and rights of the mother versus the interests and rights of the fetus, and then to determine the circumstances under which each should prevail (Robertson, 1983). In the Charleston case, both health professionals' and law enforcement officials' actions assumed what is legally and ethically controversial: that fetuses have rights and that these rights can be distinguished from those of the mother (Robertson, 1983). Rights-based reasoning of this sort fails to appreciate the fact that successful treatment should aim at restoring a healthy relationship between the mother and the yet-to-be-born child, and that punitive strategies are unlikely to foster such a relationship in the long term.

The lesson of the Charleston experience, therefore, is not so much that medicine ought to avoid involvement in difficult social problems, but that it should exercise great care in conceptualizing the problem and in tailoring intervention appropriately. Clinical approaches that individualize complex social problems are unlikely to succeed by themselves, and may involve health clinicians and administrators in external agendas that compromise the clinical encounter. If medicine is to play a constructive and responsible role in addressing problems such as cocaine use among pregnant women, it must pursue strategies that take the social and economic context of this use into account. Medical professionals need not be social reformers, but they must involve others from the community, such as community leaders, substance abuse counselors, social workers, clergy, members of the affected community, and law enforcement officials, so that the larger social and economic context will be addressed along with the individual pathology.

Although the empirical evidence is still quite limited, programs that more adequately conceptualize and address the problem of crack addiction appear to be more effective in reducing cocaine use during pregnancy (Southern Regional Project on Infant Mortality, 1993). In addition, community-based strategies provide an important opportunity for hospitals to facilitate lay participation in health care decision

making. Whether or not such participation takes the form of consultation with community groups, or more ambitious forms that enable lay
control over design and implementation, such strategies embody powerful symbols of inclusion and may help regain the trust and confidence of disaffected constituencies. Policies designed in consultation
with various community groups, and through a process of internal
review that ensures that divergent perspectives will be fully aired and
considered, will help promote accountability and discourage alienation
from the health care establishment. Policies subjected to a "test of pub-
licity" are far less likely to breach prevailing moral and legal standards,
and may avoid costly after-the-fact scrutiny from the media, courts,
and research sponsors (Bok, 1978).

POSTSCRIPT: THE REVISED POLICY ON MANAGEMENT
OF DRUG ABUSE DURING PREGNANCY

The original Interagency Policy still enjoys widespread support within
South Carolina. Both statewide candidates for attorney general in the
November 1994 elections publicly endorsed the original Interagency
Policy. One of these candidates, the Solicitor of the Ninth judicial
Circuit who initiated the policy and has been most closely identified
with it, was elected Attorney General in a landslide victory.

Nonetheless, the Interagency Policy has been revised, in large part
because of the threatened loss of federal funds by the DHHS's Office
of Civil Rights. Moreover, the OPRR has determined that the policy, as
reported in the *Journal of the South Carolina Medical Association*, constituted human subjects research that should have received prospective
IRB approval (Horger, Brown, Condon, 1990). This is because the
authors reported "preliminary" data of behavioral changes that resulted
from the policy, and also proposed plans for continued data collection
and future reporting. The OPRR determined that the policy had a
research component, and thus was subject to federal regulations governing research with human subjects. As a result, the OPRR deferred
consideration of the MUSC Multiple Project Assurance for at least 1
year, and required the development and implementation of a program
of corrective actions.

The proposed revision of the Policy on Management of Drug
Abuse During Pregnancy calls for alcohol screening as well as drug
testing. Screening tests are mandated only when a patient presents
with the following symptoms: abruptio placenta, intrauterine fetal

death, and intoxication. More care is taken to secure the informed consent of the patient. Educational efforts remain in place, and prenatal and substance abuse counseling are still made available. Arrest and the threat of arrest are not part of the proposed revision. Noncompliant patients may be given a psychological evaluation to determine whether involuntary commitment for chemical dependency is appropriate, as such patients are in Minnesota's plan, but Minnesota's plan has due process guarantees and operates within the health care system. A joint venture among the solicitor's office, the police department, and MUSC no longer exists for dealing with pregnant drug addicts.

MUSC's experience dramatically demonstrates the importance of ensuring accountability in the process of policy design and of assessing the ethical and legal standing of such policies and their empirical outcomes for patients. The proposed policy is more consistent with the legal and ethical norms of due process, informed consent, and respect for privacy. Including alcohol as a substance that triggers intervention clarifies the policy's focus as enhancing the well-being of the mother *and* the fetus, not punishing the mother for using illegal substances. Importantly, the focus is on treatment, not punishment, making the symbolic statement less disdainful and less divisive. Fewer women should feel threatened by the proposed program, as law enforcement authorities and the threat of criminal sanctions are excluded from it. Thus, the proposed policy is a true advance that avoids some of the legal and ethical pitfalls of the original policy.

The proposed policy does not, however, address some of the relatively simple but important obstacles to successful treatment, such as lack of transportation, child care, residential facilities, and neighborhood clinics. Comprehensive outreach services are no panacea, particularly because chemical dependency programs are characterized by high recidivism and the need for prolonged, regular care. Such efforts, however, would begin to take the social and economic context that gives rise to crack cocaine addiction more seriously. They would signal to the affected population a serious commitment to solving the problem.

ADDENDUM

In November, 1966, *Ferguson v City of Charleston* came to trial in federal court in Charleston, South Carolina. On January 8, 1977 the jury found that the Interagency Policy did not constitute intentional race discrimination under the Fourteenth Amendment, nor did the urine drug screening violate Fourth Amendment rights regarding consent to search and seizure for the purpose of criminal investigation. Judge Westin Houck of the U.S. District Court of the State of South Carolina ruled against other claims filed by the plaintiffs, nine African-American women and one White woman. He found no violations of their right to due process, their right to refuse medical treatment, or of a federal statute requiring confidentiality in substance abuse treatment. Judge Houck has yet to rule on three outstanding claims: that the Interagency Policy was racially discriminatory in violation of Title VI and that the women's constitutional rights to procreate and their right to privacy had been infringed. Judge Houck may also rule on whether the Interagency Policy violated the plaintiff's Fourteenth Amendment rights regarding search and seizure, in spite of the jury's finding.

On a related issue, the South Carolina Supreme Court became the first higher court in the nation to uphold a conviction for *in utero* transmission of a controlled substance. In *State v Whitner,* the High Court ruled that Cornelia Whitner could be held criminally liable for using cocaine while pregnant. The Court's decision broke with previous decisions and ruled that the state's child protection statutes apply to viable fetuses and that mothers whose behavior damages the fetus can be prosecuted under child abuse statutes.

REFERENCES

Blank, R. H. (1993). The maternal fetal relationship: The courts and social policy. *Journal of Legal Medicine, 14,* 73–92.

Bok, S. (1978). *Lying: Moral choice in public and private life.* New York: Vintage Books.

Bryant v. City of Charleston, 295 S.C. 408, 411, 368, S.E. 2d 899, 900 (1988).

Chasnoff, I. J. (1989). Drug use and women: Establishing a standard of care. *Annual of New York Academy of Science, 562,* 208–210.

Chavkin, W. (1991). Mandatory treatment for drug use during pregnancy. *JAMA, 266,* 1556–1561.

Chavkin, W. et al. (1993). Reframing the debate: Toward effective treatment for inner city drug-abusing mothers, *Bulletin of the New York Academy of Medicine, 70,* 50–68.

Colautti v. Franklin, 439 U.S. 379 (1979).

Daniels, C. R. (1993). *At women's expense: State power and the politics of fetal rights,* Cambridge: Harvard University Press.

Ferguson & Roe et al. v. City of Charleston et al., No. 2-93-26242-2 (D.S.C. filed Oct. 5, 1993).

Florida v. Johnson, No. E89-890-CFA slip op. (Cir. Ct., County, Fla., 1989).

Frank, D. A. et al. (1988). Cocaine use during pregnancy: Prevalence and correlates, *Pediatrics, 82,* 888–95.

Halpern, R. (1993). Poverty and infant development, in C. H. Zeanah Jr., Ed, *Handbook of infant mental health.* New York: Guilford Press, 73–85.

Horger, E. O., Brown, S. B., & Condon, C. M. (1990). Cocaine in pregnancy: Confronting the problem. *Journal of the South Carolina Medical Association, 86,* 527–531.

Medical University of South Carolina. (1989 Oct.). *Policy 11-7 Management of drug abuse during pregnancy.* Charleston: The Medical University.

Memorandum from Solicitor Charles M. Condon in Ferguson and Roe, No. 2-93-26242-2, at App. 1:4 (D.S.C. filed Oct. 5, 1993).

Merrick, J. (1993). Maternal substance abuse during pregnancy: Policy implications in the United States. *Journal of Legal Medicine, 14,* 57–71.

Nelson, L. J., & Milliken, N. (1988), Compelled medical treatment of pregnant women. *JAMA, 259,* 1060–1066.

Robertson, J. A. (1983). Procreative liberty and the control of conception, pregnancy, and childbirth. *Virginia Law Review, 69,* 405–464; see also Blank & C. Overall, *Ethics and human reproduction: A feminist analysis* (Boston: Allen and Unwin, 1987).

Roe v. Wade, 410 U.S. 113, (1973).

Sherman, R. (1991). Bioethics debates, *The National Law Journal, 13,* 1.

Siegel, B. (1994, Aug. 7). In the name of the children, *Los Angeles Times Magazine,* p. 15.

60 Minutes News Magazine, 1994, Nov. 20, New York.

Skinner v. Railway Labor Executives Assn, 109 S. Ct. 1402, 1413 (1989).

The Southern Regional Project on Infant Mortality, (1993, Mar.). *A step toward recovery: Improving access to substance abuse treatment for pregnant and parenting women* (Washington: Southern Regional Project on Infant Mortality).

State v. Gray, WL 124695 (Ohio App. 1990) (unreported).

Stone, D. (1993). Clinical authority in the construction of citizenship. In H. Ingram and S. R. Smith, Eds., *Public Policy for Democracy* (pp. 45–67). Washington: Brookings Institution Press.

Tolliver v. South Carolina, 90-CP-23-5178 (Cir. Ct., Manning County, S.C. 1992).

Zuckerman, F. et al. (1989). Effects of maternal marijuana and cocaine use on fetal growth, *New England Journal of Medicine, 329,* 762–768.

5

Health Care Needs of Drug-Affected Children and Their Families

Sidney H. Schnoll, M.D., Ph.D. and
Bonnie B. Wilford, M.S.

At one time, a popular belief held that a woman who used illicit drugs would significantly alter her menstrual cycle so as to preclude pregnancy. It also was believed that once a woman became pregnant, she would automatically alter her lifestyle to reduce or eliminate practices (such as alcohol and illicit drug use) that could be harmful to fetal development.

Today, we know that neither of these beliefs is true. Women who abuse and/or are dependent on alcohol or other drugs may have irregular menstrual cycles, but this does not alter their ability to conceive, nor do alcohol- or drug-dependent women stop or decrease their use of drugs during pregnancy without motivation and assistance.

In addition to the direct teratogenic risks posed by alcohol or drug use, the lifestyles of such women make them prone to numerous other medical problems that can make their care difficult and complex (Broekhuizen, Urie, & Van Mullen, 1992). These women are at increased risk for poor nutrition, psychiatric disorders, sexually transmitted diseases, hepatitis, and all of the other negative health consequences that the male substance-abusing population faces. This chapter will address the health care needs of these women and their families.

IDENTIFICATION

The problems drugs can cause in pregnancy have been recognized for some time. In the Bible, Judges 13:7 it is written, "Behold thou shalt conceive, and bear a son; and now drink no wine nor strong drink, and eat not any unclean thing . . ."

Signs and symptoms of substance abuse and the drugs that may cause them are numerous. There are no pathognomonic findings that are diagnostic for substance abuse. However, if suspicion is raised for any reason, the clinician should make a full evaluation to determine if drug use or abuse is the cause. The diagnosis will never be made if it is not considered.

The easiest patient to diagnose is the one who voluntarily presents for treatment of addiction. However, more often it is necessary to uncover a problem the patient is trying to mask. Some patients will present with physical findings that are suggestive of acute intoxication. The patient who presents with the obvious breath smell of alcohol is relatively easy to identify. Dilated pupils, or signs of withdrawal such as abdominal cramping, profuse sweating with a normal temperature, piloerection ("goose bumps"), runny nose, excessive yawning, or extreme somnolence should raise in the examiner's mind the possibility of narcotic addiction. Agitation, paranoid ideation, first seizure in a young woman, or the inability to sit still should raise the suspicion of stimulant abuse.

Quite frequently, patients do not present with such overt signs of substance misuse. A frequent, relatively subtle sign of substance abuse may be chronic inability to keep appointments. Indeed, women with drug or alcohol problems in pregnancy may not fit the usual stereotype of the alcoholic, and hence present problems in early identification and treatment. Early recognition of alcohol and drug use is particularly important in pregnancy, since alcohol and other drugs may have the capacity to affect each stage of fetal development. Screening women in the prenatal clinic with specific questions about drug and alcohol use can be effective. The diagnosis of problem drinking or drug use should be primarily based on interview and examination.

HISTORY

Every primary medical care visit should begin with a history and physical examination. This is true even of established patients. The medical history should obtain pertinent data to evaluate the patient's reason for the medical visit, but in addition should address all areas of health maintenance, including substance abuse. Patients should be asked in a concerned and nonthreatening fashion if they have ever used tobacco, alcohol, or licit or illicit drugs. The history should include questions regarding first use, frequency of use, quantity, and most recent use. In addition, a number of screening instruments have been developed to help identify patients at risk for alcohol and substance abuse problems.

A thorough mental status examination should be part of the initial medical evaluation of any woman who may have an alcohol or substance abuse problem. Patients with symptoms of drug or alcohol overdose (e.g., coma, respiratory depression, delirium, incoherence, emotional instability, hyperactivity), severe withdrawal symptoms, psychotic behavior, or suicidal threats or actions may require immediate admission and treatment for their own protection. The need for a thorough mental status examination in female substance users is underscored by the relative frequency of dual diagnosis (the cooccurrence of psychoactive substance dependence and other psychiatric diagnoses). As many as one in five women who fulfill diagnostic criteria for alcohol abuse or dependence at some time in their lives can also fulfill diagnostic criteria for depression, compared to only 1 in 20 men (Sonderegger, 1992).

In addition to depression, substance-abusing women are also at higher risk than male substance abusers of having other affective disorders, anxiety, sexual disorders, bulimia, and borderline personality disorders (Mitchell & Brown, 1990). Determining whether or not a patient suffers from one of these disorders, in addition to substance abuse, may be of utmost importance in treatment planning. It should be stressed that it is very difficult to make a psychiatric diagnosis in a woman who is intoxicated or going through withdrawal. Intoxication and withdrawal can mimic many psychiatric disorders, as well as mask disorders that may emerge later.

Once the patient's current or interim medical history and mental status examination have been obtained, it is important to focus on other historical clues that may indicate unique risk for substance abuse. A strong family history of substance abuse clearly increases an individual's risk for substance abuse problems. Numerous studies have shown that rates of alcoholism are substantially higher in relatives of alcoholics than in relatives of nonalcoholics. Children of alcoholics demonstrate a three- to fourfold increase in risk of developing the disorder themselves (Zuckerman et al., 1986).

Despite the strong influence of genetics, environment also plays a role in drug-taking behavior. A recent large study from Australia involving nearly 2,000 female twin pairs demonstrated the importance of environment in modifying hereditary influences on women's drinking patterns (Heller et al., 1988). In that study, genetic factors accounted for much less of the variance in drinking patterns in women who were married than in women who were unmarried. These findings support the notion that the male partner's drinking pattern is important in influencing the drinking patterns of women. This underscores the need for exploring not only the patient's family history for signs of alcohol or drug abuse, but also for considering the abuse patterns of a spouse. Although the genetic predisposition to the abuse of illicit drugs is less clear than that seen with alcohol, the parallel use patterns of women and their partners have long been recognized. Women are often introduced to and supplied with drugs by their male partners. Obviously, this information becomes of critical importance when attempting to treat a substance use problem in a woman. If the male partner continues to use, it is more difficult to treat the problem.

The patient's social history also may be indicative of substance use disorder. Obviously, the patient who has had frequent encounters with law enforcement agencies needs to be considered at high risk for being a substance abuser. Other less obvious clues are frequent relationship or job changes. In addition, the patient who is under a great deal of economic strain is at risk for having current substance abuse problems. The economic problems may, in fact, arise from complications of substance abuse, or the stress brought about by economic or job strains may cause a latent tendency toward substance abuse to become evident.

A thorough menstrual, sexual, and contraceptive history should be taken at the time of the initial medical evaluation, both to assess the patient's risk for sexually transmitted diseases and to confirm or exclude the possibility of pregnancy. Although it has long been accepted that alcohol and substance abusers frequently have long periods of oligomenorrhea, any woman of reproductive age with amenorrhea should be considered pregnant until a blood or urine pregnancy test indicates otherwise. At every medical interaction with sexually active females, the opportunity should be taken to review current contraceptive techniques, as well as practices designed to limit the spread of sexually transmitted diseases, especially Human Immuno-deficiency Virus (HIV) infection. All nonpregnant substance-using women should receive counseling on the importance of periconceptional abstinence from alcohol and illicit drugs to decrease the likelihood of serious birth defects.

A prior medical history of hepatitis, cirrhosis, or atypical infections should alert the clinician to the possibility that the patient has a chronic substance abuse problem. There are other, less obvious clues in the medical history. In female patients, a history of multiple sexually transmitted diseases may suggest the possibility of overt prostitution. Women engaged in prostitution are at high risk for substance use problems. Even among women who do not consider themselves to be prostitutes, the frequent practice of trading sex for drugs results in a high incidence of sexually transmitted diseases. Patients with other atypical infections, such as cellulitis or atypical pneumonias, should also be considered to be at increased risk for substance abuse problems.

A past history of physical, sexual, and verbal abuse appears to be much more common among alcoholic women than among their matched controls (Abel & Sokol, 1992). Similarly, the patient who is in a known physically or emotionally abusive relationship should be considered at high risk for alcohol or substance abuse (Finnegan, 1988).

Questionnaires that may be used include the "CAGE," a risk scoring tool that has been validated primarily in men. These questions are: "Have you ever felt the need to Cut down on your drinking? Have you ever felt Annoyed by criticism of drinking? Have you ever had Guilty feelings about drinking? Have you ever taken a morning Eye opener?" The CAGE takes from 30 seconds to one minute to administer, is efficient, and fits well into most clinical settings. It has been recommended that one positive reply to any of the four questions calls for further inquiry (Ewing, 1984). There is, however, little experience with using the CAGE for screening women.

Sokol et al. (1989) have modified the CAGE to delete the question about guilt and replace it with a question about tolerance: "Do you need more alcohol to get high now than in the past?" The mnemonic for this modified set of questions is TACE (Tolerance, Annoyed, Cut down, and Eye-opener). Many practitioners have used these tests to inquire about other drugs as well as alcohol. The tolerance question is given two points for a positive answer, the others score one point. A score of two points or more is highly correlated with risky drinking, especially during pregnancy.

Another simple set of questions to use are the questions from the Trauma Test: "Since your 18th birthday have you ever: Had any fractures or dislocations of your bones or joints (excluding sports injuries)? Been injured in a traffic accident? Injured your head (excluding sports injuries)? Been in a fight or been assaulted while intoxicated? Been injured while intoxicated?" Positive responses to two or more of these questions are highly correlated with alcohol and drug use (Centers for Substance Abuse Treatment, 1993a).

PHYSICAL EXAMINATION

After a thorough history has been taken, a careful physical examination should be performed. If the patient is presenting for a particular medical problem, obviously the examination needs to be tailored to that condition. One should not, however, fail to identify signs of an overt substance abuse problem. An enlarged, nontender liver may be an early sign of alcoholic cirrhosis. Tenderness of the liver edge may indicate alcoholic or viral hepatitis. Nearly 50% of parenteral drug abusers have a history of acute hepatitis (Abel & Sokol, 1992).

Careful inspection of the skin, not just of the extremities, should be performed in all patients in whom parenteral drug use is suspected. If intravenous or subcutaneous drug use is suspected, there should be a thorough search for needle marks or scarring from old cutaneous infections. Women will often try to hide needle marks by injecting in the axilla, under the breasts, under the tongue, and in other less obvious sites. They may try to hide injection sites by covering them with tattoos. Spider angiomata, small red skin patches composed of intermeshed fine vessels that blanch on pressure, may be a sign of liver disease. It is not unusual to find occasional spider angiomata in normal children and adults. Numerous spider angiomata often develop during pregnancy. Most patients with numerous and prominent vascular spiders, however, have some form of underlying liver disease. The finding of jaundice signals severe liver disease that requires immediate evaluation and treatment. Nasal septal irritation or even perforation may indicate chronic drug use by sniffing. Heroin addicts frequently have burns on the neck and chest from cigarette ashes falling on these areas while intoxicated. Recently, addicts are presenting with peculiar burn marks on their thumbs and forefingers from holding hot butane lighters over their crack pipes.

Enlarged lymph nodes may be suggestive of infection secondary to injection drug use, atypical sexually transmitted diseases, or advanced Human Immunodeficiency Virus (HIV) infection. All mucous membranes should be evaluated for evidence of oral thrush, which is a sign of immunodeficiency and may be the first sign of HIV infection.

Since many women with alcohol or substance abuse problems do not have annual gynecologic examinations, a thorough breast examination should be part of any medical evaluation of a patient with a suspected or confirmed substance abuse problem. She also should have a thorough gynecologic examination for sexually transmitted diseases. The practice of exchanging sex for crack cocaine has resulted in an epidemic of syphilis in the United States (Minkoff et al., 1990). There should be a careful inspection of the skin to detect the rash typical of secondary syphilis, as well as of the external genitalia to detect the characteristic lesions of primary or secondary syphilis. In addition, any lesions that may be suspicious for genital herpes should be cultured for confirmation of the disease. Sexually active patients, especially those with more than one sexual partner, should have serologic testing for syphilis at the time of any medical evaluation.

A careful speculum examination should be performed with particular attention to signs of vaginitis or cervicitis. Recurrent vaginal yeast infections may be a sign of immune compromise secondary to Human Immunodeficiency Virus (HIV) infection. Recurrent vaginal yeast infections are sufficiently common in women with otherwise asymptomatic HIV infection that they have been designated by the Centers for Disease Control as an AIDS-identifying illness in patients with HIV infection (Mitchell et al., 1990). All patients in whom chronic alcohol or substance abuse is suspected should have endocervical culture for *Neisseria gonorrhoeae* and *Chlamydia trachomatis.* Asymptomatic infection with these organisms may progress to life-threatening pelvic inflammatory disease if left untreated. Any vaginal discharge noted at the time of examination should be examined under a microscope for evidence of bacterial vaginosis or infection with *Trichomonas vaginalis.*

Many patients with substance use problems had first intercourse relatively early in adolescence and have had multiple sexual partners and multiple sexually transmitted diseases, all of which are well recognized risk factors for cervical dysplasia and ultimately for developing cervical cancer (Chasnoff, 1988). In a study of pregnant women from Detroit's Hutzel Hospital pregnant drug addict program, 24% of women admitted to the program had an abnormal Pap smear (Minkoff et al., 1990). In patients with suspected or confirmed HIV infection, however, an annual Pap smear may not be adequate evaluation. A recent investigation demonstrated that in asymptomatic HIV-positive women, the Pap smear was effective in detecting less than 10% of premalignant cervical lesions. Current recommendations are that asymptomatic HIV-positive women undergo annual Pap smears for detection of cervical dysplasia; however, given the apparent rapid progression of cervical neoplasia in HIV-positive patients, many clinicians choose to perform Pap smears more frequently (Center for Substance Abuse Treatment, 1993a).

Although the incidence of tuberculosis in the United States declined for most of the second half of the 20th century, during the late 1980s there was an increase in the incidence of this highly contagious disease. In 1992, 26,673 cases of tuberculosis were reported to the Centers for Disease Control (Center for Substance Abuse and Treatment, 1994). The increase in tuberculosis cases was disproportionate among minority groups. Although some of the increase in tuberculosis among minorities can be explained by an increased incidence of HIV infection, other contributing factors include limited access to health care, poverty, substandard housing, homelessness, and substance abuse. The medical evaluation of all patients with suspected or confirmed substance use problems therefore should include testing for tuberculosis.

Because of the reduced immune response of patients with HIV infection, the Centers for Disease Control have recommended that reactions to the standard tuberculin PPD of more than 5 mm induration should be considered positive in HIV-positive individuals, as compared to the standard 10 mm area induration considered positive for other patients (CDC, 1990). Because immunocompromised patients may not respond to the tuberculin antigen even when tuberculosis is present, the current recommendation is to test for other common antigens at the same time to determine if anergy is present. Patients with a positive PPD or patients with anergy should have chest X-rays looking for evidence of active disease and should receive appropriate treatment. A number of treatment regimens are available and with the emergence of multiple antibiotic-resistant tuberculosis strains, consultation with an infectious disease specialist regarding the current appropriate treatment should be considered.

All patients who undergo medical evaluation for possible alcohol or substance misuse should be offered HIV testing (CSAT, 1993b). Although most women contract HIV by the use of intravenous drugs or sexual relations with drug users, recent data suggest that heterosexual activity is becoming an increasingly important mode of transmission in women. Approximately one-third of the women with AIDS in the United States are presumed to have contracted the disease by heterosexual contact with infected partners. Patients who test positive for HIV infection should be counseled so they can reduce the risk of sexual transmission by practicing noninsertive sex or by consistently and properly using condoms. They should be counseled that sharing needles is an efficient way to transmit the virus to others.

Patients who test positive for HIV infection should be informed of the early clinical manifestations of HIV infection with advice to seek immediate medical attention in order to institute appropriate care for asymptomatic individuals. They should be counseled regarding the current understanding of the prognosis of HIV infection, including a period of latency estimated to be approximately 10 years at this time; that they are prohibited from donating blood products or body organs to avoid spreading the disease to others; and that they should not share toothbrushes, razors, or other implements that could be contaminated with blood. It should be suggested to the patient that all sexual and needle-sharing partners should be notified and advised of the possible need for counseling and testing (CSAT, 1993b).

LABORATORY TESTS

Patients who are thought to be at high risk for current or chronic substance abuse problems should have blood tests at the time of their initial evaluation for evidence of acute or chronic liver disease. This should include serologic testing for all forms of viral hepatitis. At least 75% of parenteral drug abusers can be expected to have serologic evidence of prior infection with hepatitis B virus (Keith et al., 1989). All types of viral hepatitis are seen in substance abusers, although hepatitis B and hepatitis C are probably the most common. Hepatitis A tends to be a self-limited disease. However, all of the other forms of viral hepatitis have the potential to cause chronic infection and chronic liver disease.

In addition, alcohol and cocaine can be hepatotoxic. For that reason, all patients with evidence of alcohol and or substance misuse should be tested for liver function at the time of the initial medical evaluation. Abnormalities in liver function can severely alter the metabolism of medications used in the treatment of addiction and other medical disorders. Patients with laboratory evidence of compromise to hepatic function may require adjustment in the dosages of relatively common medications to avoid toxicity.

A small number of parenteral drug users will develop acute or chronic renal disease. In many cases, renal disease will progress to end-stage renal failure. In addition, patients with HIV have been noted to have HIV-associated nephropathy with severe degrees of protein-uria and rapid progression to end-stage renal disease (Mitchell et al., 1990). Thus, patients should have evaluation of renal function tests at the time of their initial medical evaluation. Urine samples should be analyzed for protein. Patients with abnormally low renal function, as in the case with chronic liver disease, may require adjustments in med-ication to avoid toxicity. Patients with severe proteinuria may have specialized dietary requirements.

Patients who have cardiac murmurs noted at the time of the initial physical examination, or who have unexplained fevers, chills, pleuritic chest pain, or shortness of breath, may require echocardiographic evaluation of the heart to evaluate for endocarditis. In contrast to rheumatic endocarditis, the majority of parenteral drug abusers with endocarditis have right-sided cardiac disease, most often involving the tricuspid valve. Such patients may require prolonged intravenous antibiotic therapy to effect a cure.

The laboratory evaluation of the alcohol or substance-abusing woman also should include any testing that would be indicated in the absence of a history of alcohol or other substance abuse. For example, the postmenopausal woman with back pain may benefit from bone densitometry and spine films to determine if osteoporosis-induced compression fractures of the vertebral column may be present.

Any patient who presents intoxicated, or in whom intoxication or drug use in general are suspected, should have body fluids or breath evaluated for the presence of alcohol and/or drugs. The urine is the best fluid to check because drugs are concentrated there and can be detected long after they are cleared from blood. Although the require-ments for notification or permission needed to obtain specimens for toxicologic testing vary from jurisdiction to jurisdiction, we feel that patients should be notified of the health care provider's suspicion and asked for permission to perform toxicologic testing. To test without the patient's notification or permission may only further alienate a patient who is already having a difficult time talking about her problem with substance misuse. This is especially true in states where a positive urine drug screen in a pregnant or postpartum woman could result in prosecution and/or the child being taken away from the mother by social service agencies.

PREVENTION AND EARLY INTERVENTION

Pregnancy offers a unique opportunity to intervene with women who have alcohol and other drug use disorders. Women may be more concerned about their alcohol and drug use due to their pregnancy, and more support services may be available because of the pregnancy. However, there may be additional barriers on an institutional level, such as a lack of provision for child care, a factor that often limits accessibility of substance use programming for women. Nevertheless, since women often interact with the medical community during pregnancy, the opportunity to intervene often is present.

Contemporary prevention efforts focus heavily on educational strategies that specifically target health care providers, pregnant women, women of childbearing age, and the community. There is evidence that such community-wide educational strategies are effective in changing behavior. A significant decline in the prevalence of alcohol use was accomplished in a White, middle class, well educated sample of pregnant women through a prevention/education program (Streissguth, Darby, Barr, & Smith, 1983). Other programs have found that 35 to 88% of pregnant alcohol users decreased or discontinued their alcohol use following minimal educational intervention (Fried, Watkinson, Grant, & Knight, 1980; Heller et al., 1988; Larsson, 1983; Zuckerman, 1983). However, most of these programs focus on social drinkers or less severe alcohol users.

Prevention programs must incorporate intervention strategies with the "at risk" patient. Patient education may be a useful strategy in some alcohol-using pregnant women; however, women with a significant history of alcohol use, strong family history of alcoholism, and alcohol-related problems probably require a higher level of intervention. In this group of women, the severity of the addiction may override the desire to protect the fetus and/or their own resolve to discontinue alcohol or drug use.

Programs utilizing interventions such as supportive counseling have succeeded in reducing alcohol use of even heavy drinkers in 67 to 76% of women (Heller et al., 1988; Larsson, 1983; Rosett & Weiner, 1984; Zuckerman, 1983). Components of these particular intervention programs have included education, individual or group therapy, and case management.

Patients at highest risk for a poor outcome, unfortunately, may be those who are least likely to access the social service systems. Active outreach and case management is critical with this population.

Community agencies and organizations that are likely to come in contact with alcohol- or drug-addicted pregnant women need to help develop effective outreach strategies. Greater collaboration is needed between the medical and mental health systems of care, since drug or alcohol addicted women may be receiving one or the other such services.

Meeting the multiple service needs of addicted pregnant women requires attention to addiction treatment, mental health treatment, management of obstetric, pediatric, and other medical problems, social services, attention to family relationships, education in underdeveloped skill areas, such as parenting, and legal and vocational services. An interdisciplinary team must be engaged to provide these services through a coordinated intervention plan.

Finally, it is critical that care providers be nonjudgmental and nonpunitive in their approach to the pregnant addict. Care of such women many trigger difficult issues for the treatment team, including feelings of anger and hostility at the patient's inability to maintain abstinence. In this situation, the role of the addiction medicine specialist includes recognizing these potential problems and assisting staff with their resolution.

PRENATAL CARE

Prenatal care of addicted women is best provided under the supervision of physicians who are knowledgeable about both high-risk obstetrics and addiction medicine. However, the number of physicians with both qualifications is small. Alternatively, optimal prenatal care can be a collaborative process between an obstetrical service and addiction treatment program(s), so as to provide the best treatment for the medical disease of addiction and close monitoring of the progress of the pregnancy. Whether an inpatient or outpatient program, collaboration is essential to assure continuation of the addiction treatment after childbirth.

Certain general concepts should be kept in mind when providing obstetrical care for addicted women. Most will enter care late in their pregnancies. Their ambivalence about continuing an unintended pregnancy, their fear and guilt associated with exposing the fetus to alcohol or drugs, unpleasant past experiences with institutions and agencies, and uncertainty about the father may provide the impetus to delay seeking care. Further, because of the menstrual dysfunction often associated with addiction, addicted women may not realize that they are pregnant for many months (Mitchell et al., 1990). Others may have sought abortions but found that their pregnancies are beyond the legal time allowed or that no pregnancy termination services are available to them. These issues often prevent women from following through with appointments and prescribed treatments, especially if their motivation to seek treatment is based largely on concern for the pregnancy and not in recognition that the addictive disorder requires treatment. Similar issues also contribute to an inability to bond to the fetus during pregnancy and after birth.

The poor self-esteem often seen in addicted women may be intensified by changes associated with pregnancy, as weight gain and water retention alter appearance. Moreover, since parenting is a skill largely learned from how one was parented, the intergenerational cycle of addiction seen in many families of addicted women provides them with less than adequate preparation to be parents. Often the significant other in the woman's life also abuses drugs.

The protocol in Table 5.1 reflects information to be found in the Treatment Improvement Protocol published by the federal Center for Substance Abuse Treatment (1993), which includes a summary and review of a range of relevant issues involving medical withdrawal, use of urine toxicologies, and ethical and legal issues.

Weekly visits should include (but not be limited to) taking weight; urine dipstick for sugar, acetone and protein; and toxicology, blood pressure, fundal height, and fetal heart rate. Random blood toxicologies for alcohol are helpful as appropriate.

Women who are HIV-positive should be referred to the infectious disease clinic for initial evaluation. If they meet criteria for nonpregnant patients for treatment with antivirals or prophylaxis, consideration should be given to initiating such treatment after careful discussion with the woman of known and unknown risks/benefits.

ADDICTION TREATMENT OF THE MOTHER

Frequently, women are motivated to seek treatment for alcohol or substance abuse because of problems with their physical or emotional health or family problems. Thus, clinicians who do not necessarily consider themselves to be involved in the treatment of substance abuse should consider alcohol or illicit substance use when evaluating patients with a wide range of medical and or emotional problems.

DETOXIFICATION

The clinician must take into account the effects of withdrawal symptoms and pharmacologic agents not only on the woman, but on her fetus and neonate as well. Potential risks to offspring exposed to alcohol and other drugs *in utero* include morphologic teratogenicity (physical anomalies), behavioral teratogenicity (enduring behavioral changes resulting from alterations in the developing central nervous system); fetal or neonatal withdrawal; fetal or neonatal toxicity; and miscarriage or stillbirth (Center for Substance Abuse Treatment, 1993a). However, in research, as in clinical practice, it is impossible to separate the direct adverse effects of these substances from associated changes in lifestyle, nutrition, medical illness, and social support.

MEDICAL STABILIZATION

The initial stabilization as well as the medical withdrawal of pregnant women from their drug(s) of abuse are recognized means of reducing the acute illness associated with the use of alcohol and other drugs. The Center for Substance Abuse Treatment (1993) advises that initial stabilization of the patient should be accomplished within 10 days of first contact, or earlier if medically necessary. During the period of stabilization, caregivers need to monitor the mother and fetus for adverse signs of drug withdrawal; establish a basis for ongoing alcohol and other drug treatment and recovery; and initiate a relationship between the mother and available supportive services within the community.

Many addicted pregnant women need a period of hospitalization to be stabilized on methadone and/or for the supervised medical withdrawal (detoxification) from other drugs. If the physician is knowledgeable and experienced, and the program allows for daily monitoring, some patients can be managed as outpatients. Addiction treatment programs usually lack the expertise to monitor the fetus beyond listening to the fetal heartbeat and provide minimal education about pregnancy and pregnancy-related issues outside of addiction. Obstetrical units provide a higher level of monitoring of the pregnancy and provide programs and education specific to pregnancy, but often lack the ability to limit and monitor visitors or have programs structured to address the issues of addiction.

At a minimum, all inpatient stabilization or medical withdrawal protocols should include a comprehensive history, including drug use

TABLE 5.1 Protocol for Prenatal Care

AT THE FIRST PRENATAL VISIT:

1. Perform a complete history and physical examination;
2. Order a baseline sonogram;
3. Order baseline laboratory tests, to include but not be limited to:
   a. Complete blood count with Hgb electrophoresis
   b. Serological test for syphilis
   c. Cervical cultures for gonorrhea and chlamydia
   d. PPD with anergy panel
   e. SMA 12
   f. Pap smear
   g. Rubella titer
   h. Blood type and RH titers
   i. Hepatitis screen for B and C
4. Initiate HIV counseling;
5. Make other appropriate referrals, as for genetic counseling for women who may be age 35 or older at delivery;
6. Order an initial psychological evaluation;
7. Make a social service referral;
8. Refer the patient to a drug treatment program;
9. Refer opioid addicts for methadone maintenance for the duration of pregnancy; and
10. Establish rules, requirements and goals with the patient and her significant other(s).

AT FOLLOW-UP VISITS:

28 weeks

1. Order a follow-up sonogram;
2. Screen for diabetes;
3. Repeat the complete blood count;
4. Repeat the serological test for syphilis;
5. Establish an ongoing relationship with the patient's drug treatment providers (for obstetric personnel) or obstetrical caregivers (for addiction specialists);

TABLE 5.1 continued

6. Establish a good working relationship with the patient's significant other(s); and

7. Begin to discuss contraceptive methods.

36 weeks

1. Repeat the complete blood count and serological test for syphilis;

2. Repeat the hepatitis screen for B/C, if the initial test was negative;

3. Repeat the test for HIV, if the initial results were negative; and

4. Begin antepartum testing of women on methadone maintenance and those who have consistently positive urine toxicologies.

At labor and delivery:

1. Perform a complete history and physical (especially a recent drug history);

2. Repeat the hepatitis screen and serological tests for syphilis;

3. Order a urine toxicology;

4. Alert pediatric medical and nursing staff;

5. Alert social service personnel;

6. Provide pain management as appropriate; and

7. Select a method of delivery based solely on obstetric considerations.

During the postpartum period:

1. Encourage the patient to continue in a drug treatment program;

2. Encourage use of an appropriate contraceptive method; and

3. Remember that breastfeeding is *not* contraindicated in methadone-maintained women.

Source: Center for Substance Abuse Treatment (1993c). Treatment Improvement Protocol: Pregnant, substance-using women: Recommendations of a consensus panel (TIP No. 2). Rockville, MD: CSAT.

and physical examination, a psychosocial and mental health assessment, and discharge planning that includes followup prenatal and medical care and ongoing addiction treatment. It is important to understand that signs and symptoms of withdrawal may first manifest themselves in the fetus and thus be mistaken for normal signs of pregnancy. Ideally, case management should be initiated at this juncture.

In considering detoxification, the overriding issue is whether medications used for stabilization or medical withdrawal are harmful to the fetus. The issue requires weighing risks and benefits, and an understanding that the incidence of birth defects in the general population is about 3%. It is important to distinguish drug effects into those that cause or have the potential to cause birth defects from those that may have an effect on the infant that can be reversed (Chasnoff, 1988).

CARE OF THE NEONATE

Exposure to alcohol or drugs *in utero* can have significant effects on the fetus and newborn (as described in Chapter 2). Although it is not entirely clear what the long-term effects are on development in later life, there are data indicating that drug exposure can result in intrauterine growth retardation, prematurity, neurobehavioral and neurophysiological dysfunction, dysmorphic teratologic effects, and infections, including HIV (Kandel, 1991; Keith et al., 1989; Neerhof et al., 1989; Zuckerman & Bresnahan, 1991). In a mother who has taken drugs up to term, the newborn can experience a neonatal abstinence syndrome. This is most commonly associated with newborns exposed to opioids *in utero*, but can also be seen with exposure to alcohol and other sedative hypnotics, and to stimulants, including cocaine. Clinicians should be alert to the presence of neonatal abstinence syndrome in a woman who has a positive urine screen at term (Finnegan & Kaltenbach, 1992).

Medical assessment of the newborn should include a thorough physical examination to include weight, length, head circumference, and an assessment of gestational age. In addition, it is critical to look for the presence of congenital malformations. The mother should be assessed for the presence of sexually transmitted infections as noted above (Chasnoff, 1988). If any are present, the newborn should be screened for the presence of these infections and treated appropriately. In a mother who has adequate prenatal care, when the testing has been done prenatally, treatment should have been instituted prior to term.

Although drug withdrawal syndromes are quite distinct in adults, depending on the drug class, this is not true in the newborn. The neonatal withdrawal syndromes are all characterized by hyperactivity, irritability, increased muscle tone, difficulty with sucking, and high-pitched cries (Finnegan & Kaltenbach, 1992). If the mother has been taking long-acting drugs like methadone or diazepam, the neonatal abstinence syndrome may not appear for days or weeks after delivery and therefore may be missed. The mother or caretaker may return complaining of the infant's irritability, difficulty with feeding, or failure to thrive. At this point, urine toxicology on the infant will not provide good information, unless the child has been exposed to drugs since discharge from the hospital. It is better to refer back to the mother's urine toxicology at delivery. If this is not available, it will be very difficult to make the diagnosis and provide proper treatment.

In a newborn who has been exposed to opioids *in utero*, the Neonatal Abstinence Scale (Finnegan & Kaltenbach, 1992) can be used to determine the severity of withdrawal. This scale has been primarily developed for opioid withdrawal and has been well studied with other substances. In cases of opioid withdrawal, paregoric, methadone, or phenobarbital can be used to treat the withdrawal. For sedative-hypnotic or stimulant withdrawal, phenobarbital is the most appropriate choice. The dose of medication should be carefully titrated to the behavior of the newborn so as not to oversedate. The mother should be trained to closely monitor the child's behavior to be tolerant of feeding problems and be taught techniques to console the baby (Center for Substance Abuse Treatment, 1993c). Patience is of utmost importance in dealing with a drug-exposed newborn.

Neonates who have been exposed to drugs *in utero* should be followed in the hospital for a sufficient period of time to determine whether an abstinence syndrome might occur. This is usually by the third or fourth day after delivery. Premature neonates may require longer stays. Before discharge, the primary caregiver should be instructed in behaviors that may be associated with withdrawal, so that the child can be assessed by someone skilled in diagnosis and treatment of neonatal withdrawal (Table 5.2).

Whenever possible, a home evaluation should occur within the first few weeks of life, and follow-up appointments made for pediatric care. It is critical that the mother or other caretakers be informed of the importance of routine pediatric care and the need to keep all appointments for well-baby care and immunizations. With the shortened lengths of stay dictated by many third-party payers, it is difficult to keep the mother and neonate in the hospital long enough to assess for withdrawal and prepare the mother for the problems she may encounter.

The most critical aspect of the child's development is what happens postpartum. Does the mother remain as the primary caregiver? Does she remain in or enroll in a treatment program? Does she have a supportive, drug-free significant other at home? Does she have adequate housing and financial resources? Does she have transportation to enable her to keep her appointments? Does she want to keep the

TABLE 5.2 Follow-up and Aftercare Timeline

	Medical		Developmental		
	Exam	Immunization*	Lab	Testing	Risk Monitoring**
Week 1†	X				X
Week 2					X
Week 3					X
Week 4					X
Week 5					X
Week 6					X
Week 7					X
Week 8	X	DTP, HbCV,§ OPV			X
Week 9					X
Week 10					X
Week 11					X
Week 12	X				X
4 Months	X	DTP, HbCV,§ OPV			X
5 Months					X
6 Months	X	DTP, HbCV§	X		X
7 Months					X
8 Months					X
9 Months				X	X
10 Months	X	PPD			X
11 Months					X
12 Months			Lead	X	X
15 Months	X	MMR,¹ HbCV¶††			X
15–18 Months	X	DTP*** OPVˢ		X	X

* For all products used, consult manufacturer's package insert for instructions for storage, handling, dosage, and administration. Biologics prepared by different manufacturers may vary, and package inserts from the same manufacturer may change from time to time. Therefore, the physician should be aware of the contents of the current package insert.

** Risk monitoring to ensure the infant's continued health and safety can be provided by pediatric visit, home health visit, early intervention programs, or drug treatment programs that have a mother-child focus.

† These recommended ages should not be construed as absolute. For example, 2 months can be 6 to 10 weeks. However, MMR usually should not be given to children younger than 12 months. (If measles vaccination is indicated, monovalent measles vaccine is recommended, and MMR shoud be given subsequently, at 15 months.)

DTP = diphtheria and tetanus toxoids with pertussis vaccine; HbCV = *Haemophilus* b conjugate vaccine; OPV = oral poliovirus vaccine containing attenuated poliovirus types 1, 2, and 3; MMR = live measles, mumps, and diphtheria toxoid (reduced dose) for adult use.

§ As of October 1990, only one HbCV is approved for use in children younger than 15 months.

¹ May be given at 12 months of age in areas with recurrent measles transmission.

¶ Any licensed *Haemophilus* b conjugate vaccine may be given.

*** Should be given 6 to 12 months after the third dose.

†† May be given simultaneously with MMR at 15 months.

ˢ May be given simultaneously with MMR and HbCV at 15 months or at any time between 12 and 24 months; priority should be given to administering MMR at the recommended age.

Notes: 1. Hepatitis B immunization is now universally recommended.
  2. Children with symptomatic HIV infection should receive inactivated polio vaccine (Red Book, 1991, p. 51).

Source: Center for Substance Abuse Treatment (1993c). Treatment Improvement Protocol: Improving Treatment for Drug-Exposed Infants (TIP No. 5). Rockville, MD: CSAT.

baby? All of these questions should be answered before discharge, and assistance offered where needed, so that a healthy home environment can be provided. Those women without resources should be connected with social service agencies to assist them. When a significant other is available, this person should be assessed to determine if he or she uses drugs or alcohol and whether he or she wants to participate in raising the child. If the person uses drugs, then a referral should be made to a treatment program. If that person is interested in helping to raise the child, he or she should be included in all information and training provided to the mother. If the child is raised in a sick environment, then there will a poor outcome independent of drug exposure *in utero*.

An important question surrounded by some controversy is whether or not drug-using mothers should breastfeed (Center for Substance Abuse & Treatment, 1993c). There are many advantages to breastfeeding, including passive transfer of antibodies and increased bonding between mother and infant. If the mother is on methadone and is not using other drugs or she is in a program and has been drug free for a sustained period, breast-feeding should be encouraged. If she starts to abuse drugs again, then she should be strongly urged to stop breastfeeding. In a mother who has HIV infection or is still actively abusing drugs, breastfeeding should be discouraged.

There is an obvious need for very specialized treatment services for children and families involved in substance abuse. These services need to address all of the medical, social, and economic problems of the family. For women who are pregnant, there needs to be an integration of prenatal care, prenatal education, and substance abuse treatment to increase the likelihood of a successful pregnancy outcome.

RESEARCH NEEDS

Obtaining accurate epidemiologic data will enable us to develop more targeted prevention approaches. These approaches could then be addressed to the most vulnerable populations, and accurate data could be provided as to consequences of use and how to prevent those consequences from occurring. Accurate epidemiologic data will also enable us to test out the best treatment approaches. Recent data from treatment demonstration projects indicate that women presenting for treatment have a wide range of needs, making it more appropriate to match the treatment to the specific needs of the women and their families (Zuckerman et al., 1986). To date, we have assumed that treatment programs that are comprehensive will meet the needs of all women who are exposed. There is no evidence to support this contention. It will be necessary to develop appropriate assessment techniques that will enable us to define the precise treatment approach that will be most effective for each person. This will enable us to provide more cost-effective treatment to children and their families.

Research will help us to break down some of the ideological barriers that exist to certain treatment approaches. Current data indicate that methadone maintenance may be the most appropriate treatment for pregnant women who are addicted to opioid drugs (Wittman & Segal, 1991). However, this treatment is not universally available to pregnant addicted women (Sonderegger, 1992). Failure to provide this treatment is similar to saying that a pregnant diabetic should not receive insulin but should be able to handle her diabetes by diet alone. By placing women in appropriate treatment programs, we will be able to provide more specific treatment at lower cost.

Most current data are based on the needs of indigent inner city women (Land & Kushner, 1990), and there are few data on the needs and services required by other drug-using families (Lake et al., 1992). It is believed by some that a punitive approach to this problem will reduce drug use and therefore reduce medical consequences to both women and their children. However, no data are currently available to support this contention. To the contrary, there are emerging data that these punitive measures may keep women and children away from treatment programs and therefore provide them with less than adequate health care (Finnegan, 1991). This often results in more expensive health care needs down the road. It is clear that the health care needs of drug-affected children and their families are complex, requiring a broad array of coordinated services, both clinical and supportive (Center for Substance Abuse Treatment, 1993a, 1993c). However, these services will not be adequately provided without appropriate training of health care providers as to the nature of the problem and the most effective approaches to deal with them.

Long-term follow-up data are needed to determine the effects of prenatal exposure on later school behavior and learning, as well as later effects on health and reproductive development. Virtually no data exist on these effects beyond the first 5 years of life (Center for Substance Abuse Treatment, 1993c). In addition to looking at the specific consequences of individual drugs and groups of drugs, further research is necessary to determine whether broad public health approaches to the problems of drug use during pregnancy, and the treatment of drug-affected children and families, are more effective than drug-specific approaches to the problem.

As with any research endeavor, it is necessary to realize that the results from these studies will be difficult and costly to collect, and that it may be many years before useful applications of these results can be determined. In addition, single studies may not be reproducible. There may be design flaws that go unrecognized until the data are analyzed or new and better techniques are developed. Therefore, it may be many years, even decades, before definitive results are available.

CONCLUSIONS

The health care needs of drug-affected children and families are complex. Additional research is needed to develop targeted prevention and treatment efforts to meet the needs of this varied population. In order to do this at reasonable costs, these services must be fully integrated into the primary care health care system, and although there will be some initial start-up costs in the training of these providers, in the long run, this will probably produce better delivery of care in a cost-effective manner.

Providing care to pregnant addicted women requires the skills of a multidisciplinary team to provide all needed medical services, including appropriate treatment of alcohol and other drug problems. Assessment and appropriate treatment of psychosocial and mental health issues, as well as social services for the children also are essential.

Clinical staff should understand that the traditional approach, which often avoids setting limits for patients and regards rules loosely, can be perceived as "enabling" by addicted patients. Consistency in approaches, expectations, and the messages conveyed by all staff is critical to the successful engagement and retention of pregnant addicted women. This is best done through regular, periodic meetings of all staff or representation of staff from all sites in regular case management meetings.

On the positive side, many women may come to view their pregnancies as incentives for recovery. It is important that the obstetric and addiction programs create an environment that is supportive of these women and their needs. Understanding that the disease of addiction must be addressed first, regardless of the woman's motivation to treatment, leads to greater likelihood of success for the mother, the infant and, ultimately, the family.

REFERENCES

Abel, E. L., & Sokol, R. J. (1992). Consequences of alcohol abuse. In N. Gleicher (Ed.), *Principles and practice of medical therapy in pregnancy* (pp. 79–85). New Haven, CT, Appleton & Lange.

Broekhuizen, F. F., Urie, J., & Van Mullen, C. (1992). Drug use or inadequate prenatal care? Adverse pregnancy outcome in an urban setting. *American Journal of Obstetrics and Gynecology, 166,* 1747–1756.

Centers for Disease Control, (1990). Statewide prevalence of illicit drug use by pregnant women—Rhode Island. *Morbidity and Mortality Weekly Report, 39,* 225–227.

Center for Substance Abuse Treatment, (1993a). *Treatment improvement protocol: Pregnant, substance-using women: Recommendations of a consensus panel.* Rockville, MD: Author.

Center for Substance Abuse Treatment (1993b). *Treatment improvement protocol: Treatment for HIV-infected alcohol and other drug abusers: Recommendations of a consensus panel* (TIP No. 15). Rockville, MD, CAST.

Center for Substance Abuse Treatment (1993c). *Treatment improvement protocol: Improving treatment for drug-exposed infants: Recommendations of a consensus panel* (TIP No. 5). Rockville, MD, CSAT.

Center for Substance Abuse Treatment (1994). *Treatment improvement protocol: The Tuberculosis epidemic: Recommendations of a consensus panel* (TIP No. 18). Rockville, MD, CSAT.

Chasnoff, I. J. (1988a). Drug use and women: Establishing a standard of care. *Annals of the New York Academy of Science, 562,* 208–210.

Chasnoff, I. J. (1988b). Drug use in pregnancy: Parameters of risk. *Pediatric Clinics of North America, 35,* 1403–1412.

Chasnoff, I. J., Burns, W. J., Schnoll, S. H., & Burns, K. A. (1985). Cocaine use in pregnancy. *New England Journal of Medicine, 313,* 616–619.

Ewing, J. A. (1984). Detecting alcoholism: The CAGE questionnaire. *Journal of the American Medical Association, 252,* 1905.

Finnegan, L. P. (1991). Perinatal substance abuse: Comments and perspectives. *Seminars in Perinatology, 15,* 331–339.

Finnegan, L. P., & Kaltenbach, K. (1992). Neonatal abstinence syndrome. In R. A. Hoekelman, S. B. Friedman, N. M. Nelson, H. M. Seidel (Eds.), *Primary Pediatric Care* (3rd ed.) (pp. 1367–1368). St. Louis, MO: Mosby YearBook.

Fried, P. A., Watkinson, B., Grant, A., & Knights, R. M. (1980). Changing patterns of soft drug use prior to and during pregnancy: A prospective study. *Drug and Alcohol Dependence, 56,* 323–343.

Heller, J., Anderson, H. R., Bland, J. M., Brooke, O. G., Peacock, J. L., & Stewart, C. M. (1988). Alcohol in pregnancy: Patterns and associations with socioeconomic, psychological and behavioral factors. *British Journal of Addiction, 83,* 541–551.

Kandel, S. R. (1991). Drug abuse. In A. Y. Sweet & E. G. Brown (Eds.), *Fetal and neonatal effects of maternal disease.* (pp. 401–413). St. Louis, MO: Mosby YearBook.

Keith, L. G., MacGregor, S. N., Fridell, S., Rosner, M., Chasnoff, I. J., & Sciarra, J. J. (1989). Substance abuse in pregnant women: Recent experience at the perinatal center for chemical dependency of Northwestern Memorial Hospital. *Obstetrics and Gynecology, 73,* 715–720.

Lake, M. F., Angel, J. L., Murphy, J. M., & Poekert, G. (1992). Patterns of illicit drug use at the time of labor in a private and public hospital. *Journal of Perinatology, 12,* 134–136.

Land, D. B., & Kushner, R. (1990). Drug abuse during pregnancy in an inner-city hospital: Prevalence and patterns. *Journal of the American Osteopathic Association, 90,* 421–426.

Larsson, G. (1983). Prevention of fetal alcohol effects: An antenatal program for early detection of pregnancies at risk. *Acta Obstetrica Gynecologica Scandinavica, 62,* 171–178.

Minkoff, H. L., McCalla, M. D., Delke, I., Stevens, R., Salwen, M., & Feldman, (1990). The relationship of cocaine use to syphilis and human immunodeficiency virus infection among inner city parturient women. *American Journal of Obstetrics and Gynecology, 163,* 521–526.

Mitchell, J. L., Briggs, N., Faison, C., Brown, G. M., Loftman, P., & Williams, S. B. (1990). HIV status and the use of cocaine/crack in women delivering with little or no prenatal care. Paper presented at the Sixth International Conference on AIDS, San Francisco, CA.

Mitchell, J. L., & Brown, G. (1990). Physiological effects of cocaine, heroin, and methadone. In R. C. Engs (Ed.), *Women: Alcohol and other drugs.* (pp. 53–60). Dubuque, IA: Kendall/Hunt Publishing Co.

National Institute on Drug Abuse. (1989). National Household Survey on Drug Abuse, 1988: Population Estimates. Rockville, MD: Author.

Neerhof, M. G., MacGregor, S. N., Retzky, S. S., & Sullivan, T. P. (1989). Cocaine abuse during pregnancy: Peripartum prevalence and perinatal outcome. *American Journal of Obstetrics and Gynecology, 161,* 633–638.

Rosett, H. L., & Weiner, L. (1984). *Alcohol and the fetus: A clinical perspective.* New York, NY: Oxford University Press.

Sokol, R. J., Martier, S. S., & Ager, J. (1989). The T-ACE questions: Practical prenatal detection of risk-drinking. *American Journal of Obstetrics and Gyneology, 160,* 863–870.

Sonderegger, T. (Ed.) (1992). *Perinatal substance abuse.* Baltimore, MD: Johns Hopkins University Press.

Streissguth, A. P., Darby, B. L., Barr, H. M., & Smith, J. R. (1983). Comparison of drinking and smoking patterns during pregnancy over a six year interval. *American Journal of Obstetrics and Gynecology, 145,* 716–724.

Wittmann, B. K., & Segal, S. (1991). A comparison of the effects of single- and split-dose methadone administration on the fetus: Ultrasound evaluation. *International Journal of the Addictions, 26,* 213–218.

Zuckerman, B. (1983). Alcohol consumption by pregnant women. *Obstetrics and Gynecology, 61,* 6–12.

Zuckerman, B., & Bresnahan, K. (1991). Developmental and behavioral consequences of prenatal drug and alcohol exposure. *Pediatric Clinics of North America, 38,* 1387–1406

Zuckerman, B., Parker, S., Hingson, R., Alpert, J., & Mitchell, J. (1986). Maternal psychoactive substance use and its effect on the neonate. In A. Milunsky, E. A. Friedman, L. Gluck (Eds.), *Advances in perinatal medicine,* (pp. 125–179). New York: Plenum Press.

6

Training Health Professionals to Deliver Comprehensive Care To Drug-Affected Children and Their Families

Mary R. Haack, Ph.D., F.A.A.N.
and Janet A. Deatrick, Ph.D., F.A.A.N.

In order to provide adequate health care to drug-affected children and their families, providers of that health care must be trained in assessment, recognition, and management of the problem. It has only been within the past 20 years that medical and nursing education have recognized the need to train physicians and nurses in the problems of substance-related disorders. Despite the increase in training about substance-related disorders within medical and nursing schools, physicians and nurses in training are bombarded with the preconceived notions of those who have not yet accepted substance dependence as a treatable health problem. Substance dependence continues to be viewed as a complicating factor that is secondary to the true medical problem and is dealt with only after the others issues are treated. There also is a general attitude that substance dependence cannot be treated and that these patients and their families are hopeless.

Moreover, health professionals have difficulty coordinating prenatal services, drug treatment, psychiatric treatment, and infectious disease treatment—especially in complicated cases of substance-dependent women with HIV infection. A lack of understanding between the medical and drug treatment and psychiatric professions has led to a separatism that creates a barrier to the HIV-positive substance-dependent woman's ability to access comprehensive care. Community experiences and drug treatment have not been emphasized in medical and nursing graduate education, while substance abuse counselors lack medical treatment skills. As a result, most primary care doctors and nurses, including those handling prenatal care, are unprepared when confronted with the complex needs of the substance-dependent pregnant woman with HIV infection.

Philosophies within the primary care and drug treatment systems vary, as do clinical training programs, staffing patterns, and service delivery. All coordinate poorly with one another. The result is deficient care for pregnant women who may require a wide range of community services.

COMPONENTS OF HEALTH PROFESSIONS TRAINING

Training for medical and nursing staff, alcohol and other drug treatment providers, and others who care for pregnant, drug-using women and their children should address the following topic areas (Center for Substance Abuse Treatment, 1993):

DIAGNOSIS AND TREATMENT

- *Medical guidelines:* Basics of prenatal, labor and delivery, perinatal, and postpartum care.
- *Treatment readiness in substance-using women:* Aspects of the woman's readiness and/or motivation for treatment.
- *Assessment instruments:* Uses and benefits of various instruments to measure substance use, as well as psychosocial, psychiatric, and parental functioning.
- *Dual diagnosis:* Techniques for assessment and diagnosis and treatment planning for mentally impaired, substance-using pregnant women.
- *Women with positive toxicology screens in alcohol and other drug treatment programs:* Procedures for referral, counseling, and follow-up.
- *Follow-up care:* Approaches for relapse prevention, monitoring, and intervention.

Federal and State Guidelines and Requirements

- *Federal and state guidelines for alcohol and other drug treatment:* Techniques for assessment and diagnosis, treatment planning, monitoring, and follow-up care.
- *Confidentiality and reporting:* Requirements to report alcohol and other drug use and child abuse and neglect; federal and state confidentiality provisions.
- *Urine toxicology screening:* Procedures for and implications of screening, and the importance of informed consent.
- *Legal issues:* Approaches for coping with outstanding warrants, domestic violence, child custody, adoption, foster care, and divorce.

Population-Specific Issues

- *Child abuse and neglect:* Supportive counseling techniques for improved client functioning and healing, both for the adult or adolescent client and for her children.
- *Noncompliant patients:* Procedures for protecting the health and well-being of the mother and child.
- *Gender-specific treatment:* The special needs of women for transportation, child care, financial support, safe housing, prenatal and postpartum care, issues of sexuality and skills training regarding how to negotiate for safer sex, and sexual abuse and victimization counseling.
- *Sociocultural sensitivity:* The strengths and challenges presented by race, culture, and socioeconomic circumstances.
- *Incest, adult and child sexual abuse:* The impact of abuse and issues of anger, fear, and self-esteem.
- *Domestic violence:* Safety concerns, self-worth, independence, legal action, and alternative living environments.
- *Habilitation and rehabilitation:* Education of patients in tasks of daily living, skill development, and behavior change.
- *Child development:* Developmental stages, problems, and the special needs of children of substance-using mothers.

Case Management

- *Case management:* Definition of role and function, as well as measures of performance.

- *Coordinating medical and social services:* Conditions for referral, reporting, monitoring, and coordination of patient care.
- *Documentation:* Preparation and management of medical charts and case records.
- *Ethics:* Values and principles underlying the continuum of care, and provider responsibilities to the client and the community.

COMMUNITY NETWORKING

- *Developing cooperative agreements between medical, nursing, social work, alcohol and other drug treatment, and social service programs:* Formal and informal approaches and mechanisms to develop cooperative agreements.
- *Community services:* Types of services available, eligibility requirements, and barriers to service.
- *Outreach:* Identification and recruitment of clients into care.

STAFF DEVELOPMENT

- *Multidisciplinary team approach:* Roles, communication, conflict resolution, and team-building techniques.
- *Staff development and burnout:* Identification of the causes of and techniques to reduce stress; creation of and techniques to reduce stress; creation of professional growth opportunities.

INFECTIOUS DISEASES

- *HIV antibody counseling and testing:* Procedures for the protection of patients and program staff and approaches for supportive care.
- *Infectious diseases of drug users:* Signs and symptoms of disease, particularly sexually transmitted diseases, blood-borne infections (such as hepatitis B and C), and tuberculosis, and approaches for their prevention and treatment.

CASE STUDY: TRAINING TO DELIVER CARE TO HIV-POSITIVE INFANTS AND FAMILIES

Because most HIV-positive women acquire their disease through IV drug use or sexual contact with an IV drug user, the needs of the HIV-positive pregnant woman are far too complicated to be adequately addressed by traditional primary care and substance abuse treatment services. Through a series of National Institute of Nursing Research and Division of Nursing research and training grants, the University of Pennsylvania School of Nursing has created an innovative training model that holds promise for improving the training of advanced practice nurses to meet the needs of these families. A University of Pennsylvania team of nurse researchers and clinicians works in collaboration with an interdisciplinary team of the Special Immunology Clinic at The Children's Hospital of Philadelphia to provide what is called "Transitional Care" to HIV-positive infants and their families. Through a 6-month research treatment protocol developed by the team, the nurse practitioner is available 7 days a week by telephone and by scheduled appointments for home and outpatient visits to a group of randomly selected HIV-positive infants and their families. This "Transitional Care" research protocol also serves as a basis for a master's degree program for pediatric nurse practitioners who are educated to provide such comprehensive care to children and families with specialized health care needs.

The Transitional Care protocol is compatible with the Haack-Darnell Model of Community-Based Care (as described in Chapter 1) in that the nurse practitioner is trained to assess a wide range of health and social problems of the HIV-positive child and family and to case-manage and facilitate the amelioration of those problems through education and referral to professional and community agencies and services. The nurse practitioner assists the family by teaching members how to care for their own needs when possible and how to access appropriate agencies when necessary.

The Transitional Care nurse practitioner functions as a primary care professional who assists the child and family through a five-step process:

1. Assessment of physical problems of the mother and child, including developmental screening of the child;
2. Diagnosis of the problems;
3. Identification of a plan of care for each problem, including a prioritization of which problems should be addressed immediately and which should be addressed at a later time;
4. Designation of a therapeutic intervention appropriate for each problem, to be delivered directly by the nurse practitioner or indirectly by referral to another professional agency;
5. Evaluation of the effectiveness of the interventions, including an

appraisal of the child's or family's ability to follow through on referrals and to access the needed services.

These five steps are repeated for each level of services in the Haack-Darnell Model of Community-Based Care and are followed sequentially by the nurse practitioner in treating the affected family. Because of the immunosuppressive nature of the HIV infection, proper nutrition becomes very important to the family in minimizing the negative effects of the virus. The nurse can help identify poor dietary habits and seek assistance for the family to attain proper nutrition. For example, the family may suffer from poor nutrition due to lack of money and knowledge about diet. The nurse practitioner would first address this survival need by assisting the family in obtaining an emergency grant to pay for food. Assistance with the application for food stamps and WIC would follow.

At the same time, the nurse assesses the sick child for symptoms associated with HIV, such as diarrhea and other gastrointestinal disturbances commonly associated with HIV. If the child is severely dehydrated or running a high fever, the child may be referred to the Special Immunology Clinic at the University Hospital. If not, the nurse will teach the mother how to control the diarrhea symptoms through diet. Concurrently, the nurse will assess the mother's ability to understand the instructions and the willingness to provide the diet.

If the mother is under the influence of mood-altering drugs, the nurse practitioner will assess her physiologic need for detoxification and substance abuse treatment. Because substance abuse treatment resources for substance-dependent mothers with AIDS are limited, a successful referral is often difficult to complete; however, once the mother is in substance abuse treatment, the nurse will work with the treatment staff to establish a comprehensive plan of care after discharge.

The nurse will assess the economic status of the family and may discover, for instance, that the mother has difficulty obtaining work because of literacy problems. Due to the feelings of shame she experiences, the mother does not talk about this problem. The nurse can help the mother to improve not only her self-esteem, but also her chances of securing a job, by both discussing the feelings of shame and working with the substance abuse treatment staff to include literacy training in the mother's aftercare program. This may improve not only the mother's esteem, but also her chances of securing a job. These women may also have poor parenting skills because of factors such as their own upbringing. The nurse may play with the mother and child as a means of role-modeling good parenting. The nurse may also teach the mother how to handle the frustrations and the care of their children.

As shown in Figure 6.1, the nurse practitioner directly facilitates access to treatment for HIV disease-related problems, as well as to the limited number of substance abuse services in the Philadelphia area. The nurse practitioner helps the family to combat additional problems by linking them with other professionals and agencies. Interventions are not only aimed at the HIV-affected child, but also at other members of the family. The Transitional Care Model emphasizes the importance of addressing the health of the entire family as a means of improving the environment in which the infant grows.

As a result of a recent study conducted by York (R. York, personal communication, Sept. 1996), which found that 50% of women who received no prenatal care in Pennsylvania admitted to the use of drugs during pregnancy, a parallel University of Pennsylvania project is under development to address the need for more culturally sensitive postnatal care in the home. The educational component of this program prepares advanced practice nurses to provide prenatal and postnatal care in medically underserved neighborhoods where the incidence of substance abuse is particularly high. Prenatal care and AZT treatment have been found to be critical in reducing harm to the developing fetus, even when the pregnant mother continues to use substances.

The balance between quality of care and costs of care for infants who are HIV-positive is the goal of the University of Pennsylvania's Transitional Care Model. The nurse practitioner employed in the clinical project assesses the basic needs of babies and their families and matches those needs to appropriate care. The nurses enrolled in the graduate program are taught these skills through classroom instruction, as well as clinical placements in hospital, ambulatory, community, and home settings.

Rather than "taking care" of the family's needs, the nurse practitioner empowers the family to take care of their own needs wherever the infant and family are, across a continuum of situations—the home, community, an outpatient clinic, or in the hospital setting. Accordingly, the intervention is designed for 6 months during which the infant and families become familiar with and involved in specialty care. These 6 months are spent teaching skills and instilling knowledge that will be useful for the duration of recovery and acute episodes of illness.

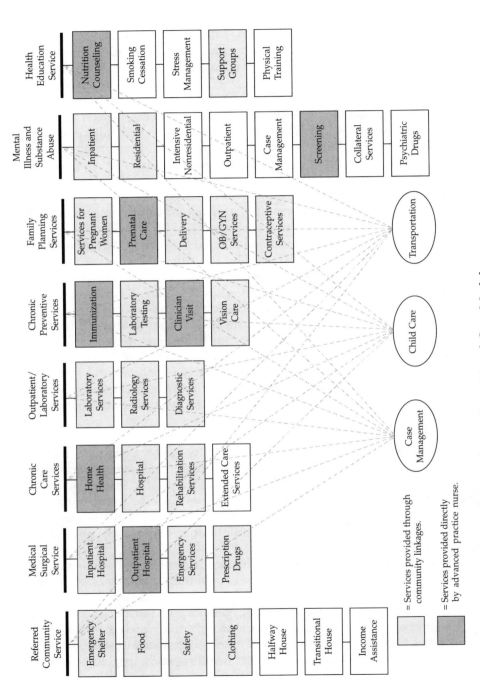

Figure 6.1 University of Pennsylvania Transitional Care Model

Sources: Adapted from Haack-Darnell Model of Community-Based Care for Drug-Dependent Mothers and Their Children, 1993. Used with permission.

Rather than provide expensive direct care that cannot be sustained over a long period, the graduate nurse specialist helps the family by teaching each member how to access appropriate health and social services, how to carry out certain procedures, and how to care for themselves and other members of their families. Direct care is provided, of course, in emergency situations, and also as a means of establishing trust with the family. The nurse specialist can provide this care vis-à-vis preparation with nurse practitioner skills.

As part of a long-term research project at the University of Pennsylvania School of Nursing, this prototype of care has been used effectively with low-birthweight babies and pregnant women with other high-risk conditions, such as diabetes. It has been shown to reduce health care costs up to 40% in some groups and to improve patient outcomes and patient satisfaction (Brooten et al., 1986; Finkler, Brooten, & Brown, 1988). Skills in assessing the comprehensive needs of families and in teaching families to care for their illness are the key factors that contribute to the success of this prototype (Brooten et al., 1991, 1995; Cohen, Arnold, Brown, & Brooten, 1991).

The University of Pennsylvania pediatric HIV-positive training project was funded by a grant from the Division of Nursing within the U.S. Department of Health and Human Services. Such training grants are provided for 3 to 5 years with the caveat that the school will devise ways to sustain the program after federal funding ceases. Schools are rarely able to obtain other funding, and the gains made by such projects can be quickly lost. Even though additional funds for the clinical project have been obtained through grants from the Pediatric AIDS Foundation and the University of Pennsylvania Research Foundation, a highly competitive funding market endangers the survival of such programs.

Graduates of the University of Pennsylvania pediatric HIV training project may also be inhibited from practicing what they have learned in the program. While third-party reimbursement policies impede the adult nurse practitioner's ability to provide care to HIV-positive adults, federal legislation mandates Medicaid reimbursement for pediatric practitioners, family nurse practitioners, and nurse midwives (Aiken et al., 1993). This regulation enables a nurse practitioner to be reimbursed for providing primary care and specialty-related care in formalized health care settings. However, graduates must successfully complete the complex and arduous tasks of obtaining approval as Medicaid providers. In addition, the "nontraditional" services, such as home visits to children who are still asymptomatic, though necessary for successful transitional care, may not be reim-bursable. Moreover, restrictions on prescriptive authority in many states would prevent nurse practitioners from prescribing drug ther-apy, which can be a critical component of treatment for HIV-infected individuals. In addition, Medicare does not reimburse nurse practi-tioners, except in designated rural areas and in nursing homes under limited circumstances.

FUTURE DIRECTIONS

Despite the progress made over the past decade in expanding research and training (see Appendix D), the immediate future does not look promising. Proposed federal budget cuts threaten to eliminate training programs in substance-related disorders. This will reduce the ability not only to train people specializing in the treatment of drug-affected children and families, but also to train generalists. As training dollars for providers are being reduced, so are funds for treatment. The cumu-lative effect of the public policies impacting drug-using pregnant women is a vicious cycle (see Figure 6.2). Lack of prevention- and treatment-oriented public policy leads to inadequate federal support for training competent providers. Without the appropriate clinical skills, providers become pessimistic and fail to recognize the health care needs of these families. Low recognition of problems leads to neg-ative obstetrical and neonatal outcomes, which support the belief that drug-using pregnant women and drug-exposed children are hopeless cases and undeserving of health care services.

Funding for demonstration research grants is being eliminated, making it difficult to carry out the research projects that are necessary to increase our knowledge in this area. This coincides with cutbacks in welfare and Medicaid funding as well as funding for such programs as Aid for Families with Dependent Children and funding for Women, Infant, and Children programs. Although this may cause some imme-diate reduction in expenditures for these programs, there are few data available to indicate how these reduced expenditures will affect other programs that may significantly increase in cost due to these program reductions. Studies in California have indicated that for each dollar spent in substance dependence treatment, seven dollars are saved in other programs, including criminal justice costs. These cutbacks do not bode well for care for this population.

One approach to cost reduction would be to integrate the health care needs of this population into the primary care health care deliv-

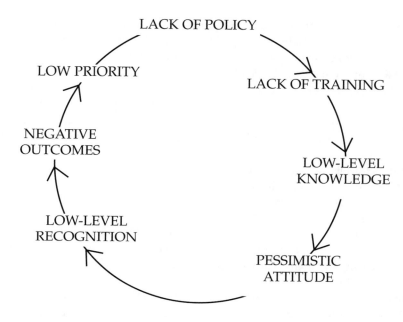

Figure 6.2 The Impact of Policy on Training: A Vicious Cycle

ery system. Although this may result in a long-term cost reduction, there will be immediate costs in training primary care providers to be able to deal with the complex needs of this population. By integrating it into the primary care system, the ability to provide comprehensive and coordinated health care services will be developed. This will also increase the capability to provide care on an as-needed basis and to adjust the intensity of that care based on the need of the individual. This will only occur when substance dependency treatment is fully integrated into the health care system and the provision of services is looked at as all other health care services.

REFERENCES

Arken, L., Lake, E., Semaan, S., Rehlman, H., O'Hare, P., Cale, S., Dunbor, D., & Frank, I. (1993). Nurse Practitioner managed care for persons with HIV infection. *Image, 25*(3), 172–177.

Brooten, D., Gennaro, S., Knapp, H., Jovene, N., Brown, L., & York, R. (1991). Functions in early discharge of very low birthweight infants. *Clinical Nurse Specialist, 5*(4), 196–201.

Brooten, D., Kumar, S., Brown, L., Butts, P., Finkler, S., Bakewell-Sachs, S., Gibbons, A., & Delivoria-Papadoupoulos, M. (1986). A randomized clinical trial of early hospital discharge and home follow-up of very-low-birth-weight infants. *New England Journal of Medicine, 315,* 834–939.

Brooten, D., Naylor, N., York, R., Brown, L., Roncali, M., Halleagourankh, A., Cohen, S., Arnald, L., Munro, B., Jacobson, B., & Finkles, S., (1995). Effects of nurse specialist transitional care on patient outcomes and cases: Results of five randomized trials. *The American Journal of Managed Care, 1*(1), 45–51.

Centers for Disease Control (1993). *HIV/AIDS Surveillance Report, 5,* 3.

Center for Substance Abuse Treatment (1993). *Pregnant, Substance-Using Women: Treatment Improvement Protocol Series, Number 2.* Rockville, MD: CSAT.

Chasnoff, I. J., Landress, H. J., & Barrett, M. E. (1990). The prevalence of illicit-drug or alcohol use during pregnancy and discrepancies in mandatory reporting in Pinellas County, Florida. *New England Journal of Medicine, 322,* 1202–1206.

Cohen, S., Arnold, L., Brown, L., & Brooten, D. (1991). Taxonomic classification of transitional follow-up care nursing interventions of low birth-weight infants. *Clinical Nurse Specialist, 5*(1), 31–36.

Finkler, S., Brooten, D., & Brown, L. (1988). Utilization of inpatient services under shortened lengths of stay: A neonatal care example. *Inquiry, 25*(2), 271–280.

York, R. (Sept. 1996). Personal communication.

PART II

Issues in Public Policy

7

Policy Choices and Legislative Mandates

Bonnie B. Wilford, M.S.

For a significant part of the late 1980s, the newspapers were flooded with heartbreaking stories about alcohol- and other drug-affected children. The plight of these children has left the headlines of our newspapers, but the children have not disappeared. . . . The problem already affects two generations: adult children of alcohol and other drug abusers are producing drug-exposed infants, and many of these disabled adults are unable to adequately care for their disabled children.

The cost of helping these people overcome their alcohol abuse and other drug use and return to being productive members of society will be high, but far less than ignoring the problem.

(Smith, 1992, pp. iii, 1).

A joint study by the Southern Governors' Association and the Southern Legislative Conference (1993) has concluded that one of the most alarming problems state policymakers and service providers face today is the long-term impact of children exposed before birth to the tobacco, alcohol or drugs their mothers used during pregnancy. This impact ripples through a host of service systems:

- *Social Services.* A study by the National Committee for Prevention of Child Abuse notes that substance abuse has become the dominant characteristic in the caseloads of child welfare agencies (Coles & Platzman, 1992). The abuse or neglect of very young children seems particularly associated with parental drug use. Some experts believe that the chaotic and often dangerous home environments in which many of these children live after being released from the hospital may do more damage than the initial drug exposure.

- *Education.* The first wave of children exposed before birth to crack cocaine—an estimated 300,000—entered the school system in 1991, along with children exposed to alcohol and other drugs (Gomby, 1991). Psychologist Vallery Wallace (1991) says that teachers are "on the front lines and often don't know how to even identify the [drug-affected] children, let alone deal with their special needs." Yet without intensive, multifaceted intervention, federal officials (Knight, 1992) predict that many of these children will grow up to be disabled adults who will strain our already overcrowded psychiatric hospitals, outpatient services and jails.

- *Medical Care.* A study by the Children of Alcoholics Foundation (Woodside, Henderson, & Samuels, 1991) also demonstrates that children of alcoholics use the medical system in much higher numbers than children from nonalcoholic families. The rate of inpatient admissions based on claims filed by 1.6 million members under a Blue Cross group policy showed that admissions were 24.3% greater for children of alcoholics than for other children and the rate of hospital days used by children of alcoholics was 61.7% greater than for other children. A high percentage of the children of alcoholics who were admitted to the hospital were diagnosed as having substance abuse problems and mental disorders.

In sum, the health, social, and educational costs of helping such children and families are significant (Hutchins & Alexander, 1990). Child welfare agencies find themselves overwhelmed by the scope of services needed to preserve these families (Jones, McCullough & Dewoody, 1992). Pregnant women particularly have a difficult time obtaining treatment for drug abuse. Few public programs are willing to accept pregnant women or mothers with children, largely because they are not equipped to deal with their related needs for health, housing, and education. The GAO has reported (1990, 1991) that a 500% increase in federal block grant funds for women who abuse drugs does not appear to have translated into an increase in the number of available treatment slots for these women, particularly those who are pregnant or who have small children.

THE ROLE OF FEDERAL AND STATE LEGISLATION

Services for children and families in crisis are provided primarily by state child welfare, mental health, and juvenile justice systems (American Bar Association, 1990). Child welfare systems are the means by which states perform their traditional function of guardianship for children reported to state protective services. Mental health systems serve emotionally disturbed children; juvenile services provide rehabilitation and treatment services for youth who commit criminal offenses. While each system is designed to handle different populations, evidence suggests that the children and families served share similar characteristics and treatment needs that may be effectively addressed by a common service (American Medical Association, 1990).

A study by the National Conference of State Legislatures (Smith, 1991) points out that, although children and families often are labeled and assigned to a system based on the incident that precipitated their entry into the public sector, their treatment needs often are multiple and cross agency boundaries. The specific services available to them typically are based on the capacity of a particular delivery system rather than on their real needs. Fragmentation of service systems results in multiple, uncoordinated, and costly interventions that fail to address underlying behavior patterns, skill deficits, and concrete needs experienced by families in crisis. Financing structures in most states are biased toward out-of-home placement, since child welfare budget line items for placement operate as open-ended entitlements, while appropriations for placement prevention alternatives are fixed. Given current fiscal conditions in most states, lawmakers are exploring programs to improve the financing, coordination, and integration of the various children and family services.

State legislatures serve a primary role in determining how well the child welfare, mental health, and juvenile justice systems function, both separately and in concert (National Governors' Association, 1992). Legislators set statutory guidelines for judicial proceedings; create, abolish, and reauthorize treatment programs and family support services; appropriate program funds, review agency budgets, and determine financial mechanisms; oversee rules and regulatory procedures; set standards and monitor performance and outcomes; advocate for constituents who face apparently hostile state bureaucracies; authorize innovative pilot programs and intersystem coordinating mechanisms; and, increasingly, determine specific aspects of programming and service delivery.

FORMULATING LEGISLATIVE RESPONSES

Experts note that policy has been difficult to formulate in response to this problem, because it requires balancing the state's interest in protecting children with the state's duty to respect the autonomy and privacy of families (Larson, 1991). Moreover, there are additional barriers. The debate over drug-exposed children is affected by other extremely volatile issues: the "war" on drugs, child abuse, and the abortion debate, and its significance to the reproductive rights of women (National Institute on Drug Abuse, 1992). These complex and emotional issues make reaching a consensus about policy toward drug-exposed infants extremely difficult.

A further impediment to policy development is the fact that the service needs of drug-exposed children fall heavily on a child protective services system that is already overburdened in many jurisdictions (McCullough, 1991). Thus, legislators concerned about drug-exposed infants quickly realize that attention must be given not only to one group of children, but to the adequacy of the child welfare system as a whole.

Finally, legislators hoping to design a response to drug-exposed infants soon confront major gaps in knowledge to guide this design. As described earlier, very little is known with certainty about what, if any, are the harmful effects on children of prenatal exposure to different amounts of illegal drugs (Weston et al., 1989). And while there is a growing body of empirical knowledge, little is yet known about what types of treatment best help pregnant women reduce drug use to maximize birth outcomes, or which treatment approaches most effectively assist new parents with drug problems so that they can maintain custody of their children.

FEDERAL POLICIES

Most legal interventions with women who abuse drugs during pregnancy are implemented locally, while the organization and funding of services to this population is addressed at the state level. It is useful, however, to point out the few relevant areas in which the federal government establishes some direction for the states to follow.

The federal Narcotic Addict Rehabilitation Act established a precedent for states interested in developing policies that offer substance abuse treatment in lieu of prosecution or punishment for a drug-related crime. In the 1970s, Congress passed the Omnibus Safe Streets Act, which created the Treatment Alternatives to Street Crime or TASC program. This program was specifically designed to offer a means of diverting drug-involved offenders into treatment, and could be adapted by states to design "treatment in lieu of prosecution" protocols (Jenks, 1992).

In 1992, Congress enacted Public Law 102–321, which reorganized the agencies of the Department of Health and Human Services that support substance abuse research and services. At the same time, PL 102–321 imposed new requirements for the administration of the federal block grant program, which is the major source of federal funds available to the states for prevention and treatment of substance abuse. With this change, funding became contingent on meeting new and expanded requirements for services to substance-abusing pregnant women. The law also authorized separate demonstration grants to fund programs designed specifically for pregnant and parenting women (Feig, 1991).

Also in 1992, the National Drug Control Strategy addressed the Bush administration's approach to pregnant women who use drugs in its section on "hard-to-reach populations" (Office of National Drug Control Policy [ONDCP], 1992). The Strategy supported the expansion and improvement of services for pregnant women and emphasized outreach to women at risk and linkage of health care and substance abuse treatment services. It expressly encouraged voluntary treatment, but also accepted coercive means to bring certain women into treatment by supporting the child protective approach that effectively makes custody of children contingent on participation in treatment. The strategy concludes that "As a rule, pregnant addicts should be diverted into treatment whenever they become involved in the criminal justice system" (ONDCP, 1992, p. 27).

STATE POLICIES

The states are free to determine whether or not to develop any policy of legal intervention specifically for women who use drugs during pregnancy (Breyel, 1992). In fact, states have adopted a wide array of policy responses to the problem of drug-exposed children (Butynski & Canova, 1990). In part, this diversity reflects the complex and controversial nature of the issue and the lack of consensus about either the prevalence or severity of the problem or what response is most likely to be effective. Further, experience to date suggests that policy responses cannot be developed without a detailed assessment of a state's resources in areas such as drug treatment, family support services, child protective services, and foster care.

A number of state legislatures have concluded that the use of legal interventions is an appropriate and necessary response to the problem of substance abuse by pregnant and postpartum women. Every state in the country has on its books a law that makes the possession, delivery, and sale of controlled substance illegal (Larson, 1991). Every state also has laws that protect children from abuse and neglect and require health and social service professionals to report suspected cases of child abuse and neglect to appropriate authorities (Moore, 1990). These laws apply to all citizens—men and women alike. In addition, many states have chosen to respond to the problem of perinatal addiction by crafting laws that specifically address women who abuse drugs during pregnancy (Smith, 1991).

PUNITIVE VERSUS REHABILITATIVE APPROACHES

Legal scholars characterize federal and state laws as taking two different and opposing approaches to the problem of illicit drug use by pregnant women and drug-exposed and drug-addicted newborns, depending on whether addiction is viewed as a criminal or a medical matter (Moore, 1990). The first approach is punitive. In this approach, the problem is defined in terms of the infant, and the goal is to reduce the number of addicted newborns. The pregnant woman is prosecuted as a drug dealer, drug user, or child abuser (English, 1990; McNulty, 1990; National Center for Prosecution of Child Abuse, 1990).

The second approach is rehabilitative. In this approach, the problem is defined in terms of the health needs of both the pregnant woman and the infant. The goal is the same—to reduce the incidence of addicted newborns (Moore, 1990). Rather than prosecution or imprisonment, this approach emphasizes medical and social interventions; monies are appropriated not for more stringent law enforcement efforts, but for the development of effective treatment programs (Smith, 1991).

While many of the laws directed toward individual pregnant women carry criminal or civil penalties, most policymakers assert that their intent is not to be punitive. Rather, they see such laws as encouraging professionals to identify women and children in need of services, as well as encouraging the women identified to seek and accept treatment (American Public Health Association, 1991). However, the intent can be difficult to ascertain from the language of the law.

Health care providers, including physicians, generally have opposed punitive action on the grounds that (1) it deters women from seeking prenatal care and thus lessens the opportunity for improving birth outcomes, and (2) it makes health care providers agents of the state when it requires them to violate a patient's trust (and their own professional oaths) by reporting a woman's behavior to child welfare or law enforcement agencies (American Academy of Pediatrics, 1990; American Medical Association, 1990). National health organizations such as the American Medical Association, the American Academy of Pediatrics, the American College of Obstetrics and Gynecology, the American Nurses Association, and the American Public Health Association all have adopted formal policies along these lines. Providers generally support legislation that expands or improves the service delivery system (see Appendix A).

The positions of child welfare agencies, including those representing private organizations, public agencies operating under state and federal laws, and groups of welfare professionals, vary with the type of legislation proposed. Most such organizations oppose criminal prosecution of maternal substance abuse. Many are overwhelmed with cases for which they are inadequately staffed (Jones, McCullough & Dewoody, 1992).

Through the end of 1992, approximately two-thirds of the states had enacted some type of legislation specifically directed to drug use during pregnancy (National Institute on Drug Abuse, 1992). Of these, a minority focus on modifying the behavior of the individual woman through punitive measures; by far the largest number attempt to modify the organization and delivery of services. About a quarter enacted laws that represent a combination of punitive and rehabilitative measures.

Defining Drug Use during Pregnancy as Child Abuse or Neglect

At least seven states have enacted legislation that specifically identifies perinatal substance abuse as evidence of child abuse/neglect, subject to civil court action (National Center for Prosecution of Child Abuse, 1990). These states have used different criteria to establish the relationship between perinatal substance abuse and potential child abuse/neglect. The relationship generally is built on one or more of the following: (1) drug exposure (as evidenced by either a positive toxicology screen or medical assessment at birth); (2) drug exposure that impairs the child or causes drug dependency or withdrawal in the child; or (3) drug use that impairs the parent's ability to adequately supervise and care for the child (English, 1990).

The intent is to criminalize drug use during pregnancy and require the reporting either of the pregnant woman, the newborn, or both to the child protective agency or the criminal justice system. Supporters of this approach argue that the threat or expectation of imprisonment or termination of parental rights will deter women from drug use (Willwerth, 1991).

Drug Screening and Mandated Reporting

State laws may require physicians to test and report pregnant women for illicit drug use, based either on a set of defined clinical symptoms or less definable "suspicion," and also may require testing and reporting of the newborn under the same circumstances (Jenks, 1990). The mother's informed consent is not required to test a newborn in these circumstances. Test results (toxicology findings) may be used as evidence in criminal charges against the pregnant woman or newly delivered woman, unless specifically noted to the contrary (National Center for Prosecution of Child Abuse, 1990). Only a few states, such as Iowa, expressly prohibit prosecution based solely on a positive toxicology.

To date, no state has required that all newborns be tested for drug and/or alcohol exposure. Minnesota has statutorily mandated testing of newborns but gives great discretion to physicians and other health care providers in deciding when to test. Doctors are required to test newborns if they have reason to believe there is drug exposure based on a medical assessment of the mother or the infant. Other states have taken a different approach: rather than address the testing issue directly, they have amended their abuse and neglect laws to include specifically a newborn who shows physical signs of drug exposure or dependency, thereby requiring reporting of child abuse laws (English, 1990).

Legislators also must consider the limitations of testing in terms of specificity and sensitivity. For example, standard urine tests for cocaine can detect metabolites for no more than 3 days after the drug is ingested. Other substances can be detected for longer periods of time but in general, a test at delivery will not disclose any drug used 3 or more weeks earlier (Chasnoff, 1990). Thus, some newborns who were prenatally exposed will not test positive at birth, while others who test positive may not actually be harmed. To lessen the risk of false positives, Minnesota requires that all positive results be confirmed by a licensed laboratory.

PROTECTION FROM PROSECUTION

Beyond the issues of definition, testing, and reporting, legislators confront the problem of defining consequences of such a report. While there is general agreement that every report of prenatal drug exposure requires some type of inquiry, there is considerable disagreement over who should perform the inquiry and what it should involve (Moore, 1990). Most states that have addressed this issue refer reports of drug-exposed infants to the state's child welfare or protective services agency for investigation (Jones, McCullough, & Dewoody, 1992). Opponents of this approach contend that cases involving prenatal drug exposure should instead be handled primarily as a medical, public health, or social services matter. They maintain that such a case should be reported to child protective services only when other factors point to a risk of child abuse or neglect (Feig, 1991).

INVOLUNTARY CIVIL COMMITMENT

Nearly every state has a law allowing the involuntary civil commitment of individuals found to pose a danger to themselves or to others as a result of a mental or physical disability (Moore, 1990). The primary goals of such laws are both to protect the public and to facilitate care of impaired individuals who may be incapable of recognizing their need for services or unable to voluntarily seek those services. Approximately 35 states explicitly permit the involuntary civil commitment of addicted persons (Garcia, 1991); only Minnesota, however, specifically addresses perinatal addiction. The law there is linked to the state's child abuse and neglect reporting law; under both, pregnant women who are assessed as drug-dependent and who refuse treatment may be involuntarily committed.

CHILD ABUSE AND NEGLECT

Legislation adopted in Minnesota in 1989 mandates that all professionals currently covered by the mandatory child abuse reporting law
(including teachers and doctors) are further required to report any
pregnant woman whom they know or have reason to believe is pregnant and has used a controlled substance for a nonmedical purpose
during the pregnancy. (Such reports may also be made voluntarily by
other than mandated reporters.) The report is made to the local welfare agency (in most counties, the Bureau of Social Services), which
then must investigate and offer services to the woman—including prenatal care and drug treatment—that are "indicated under the circumstances." If the woman refuses the services or fails to comply with the
recommended treatment, the local agency must seek an emergency
admission to a treatment program. These statutes allow emergency
and long-term commitment to treatment programs for chemically
dependent persons (Larson, 1991).

   However, the majority of states have not amended their child
abuse and neglect laws specifically to cover a fetus (Larson, 1991). In
fact, in at least two states, courts have ruled that existing abuse and
neglect statutes do not cover a fetus. In *In re Steven S.*, an appellate
court ruled that California's abuse and neglect laws did not extend to
an unborn child. Similarly, in *In re Dittrick*, a Michigan appellate court
ruled that the court had no jurisdiction over an unborn child.

COMPREHENSIVE SERVICES FOR WOMEN AND CHILDREN

Prevention and education initiatives continue to gain legislative support. A report by the Southern Governors' Association and the
Southern Legislative Conference (1992) calls on states to adopt—as
preferred methods—prevention, intervention, and treatment alternatives rather than punitive actions. Lawmakers in some states have
appropriated funds for statewide drug treatment and prevention
efforts generally, with some funds targeted to drug-dependent pregnant and postpartum women and their children; in others, they have
created programs exclusively for this population. States also have designated funds for statewide and local needs assessment and for the
development and construction of new treatment capacity (Moore,
1990).

   The National Alliance for Model State Drug Laws has promulgated
language—based on a statute adopted in Pennsylvania—that creates

treatment capacity specifically targeted to pregnant and postpartum women and their children (see Appendix B). Nine other states—Arizona, California, Hawaii, Kentucky, Massachusetts, Minnesota, South Dakota, Virginia, and Washington—have developed or expanded services for alcohol and drug-exposed infants and children. Other legislative measures aimed at drug- and alcohol-exposed children include: creating early education programs for children ages 3 to 5 (Arizona and Hawaii); developing effective teaching methods for elementary-aged children (Arizona and Massachusetts); developing a system whereby hospital and school officials can identify drug-exposed infants and children (California); expanding services for drug-exposed infants (Minnesota and Washington); and creating a Center for Perinatal Substance Exposed Pregnancies (Kentucky) (Moore, 1990).

Nationwide, drug treatment capacity falls far short of meeting the need (Butynski & Canova, 1990). Existing treatment facilities often refuse or are unwilling to admit pregnant women because of perceived medical complications and potential liability. Few existing programs are geared to female addicts, and even these often do not provide complete or appropriate services, such as pregnancy testing, prenatal care, gynecologic care, contraceptive counseling, and residential or extended care (Brown, 1992).

Responding to these deficiencies, states have prohibited discrimination on the basis of pregnancy or identified pregnant women as a priority group for local and new programs. States also have stipulated selection criteria for funding new or existing treatment programs to include a demonstrated ability to provide or arrange for the special needs of pregnant and postpartum women and their children. Other approaches to expanding services to addicted pregnant and postpartum women include expanding Medicaid coverage to include drug treatment (Alaska); giving pregnant women high priority on treatment waiting lists (Arizona); and implementing a public information campaign on the effects of prenatal exposure to alcohol and drugs (Kansas and Massachusetts). A Virginia law implements the recommendations of the state's Perinatal Drug Exposure Task Force (Moore, 1990).

TRAINING HEALTH PROFESSIONALS

A major impediment to treatment expansion is the lack of a skilled work force (Haack et al., 1993). Medical and nursing school curricula, for example, typically do not deal with the recognition and treatment of drug addiction. States have addressed these deficiencies in treatment capacity by encouraging existing treatment programs, the medical and nursing communities, and others to engage in ongoing research and evaluation of treatment modalities to determine what works, where, for whom, and why. Other states give priority to the development of special prevention and treatment programs for pregnant and postpartum women and their children. Or they require adequate alcohol and drug abuse education in the training curricula and continuing education programs of health professionals. Oregon, for example, has sought federal funds to support demonstration projects that promote continuing medical education among health care providers to improve both the identification of at-risk pregnant women and the quality and delivery of treatment services. The Oregon Health Sciences University also has been directed to implement a curriculum on drug and alcohol abuse assessment and treatment (see also Appendix D).

EVALUATING OPTIONS

The preceding discussion outlines a range of policy choices states have explored in responding to the problem of drug-exposed infants. A recent study for the National Institute on Drug Abuse (National Institute on Drug Abuse [NIDA], 1992) points out that a number of larger questions will affect these choices, and the policymaker will need to consider them.

Relative Priorities

One of the first questions is what priority legislators should give to the problem of addicted mothers and drug-exposed infants (NIDA, 1992). Such prioritization requires an understanding about the prevalence of the problem, the severity of harm caused by it, and the cost and effectiveness of various interventions. Unfortunately, much of this information is not available with respect to the problem of drug-exposed infants. As other chapters in this text make clear, there are only poor estimates of the seriousness of the problem—either in terms of the numbers of children affected, or the severity of the effect. On the other hand, clinical experience suggests that the problem is a very serious one, at least in some of the larger cities.

Policymakers must further compare the relative importance of prenatal exposure to legal drugs to other risks and needs faced by children (Zuckerman, 1991). People advocate for resources to respond to drug-exposed infants because of the fear that these infants' physical, cognitive, and/or social development has been or will be harmed. Yet, with that goal, there are other groups of infants that should also receive attention. For example, poor birth outcomes and later developmental problems also may be traced to cigarette smoking and alcohol abuse by pregnant women. In designing interventions to improve the health and development of newborns, the legislator must weigh whether these problems should receive equal or more attention and funds than the problem of illegal drug use during pregnancy (Jenks, 1992).

STRATEGIES TO INFLUENCE BEHAVIOR

Questions about the legality, wisdom, and effectiveness of alternative approaches to influencing women not to use drugs during pregnancy will also affect these policy choices. A threshold question is to ask to what extent government has a right, through prohibition or punishment, to attempt to control a pregnant woman's actions (McNulty, 1990). The legislator must consider constitutional protections, such as privacy and reproductive rights, when weighing alternative responses to the problem of drug-exposed infants.

In addition to questions of constitutionality, there is concern about the effectiveness of criminal prosecution. Proponents of criminal prosecutions believe that only the strongest measures will convince pregnant women to stop using drugs or at least get into treatment; their own freedom must be on the line (Moore, 1990). Opponents believe that the effect of criminal prosecutions will be just the opposite: fear of prosecution will deter women from seeking care, confiding in their doctors, and participating in treatment (NIDA, 1992). (Many of these opponents also believe that this deterrence will result from automatically involving the child protective services agency when a pregnant woman uses drugs.)

To date, there are no rigorous and systematic studies to help legislators select strategies for motivating or deterring behavior. There is a growing amount of anecdotal evidence, however, from communities where prosecutions or mandatory reporting have occurred (American Medical Association, 1989). Several of these communities have seen decreases in the number of women seeking prenatal care when the more punitive approaches have been publicized.

Numerous health organizations have opposed such interventions during the pregnancy period because of their belief that they will deter, not entice, women into care. They maintain that the use of criminal statutes threatens to drive women with high risk during pregnancies out of the health care system and deters confidential physician-patient communications.

ROLE OF THE PROFESSIONS

As the debate over deterrence suggests, the legislator designing a response to drug-exposed infants must also consider the proper role and qualifications of the different professional groups that might become involved in this response. The various policy choices during the prenatal and postnatal periods assign very different roles to the professions (Hutchins, 1990; Brown, 1991). Mandatory reporting by medical professionals of women who use drugs moves them into a policing role. Reporting all drug-exposed infants to child protective services agencies requires these agencies to devote resources to assessing the needs of drug-involved infants, some of whom may need health and social services but do not need the protection of child protective services. Referring all cases in law enforcement requires these professionals to deal with a group of people for whom they typically have neither training nor resources. Similarly, routinely involving the courts in these cases requires new resources for the courts and training for the judges.

Thus, the legislator considering alternative interventions must keep in mind the demands these will place on the various professions and ask whether these demands conflict with the professions' mission, training, and standards of practice (NIDA, 1992). If they do, these conflicts must be addressed and resolved.

FAMILY PRESERVATION

As discussed above, current law requires that reasonable efforts be made to keep a family together. This often requires intensive in-home or other support services to assist the parent(s) to provide proper care for the child. This focus on family preservation has great significance for developing a response to drug-exposed infants. New types of services will undoubtedly be needed to make reasonable efforts to maintain these families. Drug-exposed infants will also add to the existing caseloads of child protective services workers and juvenile court judges. Thus, in designing a response to this problem, the legislator will need to consider how well the state's system currently meets family preservation requirements, and what if any changes should be made (Consortium of Family Organizations, 1991). Included in this is an assessment of how successful the state is at finding stable, permanent placements for children in a timely manner when services and protective supervision are not sufficient to preserve the family (Feig, 1991).

RESOURCE IMPLICATIONS

Finally, there is no choice that a legislator can make in response to drug-exposed infants that will not involve questions of resources (Larson, 1991). To do nothing will continue the drain on child protective services, out-of-home care, and court resources. To adopt a more punitive approach will shift new costs to law enforcement and corrections. To provide more treatment and prevention services will also require new resources.

Ideally, funds should follow policy choices; too often, policy follows funding. Sometimes a child will be placed in out-of-home care even though the parents are capable of maintaining custody with support and treatment, because money is available for foster care but not for drug treatment. Sometimes families are referred to the court system not because they need the coercive hand of that system, but because the court order can make more services available to them. Whether public health, social services, or child protective services takes a lead role in handling these cases will likely be determined by the amount of funding available to each. Thus, the legislator designing any response to drug-exposed infants must consider not only the effectiveness of different approaches, but also any changes in existing funding structures necessary to foster the most effective approach.

Focusing policy considerations on the problem of prenatal substance exposure, the relevant economic question is: Which policies are likely to provide the greatest reduction in the adverse consequences of prenatal substance exposure for the resources expended? The spectrum of possible actions includes those designed to prevent maternal substance abuse, such as public health- and education-oriented strategies to make individuals aware of the dangers of prenatal substance exposure; prenatal care programs targeted for substance abusers; treatment programs for pregnant drug abusers; drug screening of all deliveries; increased law enforcement; and imprisonment of drug-abusing, pregnant women. Some of these policies may have broader societal effects. For example, increased law enforcement efforts also affect non-pregnant substance abusers, and may reduce crime levels.

If current policy is left unchanged, large costs will be incurred to meet the health care, foster care, and education needs of substance-exposed infants (Haack et al., 1993; Phibbs, 1991). On the other hand, programs targeted at pregnant women, with the goal of reducing low birthweight and the need for neonatal intensive care by increasing access to prenatal care, might yield a very rapid payback (Feig, 1991). For example, recent estimates suggest that prenatal care programs may come close to breaking even in the first year, with additional savings realized over time from the reduction in the long-term cost of low-birthweight births.

Educating women about the potential harm of substance use during pregnancy and treating maternal substance abuse during pregnancy may also prove to be extremely cost-effective (Magjaryi, 1991). The costs of specialized treatment programs for drug users are higher than regular prenatal care, but the potential returns appear greater. The critical fact here, however, is to identify and replicate effective programs. It is even conceivable that savings produced from successful programs that target cocaine abusers could be used to help fund programs that address other forms of substance abuse, or to fund other substance abuse-related programs, such as the child welfare system or family support programs. A reduction in the population of drug-exposed infants and children would also help reduce the burden on these programs.

CONCLUSIONS

The development and implementation of any prevention, intervention, and treatment services for pregnant women and their children may be stalled as a result of the fiscal crisis confronting many states (Moore, 1990). Chavkin asserts that "The near-bankrupt status of many states is reducing services to the poorest and highest-risk women in our communities, so that even those drug-using women who attempt to negotiate the system and seek treatment find few options. We have learned that economics has everything to do with health care and that the failure of our health care system to deal with the social and educational issues that plague perinatal medicine has everything to do with economics" (Chavkin, 1991). Yet, the preponderance of evidence is that, if alcohol or other drug use is detected and treated early in pregnancy, many of the medical and social risks to mother and child can be averted or ameliorated.

The developmental risks imposed by maternal use of drugs and alcohol are, perhaps more than any other risks, preventable. To protect the health of children and ensure that they achieve their full growth and development potential will require coordination of medical, social, and legal strategies. The evidence is now clear that better understanding of the underpinnings of risk-taking behavior, more appropriate prevention and intervention models, increased professional and public education, and new research can protect the health and improve the well-being of hundreds of thousands of infants and their families.

REFERENCES

American Academy of Pediatrics, Committee on Substance Abuse (1990): Drug-exposed infants. *Journal of Pediatrics, 86,* 639–642.

American Bar Association, Center on Children and the Law, ABA Young Lawyers Division (1990): *Drug Exposed Infants and Their Families: Coordinating Responses of the Legal, Medical and Child Protection Systems.* Washington, DC: American Bar Association.

American Medical Association (1989, December): Drug abuse in the United States: The next generation (Report of the Board of Trustees). *Proceedings of the American Medical Association House of Delegates,* Report Y.

American Medical Association (1990): Legal interventions during pregnancy: Court-ordered medical treatments and legal penalties for potentially harmful behavior by pregnant women (Report of the Board of Trustees). *Journal of the American Medical Association, 264*(20), 2663–2670.

American Public Health Association (1991, October): *Illicit drug use by pregnant women.* Washington, DC: The Association, No. 9020.

Bauer, L., & King, M. (1991): When drugs are the tie that binds. *State Legislatures, 17*(9), 12–18.

Breyel, J. M. (Ed.). (1992): *Gaining ground: State initiatives for pregnant women and children.* Washington, DC: National Governors' Association.

Brown, S. S. (Ed). (1991): *Children and parental illicit drug use: Research, Clinical, and Policy Issues—Summary of a Workshop* (National Forum on the Future of Children and Families, National Research Council, Institute of Medicine). Washington, DC, National Academy Press.

Brown, S. S. (Ed). (1992): *Including children and pregnant women in health care*

Reform—Summary of Two Workshops (National Forum on the Future of Children and Families, National Research Council, Institute of Medicine). Washington, D.C., National Academy Press.

Butynski, W., & Canova, D.: (1990): *State initiatives for women: A directory of state alcohol and drug agency resources.* Washington, D.C., National Association of State Alcohol and Drug Abuse Directors.

Chasnoff, I. J., Landress, H. J., & Barrett, M. E. (1990): The prevalence of illicit drug and alcohol use during pregnancy and discrepancies in mandatory reporting in Pinellas County, Florida. *New England Journal of Medicine, 322,* 102–106.

Chavkin, W. (1990): Drug addiction and pregnancy: Policy crossroads. *American Journal of Public Health, 80*(4), 483.

Chavkin, W. (1991): Mandatory treatment for drug use during pregnancy. *Journal of the American Medical Association, 266*(11), 1556–1561.

Coles, C. D., & Platzman, K. A. (1992): Fetal alcohol effects in preschool children: Research, prevention, and intervention. *Identifying the needs of drug-affected children: Public policy issues* (OSAP Prevention Monograph 11). Rockville, MD: Office for Substance Abuse Prevention.

Consortium of Family Organizations (1991, Winter): Drug abuse is a family issue: Family assessment of the Drug and Alcohol Treatment and Prevention Improvement Act of 1990, S. 2649. *Family Policy Report, 1,*(3).

English A (1990): Prenatal drug exposure: Grounds for mandatory child abuse reports. *Youth Law News, 11*(1), 3–8

Feig, L. (1991, January): *Drug exposed infants: Service needs And policy questions.* Washington, DC, U.S. Department of Health and Human Services, Division of Children, Youth, and Family Policy.

Fink, J. R. (1992): Advocacy on behalf of drug-exposed children: Legal perspectives. *Identifying the needs of drug-affected children: Public policy issues* (OSAP Prevention Monograph 11). Rockville, MD: Office for Substance Abuse Prevention.

Garcia, S. A., & Keilitz, I. (1991): Involuntary civil commitment of drug-dependent persons with special reference to pregnant women. *MPDLR, 15*(4), 418–437.

General Accounting Office (1990, May): *ADMS block grant . . . Women's set-aside does not assure drug treatment for pregnant women* (GAO/HRD-91-80). Washington, DC: U.S. General Accounting Office.

General Accounting Office (1990, June): *Drug-exposed infants: A generation at risk* (GAO/HRD-90-138). Washington, DC, U.S. General Accounting Office.

Gomby, D. S., & Shiono, P. H. (1991, Spring): Estimating the number of substance-exposed infants. *The Future of Children,* 17–25.

Haack, M. R., Budetti, P., Darnell, J., & Hudman, J. (1993): *An analysis of resources to aid drug-exposed infants and their families.* Washington, DC, Center for Health Policy Research.

Hutchins, E., & Alexander, G. (1990): *Substance use during pregnancy and its effect on the infant: A review of issues (HHS Region III Perinatal Information Consortium Technical Report PIC-III TRS 90-01).* Baltimore, MD: The Johns Hopkins University, Department of Maternal and Child Health.

Jenks, S. (1990, February): Drug babies: An ethical quagmire for doctors. *Medical World News,* 39–46.

Jones, R. L., McCullough, C., & Dewoody, M. (1992): The child welfare challenge in meeting developmental needs. *Identifying the Needs of Drug-Affected Children: Public Policy Issues* (OSAP Prevention Monograph 11). Rockville, MD: Office for Substance Abuse Prevention.

Knight, C. M. (1992): Educational policy issues in serving infants and toddlers born toxic-positive to drugs. *Identifying the Needs of Drug-Affected Children: Public Policy Issues* (OSAP Prevention Monograph 11). Rockville, MD: Office for Substance Abuse Prevention.

Larson, C. S. (1991, Spring): Overview of state legislative and judicial responses. *The Future of Children,* 72–84.

Magjaryi, T. (1991, September 24–26): Prevention of alcohol and drug problems among women of childbearing age: Challenges for the 1990s. Paper presented at the OSAP Conference, *Healthy women, healthy pregnancies, healthy infants—Emerging solutions in the face of alcohol and drug problems.* Miami, FL.

McCullough, C. B. (1991, Spring): The child welfare response. *The Future of Children,* 61–71.

McNulty, M. (1990): Pregnancy police: Implications of criminalizing fetal abuse. *Youth Law News (Special Issue)* 6(1).

Moore, K. G. (1990): Substance abuse and pregnancy: State lawmakers respond with punitive and public health measures. *American College of Obstetricians and Gynecologists Legis-Letter,* 9(3), 1–6.

National Alliance for Model State Drug Laws (1993). *Model laws on substance abuse.* Washington, DC: U.S. Government Printing Office.

National Center for Prosecution of Child Abuse (1990): Substance-abused infants: A prosecutorial dilemma. *American Prosecutors' Research Institute Update,* 3(9).

National Governors' Association, Center for Policy Research (1992, July): State coverage of pregnant women and children. *MCH Update,* 1–20.

National Institute on Drug Abuse, Drug Abuse Policy Center (1992): *Legal interventions directed at women who use drugs during pregnancy: What decision makers need to know* (prepared by R. L. Feldman, E. Salinsky, J. Cianci,

J. Sher). Fairfax, VA, Lewin-VHI, Inc..

Office of National Drug Control Policy/ONDCP (1992): *National drug control Strategy*. Washington, DC: U.S. Government Printing Office.

Phibbs, C., Bateman, D., & Schwartz, R. (1991): The neonatal costs of maternal cocaine use. *Journal of the American Medical Association, 266*(11), 1521–1526.

Smith, S. L. (1991): *Family preservation services: State legislative initiatives*. Washington, DC: National Conference of State Legislatures.

Smith, V. (1992): *Identifying the needs of drug-affected children: Public policy issues (OSAP Prevention Monograph 11)*. Rockville, MD: Office for Substance Abuse Prevention.

Southern Governors' Association and Southern Legislative Conference (1992): *1991–1992: The South's agenda for healthy infants and families*. Washington, DC: Southern Regional Project on Infant Mortality.

Wallace, V. (1991, July 1): And the children shall need. *Washington Post.*

Weston, D. R., Ivins, B., Zuckerman, B., Jones, C., & Lopez, R. (1989): Drug-exposed babies: Research and clinical issues. *Zero to Three: Bulletin of the National Center for Clinical Infant Programs, 9*(5), 1–7.

Willwerth, J. (1991, May 13): Should we take away their kids? *Time Magazine, 137*(1), 62–63.

Woodside, M., Henderson, B. W., & Samuels, P. N. (1991): *Parental consent: Helping children of addicted parents get help*. New York: Children of Alcoholics Foundation.

Zuckerman, B. (1991, Spring): Drug-exposed infants: Understanding the medical risk. *The Future of Children*, 26–34.

8

Financing Health Care for Drug-Dependent Women and Their Children

Julie Darnell, M.H.S.A.*

A s with health services generally, comprehensive health care for substance-exposed pregnant women and their children is financed through a variety of programs. For a number of reasons, low income women and children with substance exposure-related health care needs are less likely to be privately insured. Even when private health insurance is available, coverage is usually strictly limited to crisis- and acute care-related needs and does not cover the range of long-term rehabilitative and preventive services that are necessary for the appropriate treatment of substance abuse and its consequences. As a result, governmental programs play a central role in financing the cost of substance abuse-related care for women and children.

This chapter presents an overview of public financing of health care for substance-exposed pregnant women and their children. It begins with a discussion of the role of state and local governments in financing substance abuse-related services for pregnant women and children. It then examines the role of the federal government in financing services through discretionary health programs and entitlement programs, most notably the Medicaid program. It concludes with an examination of the Medicaid program today and prospects for its future as the largest, most stable, most flexible, and most important of

---

* I gratefully acknowledge Sara Rosenbaum who generously provided her time, technical expertise, and editorial assistance. This chapter benefited enormously from her review and comments. Most of all, I thank her for her encouragement.

all sources of public health care financing for women of childbearing age and their children.

THE ROLE OF LOCAL, STATE, AND FEDERAL GOVERNMENTS IN FINANCING COMPREHENSIVE HEALTH CARE FOR SUBSTANCE-ABUSED PREGNANT WOMEN AND THEIR CHILDREN

There is no single source of information on public funding of substance abuse-related services for women and children. Therefore, in this chapter, we assemble data on local, state, and federal funding of services obtained from a variety of sources.

STATE AND LOCAL GOVERNMENT FUNDING

State governments[1] play an important role in financing services to prevent and treat abuse of alcohol and other substances. The National Association of State Alcohol and Drug Abuse Directors, Inc. (NASADAD) estimated that in fiscal year 1994, state, county, and local agencies provided over $1.7 billion, or nearly 43% of total expenditures ($4.0 billion) for alcohol and drug abuse treatment and prevention programs (NASADAD, 1996, p. i). Additionally, states may qualify for federal funds through the federal Substance Abuse Block Grant ($1.1 billion in FY 1994 or 28% of all expenditures). In order to receive federal block grant funds, states must maintain their state expenditures at a level similar to an aggregate of expenditures during the two preceding years (NASADAD, 1996, p. 52). Additionally, states must spend not less than 5% of their block grant for treatment services designed for pregnant and parenting women, including the provision of prenatal and child care (NASADAD, 1996, p. 52). NASADAD has reported that 21,660 pregnant women received treatment in 43 states during fiscal year 1994 (NASADAD, 1996, p. 68).

FEDERAL GOVERNMENT FUNDING

Federal financing for substance abuse-related problems can be divided into two types: discretionary health programs, whose funding levels

---

[1] For a discussion of the role of states in providing comprehensive services to substance-exposed pregnant women and their families, see Chapter 7, *Policy Choices and Legislative Mandates.*

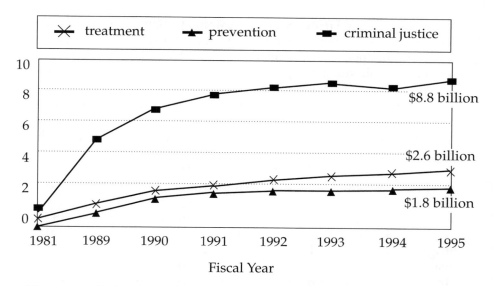

Figure 8.1 Federal Funding for Antidrug Activities
Source: Office of National Drug Control Strategy, *Fact Sheet: Drug Data Summary,* June, 1995, p. 5.

are subject to annual Congressional allocations under the appropriations process; and entitlement programs, which grow automatically as
eligible populations increase, more services are furnished, and the cost
of services grows.

Over the past decade and a half as noted in Figure 8.1, total federal
funding (including both discretionary and entitlement programs) for
antidrug activities has increased significantly from $1.5 billion in fiscal
year 1981 to $13.3 billion in fiscal year 1995 (Office of National Drug
Control Policy [ONDCP], 1995, p. 5). However, only a small proportion of these funds is spent on treatment. In fiscal year 1995, 64% ($8.8
billion) of total federal funding was spent on criminal justice activities
(e.g., interdiction, intelligence, research); 20% ($2.6 billion) was spent
on treatment; and 14% ($1.8 billion), on prevention (ONDCP, 1995, p. 5).
Moreover, even those funds that are available for treatment are subject
to significant limitations.

Discretionary Programs

The United States Department of Health and Human Services (USD-
HHS) and its agencies administer discretionary programs for substance-exposed pregnant women and their children. The Substance

Abuse and Mental Health Services Administration (SAMHSA) is the key agency responsible for federal substance abuse and mental health policy and financing. Under SAMHSA are three centers, two of which are focused on substance abuse: the Center for Substance Abuse Treatment (CSAT) and the Center for Substance Abuse Prevention (CSAP). Additionally, an Office for Women's Services addresses the special problems and prevention and treatment needs of women with substance abuse and mental disorders. SAMHSA administers the largest source of federal funding for prevention and treatment of drug abuse—the alcohol and drug abuse block grant—through CSAT. CSAT also provides demonstration and categorical funding to states, cities, and localities for a number of specialized programs, including projects for women. CSAP provides demonstration grants to communities for drug and alcohol prevention activities, including a major prevention program for pregnant women and their infants. The National Institutes of Health (NIH) provides funding for research projects. Many of the federal programs that finance treatment services are categorical in nature and are tied to specific services and activities.

In spite of significant gains in federal antidrug funding over the past two decades, it appears that funding levels for substance abuse prevention and treatment are headed downward. Congressional appropriations for fiscal year 1996 awarded SAMHSA $300 million less than its fiscal year 1995 appropriation level, representing a decrease of 14% (American Health Line, 1996). In fiscal year 1996, funding for the block grant was level-funded at the 1995 appropriation level of $1.23 billion. Federal funding for demonstration and categorical programs carried out by CSAT was $215 million in fiscal year 1995 and $106.1 million in fiscal year 1996 (Center for Substance Abuse Treatment, 1996, p. 21). Funding for CSAP was $238.6 million in fiscal year 1995 and only $89.8 million in fiscal year 1996 (Center for Substance Abuse Prevention Office, 1996, p. 1).

Even in the case of the increasingly scarce federal discretionary funding sources that do exist, investment decisions may not match funding needs and priorities or support long-term research. For example, as part of the ADAMHA Reorganization law, Congress transferred the National Institute on Drug Abuse (NIDA) to the NIH, the biomedical arm of the federal government. This transfer resulted in dismantling the NIDA research and demonstration program, and, with it, the "Perinatal 20" comprehensive therapeutic demonstration programs designed for drug-abusing women of childbearing age and their offspring. The Perinatal 20 projects provided scientific evaluation of program characteristics as they influenced treatment outcomes. Ideally, findings from these projects should have been applied to the needs of state and community-based agencies, and used to inform policymakers. But the translation of these scientific data never occurred. Moreover, once the demonstration project had expired (along with federal funding), the communities in which these programs resided could not continue the programs, because there was no stable source of funding to sustain them. The programs were not designed to identify, secure or optimize other potential sources of reimbursement (e.g., Medicaid) for services provided under the demonstration.

Beyond the issue of insufficient levels of funding is the lack of coordination among various funding sources. Even though more than three dozen federal agencies are involved in some aspect of antidrug activities, no formal relationships to coordinate activities exist among these agencies. Additionally, more than 75 congressional committees and subcommittees, both authorizing and appropriating, have jurisdiction over issues related to antidrug activities (Hogan, 1992, p. 2). Like the federal agencies, competing committees may encourage competition for resources, rather than resulting in a greater level of resources.

Entitlement Programs

There are two major entitlement programs under the Social Security Act: Medicare and Medicaid. Medicare is a health insurance program for persons 65 and older and for certain disabled persons (1994 Green Book, 1994, p. 123). While pregnant women with alcohol or drug problems could qualify for Medicare if they are receiving Social Security benefits on the basis of disability, these instances are rare. Therefore, this chapter focuses on Medicaid, the major source of public funding for maternal and child health services generally and for women and children with substance abuse problems as well. Medicaid entitles eligible individuals to coverage for a broad range of acute, preventive, and long-term medical and health-related services. As an entitlement program, Medicaid is not subject to congressional discretionary appropriations.

MEDICAID

Overview

Medicaid is a federal/state means-tested entitlement program regulated by federal law, Title XIX of the Social Security Act, and administered by the states with federal oversight provided by the Health Care Financing Administration (HCFA). Federal statutes and rules vest broad discretion in states to tailor programs to meet state needs, but also require participating states to comply with various federal standards related to eligiblity, benefits, participation, payment of providers, and other matters. States that meet the federal eligibilty and benefit guidelines receive contributions, ranging from 50 to 83% based on state per capita income, toward the cost of their programs (Kaiser Commission on the Future of Medicaid, 1995c, p. 1).

Today, Medicaid finances care for one in four American children and pays for one-third of the nation's births (Kaiser Commission on the Future of Medicaid, 1995a, p. 1). In 1988, Medicaid covered 38% of all pregnant women and children below 200% of the poverty line; by 1994, Medicaid covered 54% (Holahan, Winterbottom, & Rajan, 1995, p. 10). Medicaid represents the largest source of health insurance coverage for pregnant women and children below 200% of the poverty line. While Medicaid coverage is increasing, other sources of health insurance coverage are declining; employer-sponsored coverage declined from 37% to 30% over the same period (Holahan, Winterbottom & Rajan, 1995, p. 10).

Medicaid is uniquely positioned to serve substance-exposed women with children who are more likely to be poorer than mothers in the total population and report higher rates of drug use compared with mothers at or above the poverty line, as shown in Table 8.1. The prevalence of drug use is more than one and a half times greater for women with children below the poverty line compared with those at or above the poverty line. Furthermore, substance-exposed mothers are more likely than the overall population of mothers to have incomes below the poverty level; incomes below the poverty level are reported by 25% of past-month users and 26% of past-years users, compared with 18% of all mothers.

General Eligibility

Federal Medicaid law limits federal contributions to certain categories of individuals. Federal law also imposes strict financial limitations on who may be assisted with federal funding.

Eligibility for Children and Families.[2] States are required to provide Medicaid coverage to families receiving Aid to Families with Dependent

---

[2] See Congressional Action for changes made to this program.

TABLE 8.1 Mothers by Poverty Status and Reported Drug Use *

Family income as a Percent of Poverty	Past-Month Drug Use			Past-Year Drug Use			Total Mothers in Category	
	Number	Percent	Rate	Number	Percent	Rate	Number	Percent
0–49% of poverty	161,439	8.9	6.6	368,250	9.7	15.0	2,452,253	6.9
50–99% of poverty	282,086	15.6	7.2	627,875	16.5	16.1	3,890,855	10.9
Below poverty	**443,526**	**24.6**	**7.0**	**996,125**	**26.1**	**15.7**	**6,349,652**	**17.8**
100–299% of poverty	932,398	51.7	5.2	1,970,409	51.7	10.9	18,006,913	50.5
300–499% of poverty	222,869	12.4	2.9	546,334	14.3	7.0	7,790,268	21.8
500% and above	205,252	11.4	5.8	297,038	7.8	8.4	3,515,552	9.9
Above poverty	**1,360,520**	**75.4**	**4.6**	**2,813,781**	**73.9**	**9.6**	**29,306,190**	**82.2**
TOTAL	**1,804,046**	**100.0**	**5.1**	**3,809,906**	**100.0**	**10.7**	**3,515,552**	**9.9**

Note. NIDA, 1991 National Household Survey on Drug Abuse cited in Table 11.B.10-Distribution of women. 15–44 years of age by poverty status and family income as a percentage of poverty level according to reported drug use pattern, and rate of drug use: 1991, U.S. Department of Health and Human Services. (1994). *Substance Abuse Among Women and Parents,* p. 21.

* Table does not reflect use of alcohol or nicotine which are documented teratogens.

Children (AFDC) (Congressional Research Service, 1993, p. 5). AFDC is a federal entitlement program which provides children and families meeting federal eligibility criteria and state-set income and resource limits to cash assistance (Rosenbaum & Darnell, 1996c, p. 7). In 1994, the maximum state AFDC grant ranged from $120 per month in Mississippi (12% of the federal poverty level) to $703 in Suffolk County, New York (69% of the federal poverty level; family benefits averaged $377 per month (Burke, 1995, p. 1).

Eligibility for pregnant women and children. As a result of amendments to the Medicaid statute between 1984 and 1990, states are mandated, at a minimum, to extend Medicaid coverage to all pregnant women and children under age six with family incomes at or below 133% of the federal poverty level ($17,263 for a family of 3 in 1996). States are also required to phase-in Medicaid coverage to all children below age 19 who were born after September 30, 1983, and whose family incomes are below 100% of the poverty level; on October 1, 1996, states began providing Medicaid coverage to all children age 13 and below poverty level (National Governors' Association [NGA], 1996b, pp. 1–2). (See Table 8.2.)

States are permitted—but not required—to extend Medicaid eligibility to certain women and children beyond the minimum levels. States may extend Medicaid coverage to pregnant women and infants under age one with family incomes between 133% and 185% of the federal poverty line (Congressional Research Services, 1993, pp. 8–9). States may also use the authority under Section 1902(r)(2) of the Social Security Act to apply more liberal income and resource criteria than those used for the AFDC program to expand Medicaid coverage to pregnant women, infants, and children who would not otherwise be financially eligible for Medicaid benefits. States may also use the authority under Section 1115 of the Social Security Act to expand Medicaid eligibility to additional persons, including, but not limited to, pregnant women, infants, and children. Table 8.2 below summarizes the extent to which states have opted to expand coverage to pregnant women and children above the mandated minimum levels (NGA, 1996b).

Eligibility for disabled persons. Generally, persons who receive cash assistance under the Supplemental Security Income (SSI) program are automatically entitled to Medicaid (Congressional Research Service, 1993, p. 9).[3] SSI is a federally funded and adminstered means-tested entitlement program which provides cash assistance to low-income aged, blind, and disabled individuals (Rosenbaum & Darnell, 1996c, p. 13). Approximately 100,000 persons qualifed for SSI in 1994 because of their addiction to alcohol or other substances (Ross, 1995, p. 9).[4]

Eligibility: The Institution for Mental Diseases "IMD" exclusion. The IMD exclusion is a provision of federal Medicaid law that prohibits coverage for anyone under 65 who is an inpatient in an "institution for mental diseases" except for inpatient psychiatric services for individuals under age 21 and persons ages 65 and older. By definition, an IMD is a hospital, nursing facility, or other institution of more than 16 beds which is primarily engaged in providing diagnosis, treatment, or care of persons with mental diseases (Social Security Act §1905 (i); Reg.

---

[3] States may use more restrictive eligibility standards for Medicaid than for SSI if these standards were in effect before the enactment of the SSI program. Twelve states, known as 209(b) states, use more restrictive eligibility standards: Connecticut, Hawaii, Illinois, Indiana, Minnesota, Missouri, New Hampshire, North Carolina, Ohio, Oklahoma, and Virginia.

[4] See Congressional Action for changes made to the SSI program.

TABLE 8.2 Medicaid Coverage for Pregnant Women, Infants, and Children

State	Pregnant Women and Infants	Children Under 6	Children 6 and Older	
	Percent of poverty	Percent of poverty	Percent of poverty	Under
Alabama	133%	133%	100%	13
Alaska	133%	133%	100%	13
Arizona	140%	133%	100%	14
Arkansas	133%	133%	100%	13
California	200%	133%	100%	19
Colorado	133%	133%	100%	13
Connecticut	185%	185%	185%	13
Delaware	185%	133%	100%	19
Florida	185%	133%	100%	13
Georgia	185%	133%	100%	19
Hawaii	300%	300%	300%	19
Idaho	133%	133%	100%	13
Illinois	133%	133%	100%	13
Indiana	150%	133%	100%	13
Iowa	185%	133%	100%	13
Kansas	150%	133%	100%	17
Kentucky	185%	133%	100%	19
Louisiana	133%	133%	100%	13
Maine	185%	133%	125%	19
Maryland	185%	185%	185%	13
Massachusetts	185%	133%	100%	13
Michigan	185%	150%	150%	15
Minnesota	275%	133%	100%	13
Mississippi	185%	133%	100%	13
Missouri	185%	133%	100%	19
Montana	133%	133%	100%	13
Nebraska	150%	133%	100%	13
Nevada	133%	133%	100%	13
New Hampshire	185%	185%	185%	19
New Jersey	185%	133%	100%	13
New Mexico	185%	185%	185%	19
New York	185%	133%	100%	13

TABLE 8.2 continued

State	Pregnant Women and Infants	Children Under 6	Children 6 and Older	
	Percent of poverty	Percent of poverty	Percent of poverty	Under
North Carolina	185%	133%	100%	19
North Dakota	133%	133%	100%	18
Ohio	133%	133%	100%	13
Oklahoma	150%	133%	100%	13
Oregon	133%	133%	100%	19
Pennsylvania	185%	133%	100%	13
Rhode Island	250%	250%	250%: ages 6–7 100%: ages 8–12	13
South Carolina	185%	133%	100%	13
South Dakota	133%	133%	100%	19
Tennessee	185%	133%	100%	13
Texas	185%	133%	100%	13
Utah	133%	133%	100%	18
Vermont	200%: pregnant women 225%: infants	225%	225%	18
Virginia	133%	133%	100%	19
Washington	185%: pregnant women 200%—infants	200%	200%	19
West Virginia	150%	133%	100%	19
Wisconsin	185%	185%	100%	13
Wyoming	133%	133%	100%	13

Source: National Governors' Association, *State Medicaid Coverage of Pregnant Women and Children, Summer 1996, 1996b*. Used with permission.

§§431.431.620, 435.1009, and 440.140 reprinted in Commerce Clearing House, 1994, ¶14,601). HCFA uses the International Classification of Diseases (ICD-9) definition of mental disorders for purposes of categorizing a facility as an IMD (NASADAD, 1994, p. 2) and interprets an IMD to include residential substance abuse treatment facilities. By finding a residential substance abuse treatment center to be an IMD,

HCFA regulations have the effect of excluding from coverage persons ages 21–64; the exclusion is for all Medicaid-covered services as well as the services of the IMD (NASADAD, 1994, p. 1). The IMD exclusion effectively creates a barrier to most existing substance abuse treatment services for women of childbearing age. As a result, the IMD exclusion fosters the use of more costly crisis inpatient hospital care instead of less costly residential treatment (NASADAD, 1994, p. 4).

An important exception to the IMD exclusion is a provision declassifying as IMDs group homes of 16 or fewer beds. In addition, HCFA rules do not require that children be counted as residents if their beds are neither designed to be nor being used as treatment beds (NASADAD, 1994, p. 3). These exceptions have two important effects. First, they restore Medicaid to women and children who otherwise would lose it. Second, these rules allow homes larger than 16 persons, thereby yielding greater economies of scale.

Providers are also able to avoid the IMD exclusion by forming small residential facilities of 16 or fewer beds or by certifying discrete wings of otherwise general inpatient facilities. Despite these exceptions to the IMD rule, few states have used these options to create residential treatment programs for pregnant women.

It is recognized widely that the IMD exclusion was put in place by Congress as a means to limit federal expenditures for services in inpatient mental health facilities, long considered a state's responsibility (NASADAD, 1994, p. 2). The IMD exclusion, as it has been extended to exclude most residential substance abuse treatment centers from Medicaid reimbursement, has increased—not decreased—federal Medicaid dollars. According to a study conducted by the Center on Addiction and Substance Abuse at Columbia University, at least one in every five Medicaid hospital days are attributable to substance abuse. In fiscal year 1994, the portion of hospital care attributable to substance abuse was estimated to exceed $7.4 billion (Center on Addiction and Substance Abuse at Columbia University, 1993, p. 4).

Benefits

General Benefits. Medicaid is designed to finance services that typically fit the medical model, as specified in Figure 8.2. States must provide certain services and may provide a range of optional services. In the case of both required and optional care, states must also cover services at levels that are "sufficient in amount, duration, and scope to reasonably achieve [their] purpose." In the case of both required and optional care, states must also cover services at levels that are "sufficient in amount, duration, and scope to reasonably achieve [their] purpose" (42 C.F.R. §440.230 reprinted in Commerce Clearing House, 1995, ¶21,556). Moreover, federal regulations prohibit states from discriminating in coverage of certain conditions (42 C.F.R. §440.240 reprinted in Commerce Clearing House, 1995, ¶21,567). Federal regulations also specify that no state may "arbitrarily deny or reduce the amount, duration, or scope of a required service" (42 C.F.R. §440.230 reprinted in Commerce Clearing House, 1995, ¶21,566). A state may, however, place limits on coverage based on "medical necessity or on utilization control procedures" (42 C.F.R. §440.230 reprinted in Commerce Clearing House, 1995, ¶21,566). For adults ages 21 and above, a state may, for example, place flat limits on coverage for certain ambulatory services, such as day treatment. Under special rules applicable to children under age 21 eligible for EPSDT benefits (discussed in the description of pediatric benefits) flat limits may not be used.

Pregnancy-related benefits. Coverage extends throughout a woman's pregnancy and the last day of the month in which the 60th postpartum day occurs, even if she has a change in income which would otherwise make her ineligible. States are required to provide services related to "pregnancy (including prenatal, delivery, postpartum, and family planning services); and other conditions which may complicate pregnancy" (State Medicaid Manual reprinted in Commerce Clearing House, 1996, ¶14,231.25). Regulations have defined pregnancy-related services as "services that are necessary for the health of the pregnant woman and fetus, or that have become necessary as a result of the woman having been pregnant. These include, but are not limited to, prenatal care, delivery, postpartum care, and family planning services" (42C.F.R. §440.210 reprinted in Commerce Clearing House, 1995, ¶440.210). Furthermore, "services for other conditions that might complicate a pregnancy include those for diagnoses, illnesses, or medical conditions which might threaten the carrying of the fetus to full term or the safe delivery of the fetus; and . . . all services under the plan that are pregnancy-related for an extended postpartum period" are required (42C.F.R. §440.210 reprinted in Commerce Clearing House, 1995, ¶440.210). As such, any service or treatment (including substance abuse-related services) for a pregnant woman is covered as a mandatory benefit through the end of the month of the 60th postpartum day if such service is provided at a level that is sufficient in amount, duration, and scope to reasonably achieve its purpose and is medically necessary.

Mandatory Services for Categorically Needy Individuals
- Inpatient hospital services
- Outpatient hospital services
- Rural health clinic services
- Federally qualified health center services
- Other laboratory and x-ray services
- Nursing facility services (age 21 or over)
- Home health services for individuals entitled to nursing facility services
- Early and Periodic Screening, Diagnosis, and Treatment Services (EPSDT) (under age 21)
- Family planning services
- Physicians' services
- Nurse-midwife services
- Certain pediatric and family nurse practitioners' services

Mandatory Services for Medically Needy
- Prenatal and delivery services
- Ambulatory services
- Home health services for persons entitled to nursing facility services
- In states choosing to cover the medically needy in intermediate care facilities for the mentally retarded (ICF/MR) or in institutions for mental diseases (IMDs), broader requirements apply

Optional Services
- Podiatrist services
- Optometrist services
- Chiropractic services
- Other physician services
- Private duty nursing
- Clinic services
- Dental services, including medical and surgical services
- Physical therapy and related services
- Occupational therapy
- Speech, health, and language disorder
- Prescribed drugs
- Dentures
- Prosthetic devices

Figure 8.2 List of Services for Which Federal Matching Payments Are Available under Medicaid

Optional Services (continued)

- Eyeglasses
- Other diagnostic, screening, preventive, and rehabilitative services
- Inpatient hospital services for persons age 65 or over in mental institutions
- Nursing facility services for persons age 65 or over in mental institutions
- Nursing facility services for persons under age 21
- IMD services for persons over age 65 or under age 21 and ICF/MR services
- Inpatient psychiatric hospital services for persons under age 21
- Christian Science nurses/sanatoria
- Emergency hospital services
- Personal care services
- Transportation services
- Case management services
- Hospice services
- Respiratory care services

Source: Congressional Research Service, 1993, p. 3.

Figure 8.2 *(continued)*

Pediatric benefits. The EPSDT (Early and Periodic Screening, Diagnosis and Treatment) program is a mandatory benefit package for anyone less than 21 years of age who is eligible for Medicaid. At a minimum, EPSDT services include: periodic screens; interperiodic screens; vision, dental, and hearing care; diagnostic services; and treatment services. Most significantly, the EPSDT program must cover all services allowed under federal Medicaid law when needed by eligible children, whether or not they are covered for adults (Perkins, 1993, p. 1).

Institutional services. Medicaid covers nearly all hospital-based services as noted in Figure 8.2. However, most substance abuse treatment services are provided within nonhospital (freestanding) residential treatment institutions, which are the most difficult to cover under Medicaid because of the IMD (Institution for Mental Diseases) exclusion described previously.

Substance abuse services. While there is no specific mention of substance abuse treatment in the Medicaid statute, the legislative history and amendments made to the Medicaid statute by the Ominibus Budget Reconciliation Act of 1990 (P.L. 101–239) clarify Medicaid's role in financing substance abuse services. The sentence, "no service (including counseling) shall be excluded from the definition of 'medical assistance' solely because it is provided as a treatment service for alcoholism or drug dependency" was added to §1905(a) of the Social Security Act. This policy clarification appears to open the doors for states to use Medicaid to finance a wide range of inpatient and outpatient drug treatment services (Gates, 1991, pp. 22–23).

Despite the fact that Medicaid was not designed to fund alcohol and drug treatment, an increasing number of states are using it for that purpose however limited. The National Drug and Alcoholism Treatment Unit Survey (NDATUS) reports that Medicaid reimbursements for substance abuse treatment doubled between 1982 and 1987. However, obtaining Medicaid dollars for substance abuse treatment can be a complicated process. In fiscal year 1994, it is estimated that federal/state Medicaid expenditures for substance abuse totaled $1.4 billion, of which $405 million ($230 million federal; $175 million state) was for drug abuse services and $1 billion was for alcohol abuse services ($570 million federal; $435 million state) (United States Department of Health and Human Services, 1996, p. 1). The individual, the service, and the provider institution are all required to meet a complex set of qualifying criteria. States participate in the Medicaid program on an optional basis and administer it within broad federal requirements and guidelines which allow considerable discretion in determining eligibility, covered benefits, and provider payment mechanisms. Therefore, very little uniformity exists from one state to the next. In some states Medicaid plays an important role in financing drug and alcohol abuse treatment; in others, Medicaid's role is negligible (Gerstein and Harwood, 1990, p. 267). A study conducted by the Southern Regional Project on Infant Mortality of 97 substance abuse treatment programs in four states (Virginia, Oklahoma, Kentucky, and Puerto Rico) found that although 61% of women interviewed were covered by Medicaid, only 14% were using Medicaid to finance their substance abuse treatment. A majority of the programs were not eligible for Medicaid reimbursement for services, even though federal Medicaid law would allow it, since these services were not included in their state Medicaid plan (Southern Regional Project on Infant Mortality, 1993, p. 7).

In practice, most states cover only short-term hospital treatment for a 3- to 6-day inpatient detoxification stay and one to three outpatient counseling visits, and very few provide long-term substance abuse treatment options for Medicaid patients (S. Becker, personal communication, 1993). The result is a cycle of relapse and return to detoxification. Access to long-term care is critical if treatment for addicted pregnant women is to be successful.

Congressional Action

During the 104th Congress President Clinton signed into law two bills which could have a significant impact on access to substance abuse coverage for women and their children. Congress also considered a Medicaid reform bill, but because of a threat of presidential veto, Congress dropped provisions to overhaul the Medicaid program.

Legislation Restricting SSI for "Alcoholics" and "Drug Addicts," H.R. 3136, the Contract with America Advancement Act, was signed by President Clinton on March 29, 1996, and it became P.L. 104-121 (United States Congress, P.L. 104-121, 1996). This new law terminates Social Security Disability Insurance (SSDI) and Supplemental Security Income (SSI) for any individual for whom drug addiction or alcoholism is a contributing factor to their disability (United States Congress, P.L. 104-121, 1996). Previously, persons could qualify for SSI for up to 36 months if they complied with drug or alcohol treatment and had a representative payee manage their monthly benefit payments (Ross, 1995, p. 9). Approximately 100,000 persons in 1994 received SSI because of their addiction to drugs or alcohol; this number was projected to grow to over 200,000 by the year 2000 (Ross, 1995, pp. 9–10).

Because of the link between SSI and Medicaid (i.e., persons who receive SSI generally qualify for Medicaid coverage automatically), this new law could potentially reduce the number of persons eligible for coverage of substance abuse services under the Medicaid program. While substance-exposed pregnant women may qualify for Medicaid independent of their addiction under the eligibility pathway created especially for pregnant women and children, nonpregnant women with addictions may not have an alternative basis of eligibility other than receipt of cash assistance under the SSI program. For them, loss of SSI may mean the loss of Medicaid (Rosenbaum and Darnell, 1996a, p. 4).

Welfare Reform Legislation. The Personal Responsibility and Work Opportunity Reconciliation Act of 1996 disproportionately impacts women, who represented 86% of all adult recipients of cash assistance under the Aid to Families wih Dependent Children (AFDC) program in fiscal year 1995 (P. Brannen, personal communication, September, 1996). Receipt of cash assistance (AFDC) is a critical but largely overlooked route to health insurance coverage (i.e., Medicaid) for low-income women. As such, it has broad implications for the continued coverage of substance abuse and other services for substance-exposed women and their families. The legislation was passed by Congress on July 30, 1996, and signed by the President on August 22, 1996 (United States Congress, P.L. 104-193, 1996).

The new law replaces the AFDC entitlement with a cash welfare block grant, Temporary Assistance for Needy Families (TANF). Previously, families who received AFDC were automatically eligible for Medicaid. Because the block grant eliminates the cash entitlement, the bill could have resulted in a significant loss of Medicaid coverage among former AFDC recipients. To prevent this result, the new law requires states to provide Medicaid to any individual who meets the state's July 16, 1996 AFDC eligibility rules. While it may appear that the new welfare reform law makes few changes in Medicaid, it will have major direct and indirect effects on Medicaid eligibility for millions of women and children (Rosenbaum and Darnell, 1996a, pp. 3–4).

Three core aspects to Medicaid's relationship with welfare will be directly affected by the new welfare law. First, the receipt of welfare has been in and of itself an eligibility category for Medicaid. Under the new welfare law, eligibility for cash welfare under the block grant no longer entitles families to Medicaid coverage; as noted previously, only persons meeting July 16, 1996 AFDC eligibility rules will continue to be eligible for Medicaid (Rosenbaum and Darnell, 1996a, pp. 1–2).

Second, Medicaid has operated as a "piggyback" program, provided automatically to AFDC recipients without separate application. Thus, Medicaid enrollment rates may be affected as a result of separate application procedures and eligibility standards. Enrollment is lower for persons who must apply separately compared with persons who automatically qualify for Medicaid. Furthermore, separate enrollment tends to occur at the point at which there is medical care need rather than at a time when the only health care needs are primary and preventative (Rosenbaum and Darnell, 1996a, p. 2).

Third, the implementation of welfare reform will be a time of administrative upheaval for most states as eligibility rules are changed, new application forms developed, workers retrained, and information systems redesigned. Because the Medicaid eligibility process is part of state AFDC administrative systems, it is inevitable that the start-up of welfare reform will lead to changes in the process of eligibility determination and enrollment in Medicaid (Rosenbaum and Darnell, 1996a, p. 2).

As a practical matter, it may be impossible to reduce the number of welfare recipients without reducing the number of substance-exposed women and their families with access to substance abuse and other services under the Medicaid program (Rosenbaum and Darnell, 1996a, p. 3).

Medicaid Reform Legislation. Although historically Medicaid has provided perhaps the most stable funding source for services provided to substance-exposed women and their families, the future of the Medicaid program as an entitlement (with guaranteed funding for eligible populations) is unclear. During the 104th Congress the House and Senate recommended converting Medicaid into a block grant program and reducing federal expenditures by $133 billion over seven years in their budget agreement. The budget agreement passed both chambers but was ultimately vetoed by the President (United States Congress, H.R. 2491, 1995). Subsequently, Congress attached provisions to convert the program into a block grant to their budget reconciliation bill (United States Congress, H.R. 3507/S. 1795, 1996). After objections from President Clinton, Congress dropped the Medicaid reform provisions from the reconciliation bill, retaining only the welfare reform provisions which were eventually signed into law. Since no agreement on Medicaid was reached, it remains unclear what the future holds for Medicaid generally and for the funding stream for substance-exposed women and their families in particular. It is likely that pressures to contain the growth of spending by entitlement programs, including Medicaid, will not only continue but will exacerbate, especially in light of the changes made to the welfare programs. As a result, states will likely be forced to survive with fewer federal and state dollars for their Medicaid programs. If the recent budget cuts directed toward the Substance Abuse and Mental Health Services Administration, which sustained a $300 million or 14% decrease in its fiscal year 1996 appropriation level, are any indication of congressional priorities for behavioral health, substance abuse service may be in serious jeopardy (American Health Line, 1996).

Medicaid Residential Substance Abuse Treatment Legislation. Residential substance abuse treatment centers did not exist when Congress enacted the Medicaid program in 1965. Thus, Congress could not have had such facilities in mind when the IMD exclusion was passed (NASADAD, 1994, p. 3). To address the resulting difficulties of covering residential substance abuse treatment services for substance-exposed pregnant women and their families, Senator Daschle has introduced legislation in the 102nd and each subsequent Congress to provide for coverage of alcoholism and drug dependency residential treatment services for pregnant women and certain family members under the Medicaid program (United States Congress, S. 171, 1995).

The Congress, however, has neither considered nor passed legislation to amend the Medicaid statute to exempt these facilities from the effects of the policy.

Managed Care

Despite little consensus over what to do with the Medicaid program at the federal level, the Medicaid program is undergoing significant changes at the state level. These changes are manifesting themselves by an abrupt departure from the way services have been delivered traditionally (i.e., fee-for-service) to a new delivery system fashioned around managed care arrangements, such as Health Maintenance Organizations (HMOs) and primary care case management (Kaiser Commission on the Future of Medicaid, 1995b, p. ix). In recent years, Medicaid's use of managed care has grown exponentially, from 800,000 beneficiaries in 1983 to 11.6 million beneficiaries in 1995 or approximately one-third of all Medicaid beneficiaries, most of whom are women and children (Kaiser Commission on the Future of Medicaid, 1996, p. 1). The advent of Medicaid managed care could have a potentially significant impact on the availability and quality of substance abuse services for women and dependent children.

Federal waivers. While the Medicaid statute offers states substantial flexibility concerning the size and scope of their Medicaid programs, current Medicaid law prohibits states from mandating enrollment in managed care plans. In order to establish Medicaid managed care programs, states must obtain one of two types of federal waivers (compared in Table 8.3) from the Health Care Financing Administration: (1) freedom-of-choice waivers authorized under Section 1915(b) of the Social Security Act; and (2) research and demonstration waivers authorized under Section 1115 of the Social Security Act (Kaiser Commission on the Future of Medicaid, 1995d). These federal waivers are becoming important vehicles by which states are providing substance abuse services for their Medicaid beneficiaries (Policy Resource Center and Center for Health Policy Research, 1996). Forty-three states and the District of Columbia have waivers mandating beneficiaries enroll in managed care plans; of these, seven states include substance abuse treatment in their waivers (United States Department of Health and Human Services, 1995).

Most waivers granted by HCFA are program waivers under Section 1915(b) that allow states to waive basic Medicaid requirements (e.g., freedom-of-choice, uniform statewide operation, and comparability of benefits). Frequently, these waivers are used to limit a Medicaid bene-

TABLE 8.3 Comparison of Section 1915(b) and 1115 Waiver Authority

Federal Requirements	Section 1915(b)	Section 1115
	Federal Requirements May Be Waived	
Eligibility	NO	YES
Minimum benefits	NO	YES
Freedom-of-choice	YES, with certain exceptions	YES
Federal standards for full-risk managed care plans	NO	YES
Provider reimbursement rules	YES, in limited circumstances	YES
State administration requirements pertaining to eligibility determination, quality control, and other administrative activities	YES, in limited circumstances	YES

Note. From *Medicaid Section 1115 Demonstration Waivers-Approved and Proposed Activities,* by S. Rosenbaum and J. Darnell, 1995, p. 3. Washington, DC: Kaiser Commission on the Future of Medicaid. *Used with permission.*

ficiary's choice of providers to primary care case management or HMOs. These waivers are granted for 2 years and may be renewed. The growth of Medicaid managed care is attributed chiefly to the use of Section 1915(b) waivers (Kaiser Commission on the Future of Medicaid, 1996, p. 3).

In 1993, the Department of Health and Human Services initiated a series of substantial revisions to Section 1115 of the Social Security Act. This section waives conditions of federal financial participation for certain programs, including Medicaid. Under Section 1115 authority, states may carry out research and demonstration projects which change fundamentally the Medicaid program as it is under current law. Before 1993, only one state had received a statewide Section 1115 Medicaid waiver: Arizona (Rosenbaum and Darnell, 1995, p. 1). Over the past few years, several states have opted to take advantage of this authority. As of July 1996, ten states (Arizona, Delaware, Hawaii, Minnesota, Ohio, Oklahoma, Oregon, Rhode Island, Tennessee, and Vermont) have implemented their Medicaid demonstration programs under Section 1115. Furthermore, implementation is pending in five states and an additional six states are waiting for approval from HCFA. Since the Clinton Administration reinterpreted the rules and procedures, making it easier for states to develop demonstration projects, only two states have received disapproval for their waiver: (1) Louisiana and (2) Montana for its behavioral health program. (Rosenbaum and Darnell, 1996b).

The waivers have important implications for substance abuse services for pregnant women and infants. In a number of states with Section 1115 waivers, certain federal Medicaid payment restrictions have been relaxed, making coverage of substance abuse services possible and more flexible. For example, eight states (Maryland, Massachusetts, New Hampshire, New York, Ohio, Rhode Island, South Carolina, Vermont) have requested waivers of the Institution for Mental Diseases (IMD) exclusion (Rosenbaum and Darnell, 1996b, pp. 13, 17). As a result, states may provide substance abuse services and any other covered Medicaid services to individuals age 21 to 64 who reside in a free-standing residential substance abuse treatment center when such services are a direct substitute for inpatient services. More generally, the twin goals of managed care are prevention and early intervention to avert long-term health costs. Thus, managed care plans have incentives to offer benefits which prevent or treat substance abuse before more costly interventions are required.

The irony is that when granted this new flexibility, only a few states have chosen to exercise their option to waive the IMD exclusion or to provide substance abuse treatment in residential settings. Instead, states have used their 1115 authority to cover short-term, acute mental illness and substance abuse treatment.

Options for Medicaid Coverage of Comprehensive Care for Substance-Exposed Pregnant Women and Their Children

Despite the inherent limitations of Medicaid, the failure of legislation to provide substance abuse treatment in residential settings for pregnant women and their children, and the failure of states to optimize the use of their Section 1115 authority to waive the IMD exclusion, Medicaid offers significant opportunities to finance many components of a comprehensive treatment program for substance-exposed infants and their families.

Using the model of comprehensive care for substance-exposed children and their families described by Haack in Chapter 1, Figure 8.3 shows Medicaid's potential role in financing services in the comprehensive model. While no one funding source can support all components of

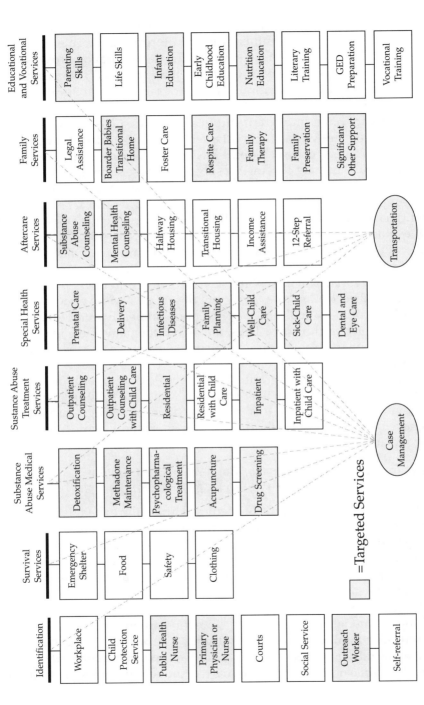

Figure 8.3 Medicaid as a Source of Financing for the Community-Based Model of Care for Drug-Dependent Mothers and Their Children

Sources: Haack-Darnell Model of Community-Based Care for Drug-Dependent Mothers and Their Children, 1993. Used with permission.

a comprehensive treatment program for substance-exposed children and their families, Medicaid can provide partial funding of a component, and, in combination with other funding sources, can together finance many of the components of the comprehensive model of care.

Identification. Medicaid may be used to finance many services which would aid in the identification of substance-exposed women and their children by practitioners (e.g., public health nurse, primary care physician or nurse, outreach worker). Medicaid covers medical exams (including drug history assessment); psychiatric histories; psychosocial evaluations, if performed by a licensed psychologist or other treatment professional licensed under state law; psychosocial evaluations, performed by licensed personnel and if provided as a component of case management; drug history assessments, provided as a component of case management; and medical screening for children under age 21 through the EPSDT program.

Survival services. Medicaid may not be used for basic survival services.

Medical substance abuse services/substance abuse treatment services/ special health services. Because Medicaid services are designed to fit the medical model, they may used to finance the required medical substance abuse services, including detoxification, methadone maintenance, psychopharmacological treatment, acupuncture, and drug screening; and many of the substance abuse treatment services (e.g., outpatient counseling, residential treatment in facilities with 16 or fewer beds, and inpatient care) and special health services (e.g., prenatal care, delivery, family planning, well-child and sick-child care, and dental and eye care) needed by women with dependent children. Additionally, if preventive and primary health care provided by federally qualified health centers or rural health clinics is combined with alcohol and other drug dependency treatment programs or with outpatient hospital clinics or free-standing medical clinics, on-site primary and preventive medical care can be covered easily.

Aftercare services. Aftercare services may or may not be covered by Medicaid. Outpatient counseling as aftercare following residential treatment can clearly be covered, but support group activities may not be covered. Inpatient substance abuse counseling, psychological counseling, psychiatric counseling, and family or collateral counseling are all covered by Medicaid unless the residential treatment program is considered an IMD, and therefore would be subject to the IMD exclusion. At a hospital, these services must be categorized as an inpatient or outpatient hospital service. If provided by a free-standing clinic on an outpatient basis, they are covered as a clinic service. They may be covered if provided by a psychologist or other licensed mental health practitioner under the category of medical or remedial care, or, if it is in a community health center, under the clinic option or by a physician agreeable to reimbursement rates.

Family services. Family or collateral counseling is limited to only eligible persons.

Educational and vocational services. Although vocational and educational training are vital to substance-exposed pregnant women, these services are not covered under Medicaid. Assessments and referrals to vocational and educational services, however, may be covered under Medicaid as a component of case management. Life skills counseling and training may be covered as a rehabilitation service if it is designed and billed as a component of the alcohol and drug dependency counseling.

Case management and transportation. These services are explicitly covered by Medicaid and are critical components of the service delivery model and allow the substance-exposed woman and her children to make the transition from one stage to the next.

CONCLUSION

Despite the potential for Medicaid as a funding stream for substance abuse treatment, states and treatment providers often become discouraged by complex regulations and the waiver application process prescribed by federal requirements. Additionally, states are generally unwilling to spend more of their state dollars on the Medicaid program. During the Medicaid reform debate during the 104th Congress the governors sought to further limit state dollars by reducing their state's maximum matching contribution from 50 to 40% (National Governors' Association, 1996b, p. 1).

Thus, there remains a wide discrepancy between the potential of Medicaid as a source of funding for substance-exposed pregnant women and their children and the ability and willingness to access those funds for these purposes.

REFERENCES

American Health Line. *Some Win, Some Lose.* (April 26, 1996). Alexandria, Virginia: Author.

Brannen, P. Administration for Children and Families. United States Department of Health and Human Services. (September 1996). Personal Communication.

Burke, V. (1995). *Welfare reform: Issue brief.* Washington, DC: Congressional Research Service.

Center for Substance Abuse Prevention Budget Office. *Budget Request Historical Table.* Rockville, MD: Substance Abuse and Mental Health Services Administration.

Center for Substance Abuse Treatment. (1996). *General statement.* Rockville, MD: Substance Abuse and Mental Health Services Administration. United States Department of Health and Human Services.

Center of Addiction and Substance Abuse at Columbia University. (1993). *The cost of substance abuse to America's health care system report 1: Medicaid hospital costs.* New York: Author.

42 C.F.R. §440.230. reprinted in Commerce Clearing House, Inc. (1995). Chicago, IL: Author. ¶21,566.

Commerce Clearing House, Inc. (1994). *Medicare and Medicaid guide.* Chicago, Illinois: Author. ¶14,601.

Commerce Clearing House, Inc. (1995). *Medicare and Medicaid guide.* Chicago, Illinois: Author. ¶14,231.25.

Congressional Research Service. (1993). *Medicaid source book: Background data and analysis* (A 1993 Update). Committee Print 103-A. Washington, DC: U.S. Government Printing Office.

Falco, M. (1992). *The making of a drug-free America: Programs that work.* New York, NY: Times Books.

42 C.F.R. §440.210 reprinted in Commerce Clearing House, Inc. (1995). *Medicare and Medicaid guide.* Chicago, Illinois: Author. ¶440,210.

42 C.F.R. §440.230 reprinted in Commerce Clearing House, Inc. (1995). *Medicare and Medicaid guide.* Chicago, Illinois: Author. ¶21,566.

42 C.F.R. §440.240 reprinted in Commerce Clearing House, Inc. (1995). *Medicare and Medicaid guide.* Chicago, Illinois: Author. ¶21,567.

Gates, D. (1991). *An introduction to Medicaid for alcohol and drug abuse agency staff.* Washington, DC: National Health Law Program.

1994 Green Book. (1994). Overview of Entitlement Programs. Washington, DC: Committee on Ways and Means, U.S. House of Representatives.

Gerstein, D. R. & Harwood, H. J. (Eds). Institute of Medicine. (1990). *Treating drug programs Volume 1. A study of the evolution, effectiveness, and financing of public and private drug treatment systems.* Washington, DC: National Academy Press.

Hogan, H. (1992). *Drug control: Issue brief.* Washington, DC: Congressional Research Service.

Holahan, J., Winterbottom, C., & Rajan, S. *The changing composition of health insurance coverage in the United States* (1995). Washington, DC: Kaiser Commission on the Future of Medicaid.

Kaiser Commission on the Future of Medicaid. (1995a). *Medicaid: Covering the basics.* Washington, DC: Author.

Kaiser Commission on the Future of Medicaid. (1996). *Medicaid and managed care.* Washington, DC: Author.

Kaiser Commission on the Future of Medicaid. (1995b). *Medicaid and managed care: Lessons from the literature.* Washington, DC: Author.

Kaiser Commission on the Future of Medicaid. (1995c). *The Medicaid program at a glance.* Washington, DC: Author.

Kaiser Commission on the Future of Medicaid. (1995d). *Medicaid section 1115 demonstration waivers: Overview and policy implications.* Washington, DC: Author.

Legal Action Center. (No date). *Integrating the existing public and private alcohol and drug treament and prevention systems into a managed competition model.* New York, NY: Author.

National Association of State Alcohol and Drug Abuse Directors, Inc. (1994). *Institution for mental disease (IMD) exclusion: A barrier to substance abuse treatment.* Washington, DC: Author.

National Association of State Alcohol and Drug Abuse Directors, Inc. (1996) *State resources and services related to alcohol and other drug problems for fiscal year 1994.* Washington, DC: Author.

National Governors' Association. (1996a). *Restructuring Medicaid.* Washington, DC: Author.

National Governors' Association. (1996b). *State medicaid coverage of pregnant women and children—summer 1996.* Washington, DC: Author.

Office of National Drug Control Policy. (1995). *National drug control strategy budget summary.* Washington, DC: The White House.

Perkins, J. (1993). *An advocate's Medicaid EPSDT reference manual.* Chapel Hill, North Carolina: National Health Law Program.

Policy Resource Center and Center for Health Policy Research, The George Washington University Medicaid Center. (1996). *First quarterly report: Public sector moves managed care to forefront of behavioral health services.* Washington, DC: The Substance Abuse and Mental Health Services Administration, United States Department of Health and Human Services.

Rosenbaum, S. & Darnell, J. (1995). *Medicaid Section 1115 Demonstration Waivers: Approved and proposed activities.* Washington, DC: Kaiser Commission on the Future of Medicaid.

Rosenbaum, S. & Darnell, J. (1996a). *An analysis of the Medicaid and health-related provisions of the personal responsibility and work opportunity reconciliation act of 1996.* Washington, DC: Kaiser Commission on the Future of Medicaid.

Rosenbaum, S. & Darnell, J. (1996b). *Medicaid Section 1115 Demonstration Waivers: Approved and proposed activities.* Washington, DC: Kaiser Commission on the Future of Medicaid.

Rosenbaum, S. & Darnell, J. (1996c). *Welfare reform: Description of current law and H.R. 4, The Personal Responsibility and Work Opportunity Act of 1995.* Washington, DC: Henry J. Kaiser Family Foundation.

Ross, J. L. (1995). *Supplemental security income: Recent growth in the rolls raises fundamental program concerns.* Testimony before the Subcommittee on Human Resources. Committee on Ways and Means. U.S. House of Representatives. (GAO/T-HEHS-95-67). Washington, DC: United States General Accounting Office.

Social Security Act §1905(i); Reg. §§431.431.620, 435. 1009, and 440.140 reprinted in Commerce Clearing House, Inc. (1994). *Medicare and Medicaid guide.* Chicago, Illinois: Author. ¶14,601.

Southern Regional Project on Infant Mortality. (1993). *A step toward recovery.* Washington, DC: Author.

State Medicaid Manual, HCFA-Pub. 45-3, §3306, Transmittal No. 56 (June 1991) reprinted in Commerce Clearing House, Inc. (1996). *Medicare and Medicaid guide.* Chicago, Illinois: Author. ¶14.231.25.

United States Congress. House. (1996). *Contract with America Advancement Act of 1996.* P.L. 104-121. 104th Cong. 2nd sess. H.R. 3136.

United States Congress. House. (1996). *Personal Responsibility and Work Opportunity Reconciliation Act of 1996.* P.L. 104-193. 104th Cong. 2nd sess. H.R.3734.

United States Congress. House. (1995). *Seven-Year Balanced Budget Act of 1995.* H.R. 2491. 104th Cong. 1st sess.

United States Congress. House. Senate. (1995). *Medicaid Restructuring Act of 1996.* H.R. 3507/S. 1795. 104th Cong. 2nd sess.

United States Congress. House. Senate. (1995). *Medicaid Substance Abuse Treatment Act.* S. 171. 104th Cong. 1st sess.

United States Congress (1990). Omnibus Budget Reconciliation Act of 1990. P.L. 101–239 101st Congress.

United States Department of Health and Human Services. (1995). *Section 1915(b) Waivers—Quarterly Report.* Baltimore, Maryland: Health Care Financing Administration.

United States Department of Health and Human Services. (1996). *Federal Medicaid Expenditures by Various Categories for FY97 Budget Cross-Cutting Tables, Medical Assistance Payment Only.* Baltimore, Maryland: Health Care Financing Administration.

United States Department of Health and Human Services. (1994). *Substance Abuse Among Women and Parents.* Washington, DC: Public Health Service, National Institutes of Health, National Institute on Drug Abuse, Office of the Assistant Secretary for Planning and Evaluation.

United States General Accounting Office. (1991). *ADMS Block Grant: Women's Set-Aside Does Not Assure Drug Treatment for Pregnant Women.* (GAO/HRD-91-80). Washington, DC: Author.

9

The Role of the Courts

Judith Larsen, J.D.

The widest gate into the treatment environment is the courthouse door. Relatively few drug-involved people come to treatment voluntarily. Most are prodded into it, and a judge can offer the strongest inducements: "Go to treatment or lose your child" is one; "Go to treatment or go to jail" is another.

Court actions involving parents can be of two basic types: civil or criminal. Civil cases typically do not involve imprisonment. Their aim is not to punish, but to ameliorate unacceptable social conditions by providing services (as in child neglect cases), assuring that disputes are peaceably settled (as in domestic violence cases), and fairly settled (as in divorce cases). In criminal cases punishment (for example, imprisonment) and rehabilitation (for example, acquisition of job skills) are major purposes of the laws.

NEGLECT-ABUSE CASES

The number of people who enter treatment for alcohol and other drugs (AOD) abuse is affected more by child neglect-abuse cases (also known as dependency cases) than by any other kind of court case. In 1994 the U.S. General Accounting Office estimated that 78% of children in foster care had at least one drug-involved parent (GAO, 1994, p. 2). In urban courts, even higher estimates are heard. The number of child abuse cases has risen every year, either because of greater drug use, or because more children are identified by better-trained professionals (including teachers, nurses, doctors and social workers), or both.

196

Every state has both a reporting law and a court-process law. The reporting law lays out the criteria for identifying neglected and abused children: usually it contains a definition of neglect and abuse, lists those persons who must report child abuse, and extends to these reporters both confidentiality and immunity. The court-process law describes how the case shall proceed through the courts after a legal complaint is filed. The court process law describes which parties shall have legal representation, who has the burden to prove the case, what the time parameters are for trying the case, and so forth. The chronology of a case usually is laid out like this:

1. *Petition and complaint* drawn up.
2. *Initial hearing* to decide whether the court has "probable cause" to take the case, that is, whether there is enough evidence to make it seem likely that there has been neglect or abuse.
3. *A trial* (some states have a "speedy trial" provision).
4. *Disposition of the children,* that is, whether the children will go into foster care, be placed with a relative, or go home.
5. *Reviews.* These court or administrative reviews continue for the duration of the case.

State laws reflect not only local concerns, but national priorities. One of the most powerful federal laws affecting neglect and abuse cases is the Adoption Assistance and Welfare Act of 1980 (PL 96–272; 42 U.S.C. sec. 670 *et seq.*). It generously subsidizes the cost of a state's foster care program in return for the state complying with its standards on extending services to families. The underlying assumption of that law is that a child's "best interests" usually coincide with being raised by the child's own family, if the parents can provide a safe environment. Child protection agencies are required to make "reasonable efforts" to provide services that make family reunion a possibility. These services can include drug treatment for the parents. Thus, a family court judge is under the twin imperatives to reunify the family if at all possible, and to make certain that the child is safe. It is very difficult to walk the middle ground between these two standards. Some courts lean more toward reunification (thus saving foster care costs, but often putting the child's life at peril unless strong supportive services are offered to the family); other courts lean toward safety (which can mean that children are separated from their families and rapidly moved into adoptive homes, or worse, linger in foster care).

Neither case law nor statutory law lays down time parameters for treatment.

Which services are offered in a neglect-abuse case, and whether those services include drug treatment, is very much in the hands of the judge. Some judges simply accept the recommendation of the social worker. Other judges "micromanage" their cases, educating themselves about AOD treatment, touring the local treatment facilities, and monitoring the progress of the parents.

The same diversity exists in payment for services. Some jurisdictions pay virtually all of the costs for all of the services offered (in conjunction, of course, with Medicaid, Temporay Aid for Needy Families, Supplementary Social Security, and so on). Other courts are strict about the adults assuming the costs of their own services: the parent is ordered to pay for the services unless it is demonstrated that there is no way at all for that to be accomplished. While that eases the taxpayers' burden, it often means that the parent goes without the services.

How do courts enforce their orders in neglect-abuse cases if imprisonment typically is not available as a remedy in civil cases? Family court judges hold the strongest of all inducements: the child. A neglect-abuse case is "about" the child—it is only "about" the parents to the extent that the court may seek to remedy the child's problems by improving the skills and resources of the parent. The court has total jurisdiction over the child, in the sense that the court can even take a child away from the care of the parent—despite the fact that the ability to raise one's own child is a constitutionally protected right with a rich history of case law to back it up. That power to remove a child is the court's enforcement power. Parents seldom are willing to relinquish such a precious being. Many women have said that it is only the fear of losing their children that brought them into treatment at last.

DIVORCE-CUSTODY CASES

Typically, treatment issues arise in a divorce case only if one of the two adults accuses the other of AOD involvement. Only rarely would a court-appointed guardian for a child, or the judge alone, raise the issue in the absence of it having been raised by the divorcing parties. That means that in divorces that are consented to by both parties, or that bring only specified narrow problems before the court like property division, a substance abuse problem may never come to the attention of the judge.

In divorce cases where custody of the child is at issue, and where one or both adults raise the issue of the other partner's AOD involvement, the judge has the same power as in a neglect-abuse case: the power to keep the child away from the substance-involved parent until treatment occurs. Often, if such a serious allegation is raised, the judge will appoint a guardian for the child, and ask for an independent investigation and recommendation.

Since many issues in divorce cases are settled out of court, and statistics on drug involvement of the parties are not systematically collected by courts, it is difficult even to estimate what percentage of people are brought into treatment through judicial orders in divorce cases. Certainly, divorce-custody cases do not provide the highway to treatment that neglect-abuse cases do.

DOMESTIC VIOLENCE CASES

Domestic violence cases in family court, as distinct from those that arise as assault cases in criminal court, usually are initiated with a petition for a restraining order. That is, the judge is presented with allegations and evidence of spousal abuse. If these convince the judge that abuse occurred, the court may issue a "stay-away" order and attach conditions to that. If allegations of substance abuse have been made and substantiated, the judge might order drug testing and state that the abusing spouse could not return to the household until there is evidence of successful completion of drug treatment.

The main focus of most courts in domestic violence cases is to stop partner battering. Typically, the case does not last long enough, and is not closely enough monitored, to produce a treatment result. While many women enter treatment through services offered at shelters for battered women, the court often is not involved in enforcing treatment. As with divorce-custody cases, there is no wide highway to treatment through domestic violence cases.

JUVENILE DELINQUENCY

There is more leeway to design treatment programs for substance-abusing juveniles than there is to design programs for adults under criminal laws. The judge in a juvenile case retains some of the "fatherly" discretion (the legal term is *parens patriae*) on which separate courts for juvenile offenders originally were founded.

A problem that a young pregnant woman offender would face in the juvenile system is that a stern atmosphere of punishment is likely to prevail in any teen treatment center to which she is sent. It is unlikely that a pregnant teenager who is charged with shoplifting or drug distribution or assault would succeed in obtaining diversion to a drug program specifically designed for pregnant women. Therefore, her larger needs for parental training, medical care, and social services support might well go unmet.

The best strategy for pregnant teen offenders who want drug treatment would be to seek placement through the neglect-abuse system. In some states, such a crossover could be accommodated.

CRIMINAL CASES

Enraged by the afflictions that newborns suffered as the result of their mothers' use of alcohol or drugs during pregnancy, prosecutors, legislators, and judges began to apply criminal laws to perinatal substance abuse in the late 1980s. There was no one strategy in this effort: prosecutors would look at the language of the local criminal laws and try to fashion a crime. Inventiveness in interpreting the laws was required for two reasons. First, that none of the criminal laws had been written with fetal alcohol and drug effects in mind. Second, plenty of constitutional case law held that a fetus is not a "person" in the eyes of the law: that is, the fetus cannot be considered as a human being separate from the mother with separate rights. The foundation case for the principle that the fetus does not have "personhood" separate from the mother—at least until it becomes viable—is *Roe v. Wade,* 410 U.S. 113 (1973).

In order to get around the concept of the inseparability of fetal rights from maternal rights, prosecutors did such things as charging the mother with "delivering drugs" to an infant at the moment of birth, just before the umbilical cord was clamped. The Florida criminal statute under which a mother was so charged reads:

> Except as authorized by this chapter, it is unlawful for any
> person 18 years of age or older to deliver any controlled sub-

stance to a person under the age of 18 years, or to use or hire a person under the age of 18 years as an agent or employee in the sale or delivery of such a substance, or to use such a person to assist in avoiding detection or apprehension for a violation of this chapter" Fla. Stat. sec.893.13(1)(c)(1989). Uniform Controlled Substances Act.

The case, *Johnson v. State,* was reversed by the Florida Supreme Court, 602 So.2d 1288 (1992).

For a while, between 1987 and 1989, it looked as if criminal prosecutions of pregnant women were sweeping the country, but one by one those cases began being overturned on appeal. Meanwhile an outcry arose against criminal prosecution from many groups. Physicians, nurses, and treatment providers said that women were refusing prenatal care and were hiding during birth, rather than risking imprisonment and loss of their children. Women's rights groups said that never before had the government sponsored the development of hostility, instead of nurturing, between women and their fetuses. People concerned about discrimination and equal rights noted that pregnant women were being sentenced as status offenders and men were not. For example, if a pregnant woman came before the court on a first-time shoplifting charge, or a bad check charge, and the judge noticed that she was pregnant and there was reason to believe that she was drug-involved, the judge might sentence her to jail to enforce her sobriety, whereas a drug-involved man coming before the court on the same first-time shoplifting charge might receive probation. People who were familiar with the criminal justice system were able to point out that seldom were AOD treatment programs available in jails or prisons, and that in fact drugs could be obtained there almost as readily as they could on the street. They argued that the effect of the criminal prosecution statutes was to interfere with AOD treatment.

Criminal prosecution for perinatal substance abuse has lessened as of this writing. Legislators are trying to reach the problem in other ways: by assigning treatment priority to pregnant women, revised code of Washington 70. 83C.005 *ex seq.* (Maternity Care Access Bill); by placing the burden of discovering, reporting, and treating substance-abusing pregnant women on the medical profession, California Health and Safety Code §§123600 and 23605; and by forcing parents to make fast hard choices about entering treatment or losing their children (for example, the laws of the State of Florida have been revised to permit parental rights to be terminated quickly, and without a contract offered, if the parent even once commits "egregious abuse" Sec.39.464(4) The Juvenile Justice Act, Florida Statutes; it is under this law that drug-involved parents now tend to lose their children).

Pregnant women who find themselves in jail or prison on an unrelated criminal charge seldom will have access to consistent and effective treatment. Many judges believe that a drug-involved person benefits from enforced sobriety behind bars, but there is convincing testimony from inmates that access to drugs continues inside prisons. While 12-step group therapy may be available, actual treatment usually is not.

Drug treatment may be available for first-time offenders as an alternative to court, or to convicted persons released on probation. Access to treatment for them often depends on the skill of their lawyer or probation officer in advocating for their needs, as well as the degree to which the judge is informed about the efficacy of treatment.

SUMMARY: THE COURT AS A TREATMENT ENFORCER

Only in neglect-abuse cases does the court have a continuing opportunity to bring adults into AOD treatment. That opportunity is great, in terms of numbers. By far the majority of parents in neglect-abuse cases have AOD involvement as an underlying issue. The court's enforcement is powerful: the ability to take away the child. Moreover, most of these cases have a long life, extending over years, giving the court an opportunity to monitor the parents' progress in treatment. What is lacking are sufficient treatment programs to meet the needs, and a thoroughly educated social service and judiciary which can match adults to appropriate treatment and deal with issues such as relapse from treatment in an informed manner.

CRITICAL QUESTIONS

SUSCEPTIBILITY OF DRUG-RELATED CASES TO MEDIATION

So often, success in treatment depends on making it available when the drug-involved person is ready to accept it. This issue, particularly, is difficult in court cases, because case backlogs and lawyers' strategies may mean that there is a great time lag between the time that treatment is recognized as a need, and the time when the need can be satisfied. It is no exaggeration to say that the children may have grown up, and the parents may have dropped out of both the court system and the family, before the court is ready to order services that would reunite the family. Therefore, many critics of our court system have suggested that we look toward pretrial mediation to bring treatment to families when they need it.

An unresolved problem in mediation has to do with drug-caused violence. Are there certain drugs that are so likely to cause the abuser to become violent that it is unsafe to allow the case to be mediated without the enforcement power of the court? Are there certain family constellations, or family dynamics, which, when put together with drug-alcohol use, hold too great a potential for violence to risk leaving children with their parents while services are obtained? These are questions that need study. If a protocol could be developed that reliably predicted which cases with AOD issues were amenable to mediation, treatment could be offered to afflicted families at a much earlier stage.

DISCRIMINATION AGAINST THE POOR

Having noted that neglect-abuse cases are the greatest gateway to treatment through the courts, it must also be noted that the great majority of people who come into neglect-abuse court are poor. That is not because only the poor take drugs and neglect and abuse their children. There are plenty of studies that refute that notion (Chasnoff, Landress, & Barrett, 1990; Roberts, 1991). It is because the poor are easy to find. Being stripped of resources, their problems cannot be hidden away in great estates bordered by spacious lawns: these are people who are on the streets, who are visible. If they accept welfare payments, most details about their living arrangements are known. If they enter an emergency room for health care, they are categorized according to their profile: being characterized as shabby, wearing unclean clothes and lacking a fixed address may well lead to drug testing. Such profiles affect the poor negatively in every social system: teachers, police, social workers, and other middle-class professionals often are quick to make judgments about drug use among the poor that they would hesitate to make about well-dressed families.

If the sole effect of a neglect-abuse case were to bring services like drug treatment to families, there might be no quarrel with the unequal way that people are selected to enter the court system. But in fact, there is a cruel element of punishment: one's children can be taken away unless treatment is accomplished swiftly and successfully. The middle-class and the rich seldom have their children taken away in neglect-abuse actions, because they seldom enter neglect-abuse court.

LENGTH OF TREATMENT AND AGE OF THE CHILD

The Adoption Assistance and Welfare Act of 1980, P.L. 96-272; 42 U.S.C. §670 *et seq.*, requires courts to set a goal of 18 months within which to obtain a permanent placement for a child in foster care. The idea is that if a child is not well on the way to family reunion after 18 months of displacement into foster care, then adoption should be considered. Foster care is not supposed to be a long-term solution for neglected and abused children.

Underlying Congress' concern that every child have a home to call its own was the work of mental health experts, who have pointed out that a child has a sense of time quite different from that of an adult (Goldstein, Freud, & Solnit, 1973). To an infant who does not know if mother will ever return, an absence of days can be traumatic. For a young child, a year can seem like forever.

Crack cocaine, of course, changed American patterns of drug use and consequently of drug treatment. More women than ever before became drug-involved, probably because smoking was not the barrier that injection had been. More children, therefore, lost their mothers to years of drug use. The most effective treatments have required years of behavior modification. While that can be accomplished in a facility that accommodates mother-child relationships, there have not been enough of those to meet crack cocaine treatment needs. Even women who are lucky enough to enter such treatment centers usually can bring only their youngest children, leaving other children to find other homes.

Judges have had either to ignore the 18-month placement standard of the federal law, leaving children in foster care for an unconscionably long time, or to place more and more children for adoption while their parents seek treatment. It is this uncomfortable bind that has encouraged certain states to move toward fast-track adoption, orphanages, and other solutions.

INFORMED CONSENT AND DRUG TESTING

A matter of high concern for health care workers is the extent of information which must, by law, be given to a pregnant woman before she is drug-tested. Traditionally, in many hospitals, drug tests simply are included in the routine health care tests. The patient is given a document to sign when she enters the clinic or hospital which gives permission for all medical tests that the physician or other staff deem necessary. Because good health care is the goal of health professionals, that seems to them to be a sensible approach.

Lawyers look at this issue much differently, however. Two factors in particular suggest the need for a higher level of information. First, a drug test is an invasive procedure which yields information about an illegal activity. Our long history of criminal case law makes the point that if privacy is to be breached by an invasion of the body, there must be a good reason for it: the agency that wants that information must have either the person's informed consent, or be able to demonstrate "probable cause" to believe that the person has taken illegal drugs (*Schmerber v. California*, 384 U.S. 757, 1966). Second, there is a long history of cases that protect the right of parents to raise their children (*Meyer v. Nebraska*, 1923; *Pierce v. Society of Sisters*, 1925). While health care workers may not want to think about this, the end result of a drug test could be that the pregnant woman's child will be removed from her care. When constitutionally protected rights are breached, special legal processes go into effect. There must be "due process of law."

In fact, very few informed consent cases relating to drug tests of pregnant women have come to court. Why is that? The major reason stems from another failing of our health care and legal systems: discrimination against the poor. For the most part, the pregnant women who are drug-tested are poor. Unless a hospital drug-tests every woman who comes into it for prenatal care, the women who are tested will be selected by some procedure. Usually they are selected according to a hospital protocol that has a built-in profile—one that describes certain risk factors. Those risk factors often coincide with poverty: lack of previous care, no fixed address, appearance unclean or ragged, and so forth. That brings poor women into court. Poor people generally are not empowered to advocate for their rights, and lawyers whose daily cases are in family or criminal court generally do not think of the informed-consent issue, outside of typical "stop and search" criminal cases.

As hospitals become more aware of the legal dimensions to various tests—including not only drug tests but also screening for HIV, TB, and STDs (sexually transmitted diseases)—the consent forms gradually are becoming more specific. In a nutshell, the dilemma is how to respect a patient's privacy while bringing her into the ambit of health care.

Monitoring and Aftercare

A weakness in most states' family court systems is the lack of follow-up in social services once the main parts of the case—the trial and the initial placement of the child—have been accomplished. This probably parallels a similar lack of follow-up for adults who have been discharged from treatment centers. At the beginning of a court case, there is heightened interest by the professional staff in all of the details. Is the home safe? Are the parents receiving drug treatment? Are the children in therapy? The judge is demanding answers to these questions, and laws require that services be rendered to bring about family reunion.

After the trial has been held, however, and court reviews have tracked the fate of the children for 18 months, the case either is discharged from the court system, or it slips into a kind of inactive status, often with court or administrative attention just once a year. If the children do not have advocates—or if the parents either do not have lawyers or do not instruct their lawyers to push for resolution—the family easily can drift back into drug-using chaos. Americans seem to specialize in emergency interventions without developing skills for prevention and maintenance. That is as true in the court system as it is in health systems. Consequently, it is not unusual for families to have multiple and repeated neglect-abuse, domestic violence, and criminal cases, with alcohol and drug problems underlying them all.

FUTURE DIRECTIONS

Faster Separation of Children from Drug-Involved Parents

There is a strong feeling among both state and federal legislators—and indeed, among family court judges—that too much attention has been paid to the treatment needs of adults, and too little attention has been paid to the needs of their children. This frustration contains several elements:

- While professionals in the health field generally understand relapse from treatment to be an expected part of recovery, that understanding does not extend to professionals in the legal field. Judges tend to look at relapse from treatment as failure, on the criminal-law theory that a person deserves one chance, but only one chance, to succeed. Therefore, judges tend to think that the high rate of "failure" means that successful treatment is an illusion—or at least unlikely. They think children are likely to be better off if permanent adoptive homes are found for them right away, rather than being "warehoused" in foster homes in the hope that parents will recover enough to resume parenting responsibilities.

- Foster care is expensive. Treatment also is expensive, and it is a service that states arguably are obligated to provide as part of the "reasonable efforts" to keep families together. If children are put into adoptive homes within the first 6 months or a year of removal from their homes of origin, the community will not have to carry the costs of foster care and treatment.
- Many children of drug-involved parents have developmental delays and handicaps, particularly in their earliest years. Recent studies indicate that many of their problems will diminish if they are raised in good homes with a stable environment and nurturing parents (Howard et al., 1989). The perception is that the homes of current or even former drug users are not the environments within which troubled children can succeed. Many legislators and judges think that the faster that children can be severed permanently from bad homes, the better for the children.
- Treatment for developmental delays in children is complicated. Courts can be a helpful mediator in administering treatment, because there is an excellent law that makes many services available: the Education of the Handicapped Act, 20 U.S.C. §§1400 *et seq.* The social worker in a neglect-abuse case can act as a case manager to bring these services to a child. However, many lawmakers are thinking that if children are placed in adoptive homes, the new parents can take on these case management tasks, freeing government resources.

As a result, it is likely that more and more states, and possibly the federal government as well, will move toward fast-track adoption as a quick-fix for social and economic problems.

Less Time to Accomplish Treatment

Concomitant with faster separation of children from drug-involved parents is the requirement that parents demonstrate sobriety if they want to keep their children. In order to meet this expectation on the part of the court, treatment providers may begin to emphasize shorter interventions.

One obvious problem with this trend is that unless there is excellent case management, and actual access to effective treatment programs, treatment may not succeed. Parents may be able to "hold it together" long enough to appear in court and pass a drug test or two, but may not be able to change their behavior without careful follow-through. This could endanger both the children and their parents.

Another problem is that parents and children may be separated permanently if parents fail to demonstrate sobriety within a short period of time. Loss of children further detaches an adult from healthy social ties and a powerful motivation to seek treatment.

A third problem is that many family court judges—and, indeed, the caseworkers from the child protection agency—do not understand what "treatment" is. It is not unusual to hear a judge order a parent into a twelve-step program for "treatment." This fosters an illusion in court that treatment is occurring if the parent can demonstrate attendance at Narcotics Anonymous meetings.

The consequence of this is that there may be a trend toward shorter interventions to prevent immediate loss of children in neglect-abuse cases. Such interventions might consist of 28-day in-residence care (which can be covered by insurance), combined with day programs that allow the parent to continue to live at home and mandatory attendance at twelve-step programs.

MORE DRUG-SPECIFIC LANGUAGE IN THE LAWS

Traditionally, definitions of neglect and abuse in states' reporting laws and the court-process laws have been very broad. For example, they might state that a child is neglected if the child lacks food, clothing, shelter, education, medical care, or a supportive environment. Those kinds of definitions were sufficiently comprehensive to embrace almost any kind of incident, including parental drug use. However, beginning in the 1970s, legislators felt the need to demonstrate to their constituents that they were concerned about children by inserting language into definitions that referred to current social problems. In the 1970s, sexual abuse was the topic of the day, and many laws became packed with references to the kind of evidence required to prove those cases. When drugs then became the main issue, drug-specific language often was added to the definitions of neglect and abuse. This created a number of problems in the 1980s, because the specific language often was an evidentiary trap. For example, if a neglected child is defined as one whose parents test positive for drugs, then it can be difficult to prove that parents have a drug problem if they test negative for drugs.

A number of states, such as Illinois and Florida, went through several permutations of drug-specific definitions of neglect and abuse until they found formulas with which they could work. Illinois lawmakers finally settled on the following addition to the definition of a neglected child: "any newborn infant whose blood or urine contains any amount of a controlled substance . . . or metabolite of a controlled substance, with the exception of controlled substances or metabolites of such substances, the presence of which in the newborn infant is the result of medical treatment administered to the mother or the newborn infant", 325 Illinois compiled Statutes 5/3 §3 (Abused and Neglected Child Reporting Act). Legislators are continuing to find ways to express their constituents' anger about drugs, by inserting descriptive language into the laws. Recently, the focus has been on describing the environments where parental drug use often takes place. For example, the District of Columbia amended its definition of "abuse" to include a child whose caretaker inflicts "an injury that results from exposure to drug-related activity in the child's home environment" (D.C. Code §16-1201 [23]).

Resulting laws are likely to carry an ever-greater freight of drug-specific words to describe the kind of parents and the kind of homes that are unacceptable for children.

Coordination of All Cases Relating to One Family

Currently, a great gap in the court system is the failure to account for one family's cases that are located in different parts of the court. A family's legal problems may be so fragmented that no judge can see how drug problems underlie all of them. In large urban courts, it is not unusual for a family to come before one judge on a neglect-abuse case, and another judge in a domestic violence case, while the father may have an adult criminal case, and the teenage son is facing juvenile charges. All of those cases not only may concern drugs, but they might concern the *same* drug event. That is, drug use may have caused the violence that brought both the child abuse and domestic violence cases into court, while the father's criminal case may be for drug possession and the teenager's charge may be for drug distribution.

Very few courts have worked out an administrative way to coordinate one family's cases—or one individual's cases, for that matter. Part of the problem is that family cases—including both neglect-abuse and juvenile cases—are to be handled confidentially, because of the tender years of the youths, whereas criminal cases and other kinds of civil cases are matters of open record. Another reason for the lack of coordination is that most courts do not have very sophisticated information systems. Civil, criminal, and family divisions may be run as separate kingdoms, with separate records departments. The dominant reason for the failure to coordinate, however, is that courts simply have not looked at these problems in a systemic way, with drugs as the common thread. Rather, the court has looked at each case as generated by a specific event: a mother who beat a toddler; a son who stole a car; a man who beat up the woman he lives with; a woman who shoplifted; and so forth. The sentences handed down are equally fragmented.

Under federal pressure to reform family court practice, analysts at last are beginning to look at court administration in a different way. They are asking: what is the root cause of this family's dysfunction? Is there a way that we can cure the family system, rather than just punish one person? Indeed, unhappy with the failure of states to meet federal standards for providing services to families with children in foster care, federal lawmakers passed the Family Preservation and Support Act of 1993, P.L. 103-66, which amends the Adoption Assistance and Welfare Act of 1980. The new act provides funds to courts to examine how well local laws are working, and to reform their practices over a 5-year period.

As a consequence of this activity, there will be a greater attempt to coordinate all of the cases in court that relate to one family. This will occur as information transfer systems become more sophisticated and case flow and social services change in response. Changes, however, will be slow.

EARLY INTERVENTION FOR DRUG-EXPOSED CHILDREN

Armed with excellent recent laws, courts can use their enforcement powers to issue orders for services to drug-exposed children. The Education of the Handicapped Act, 20 U.S.C. §§1400 *et seq.* serves children who are afflicted with mental retardation, visual or hearing impairments, specific learning disabilities and multiple handicaps, 34 C.F.R. §300.16. Children as young as those who are experiencing developmental delay may also be found eligible. These individuals are entitled to a broad array of services—occupational therapy, psychological, home visits, and family counseling, to name just a few. People who receive Medicaid are among those who can qualify to receive these vital supports.

All states have incorporated that provision from the federal law into their state laws. In addition, many states have taken the next discretionary step, and included children who are "at risk" for developmental delays.

A problem remaining is how to identify the children who would qualify for services that address developmental delays. Family courts that handle neglect-abuse cases can help this identification process. By ordering diagnostic tests for drug-exposed infants, and then assuring that a case management system is in place that will bring the services to qualifying families, judges can affect positively the lives of thousands of children that pass before them. Most courts currently are unaware that they have this power, and most lawyers have not been educated to advocate for these services.

It seems clear that, in coming years, more attention will be focused on early intervention for drug-exposed children. To make the best use of court enforcement powers, two areas require work: the bench and the bar must be educated about their power, and professionals in the health care and legal systems must work more closely together to help one another.

Development of Out-of-Court Mediation

The great influx of neglect-abuse cases, as well as domestic violence, criminal, and juvenile cases, has sent courts scurrying for alternatives to lengthy trials. Mediation is an increasingly popular means to deflect cases from the mainstream court process—or at least to resolve certain issues, leaving only those problems that truly are "in controversy" for the judges or juries to decide. Mediation has worked extraordinarily well in divorce cases—especially to resolve custody and visitation issues, and to divide property. However, where physical violence is a problem, where there is an obvious power imbalance between the bargaining parties, experts agree that court enforcement is necessary.

For neglect-abuse cases involving drugs, it would seem that mediation would be the best way to bring drug-treatment services quickly to families. Otherwise, they may have to wait until the end of a trial to acknowledge their drug-use problem. In states that do not have a speedy trial provision, a trial can take a year or more to occur—by which time a feeling of hopelessness can set in for the drug user. There is a problem with mediation for drug users, however, and that is the potential for violence with which some drugs may be associated. Questions currently unresolved include whether the potential (or existence) of violence in a home can be detected, or predicted, and if so, whether court enforcement is necessary to assure safety of the child. There is need for development of a good protocol to help sort out questions of violence in mediated neglect-abuse cases.

In juvenile cases, mediation already exists in a number of courts in several states. In fact, if one considers court diversion programs to be a form of mediation, one could say that its use is widespread. The rationale for using mediation in juvenile cases is similar to that for neglect-abuse cases. It brings needed services—drug treatment, job training, education—to a youth at a moment of great need when motivation is high to make use of these services.

Mediation is not used widely in domestic violence cases because of the power imbalance that exists between a battered spouse and the batterer. Court enforcement in the form of a "stay-away" order is required to stop the abuse.

Adult criminal cases are not as amenable to mediation. The application of court process and strict sentencing guidelines is nearly implacable. There is some room for diversion for first-time offenders, and it is there that drug treatment is often made an opportunity to avoid the stigma of a criminal record. A new trend toward "drug courts" and "community courts" is making growing use of diversion for first-time offenders.

It seems reasonable to assume that courts will move more completely and with greater certainty into mediation as an alternative to full court process. Successful experience with mediation in divorce cases is being applied in some other kinds of family cases. However, where violence is a threat, court enforcement often is necessary, making mediation inappropriate for domestic violence cases, and only to be cautiously applied in neglect-abuse cases where drugs are the dominant cause of family dysfunction. Nevertheless, mediation will develop as an important court-diversion.

REFERENCES

Chasnoff, I. J., Griffith, D. R., Freier, C., & Murray, J. (1992). Cocaine/polydrug use in pregnancy: Two-year follow-up. *Pediatrics, 89,* 284–289.

Chasnoff, I. J., Landress, H. J., & Barrett, M. E. (1990). The prevalence of illicit-drug or alcohol use during pregnancy and discrepancies in mandatory reporting in Pinellas County, Florida. *New England Journal of Medicine, 322,* 102–106.

General Accounting Office (GAO) (1994). *Foster care: Parental drug abuse has alarming impact on young children* (GAO/HEHS–94–89).

Goldstein, J., Freud, A., & Solnit, A. (1973). *Beyond the best interests of the child.* New York, NY: Macmillan.

Howard, J., Beckwith, L., Rodning, C., & Kropenski, V., (June, 1989). The development of young children of substance-abusing parents: Insights from seven years of intervention and research. *Zero to Three,* 8–12.

Roberts, D. E. (1991). Punishing drug addicts who have babies: Women of color, equality, and the right of privacy. *Harvard Law Review, 104,* 1419–1482.

Zuckerman, B., & Frank, D. A. (1992). "Crack-Kids" not broken. *Pediatrics, 89,* 337–339.

CASES

Johnson v. State, 602 So.2d 1288 (Fla.S.Ct. 1992)

Meyer v. Nebraska, 262 U.S. 390 (1923)

Pierce v. Society of Sisters, 268 U.S. 510 (1925)

Roe v. Wade, 410 U.S. 113 (1973)

Schmerber v. California, 384 U.S. 757 (1966)

FEDERAL STATUTES

Adoption Assistance and Welfare Act of 1980, P.L.96-272; 42 U.S.C sec.670 *et seq.*

The Family Preservation and Support Act of 1993, P.L. 103-66.

The Education of the Handicapped Act, 20 U.S.C. secs.1400 *et seq.* Federal regulations are found at 34 C.F.R.secs. 300 *et seq.*

STATE STATUTES

California Health and Safety Code secs.123600 and 123605 (Perinatal Health Care)

District of Columbia Code sec. 16-1201 (Family Division Proceedings)

Florida Statutes sec.39.464(4) (1990) (The Juvenile Justice Act)

Florida Statutes sec.893.13(1)(c)(1989) (Uniform Controlled Substances Act)

325 Illinois Compiled Statutes 5/3, sec.3 (Abused and Neglected Child
    Reporting Act)
Revised Code of Washington sec.70.83C.005 *et seq.* (Maternity Access Bill of
    1989).

10

The Role of Child Welfare

Laura Feig, M.P.P. and Charlotte McCullough, M.Ed.*

E ach state has a system in place designed to investigate reports of child abuse or neglect and to intervene if a child is being endangered by a parent or other person. Collectively known as the child welfare system, the agencies performing these functions may be state or locally based, and are generally either public or private, nonprofit agencies. Usually the investigative functions, referred to as child protective services or "CPS" in most communities, are conducted separately from service delivery activities.

However this system is organized, the child welfare system is designed to perform several tasks:

- It receives and investigates reports of child abuse or neglect.
- It makes decisions about whether there is evidence that abuse or neglect has occurred and whether the child in question is in ongoing danger.
- If a child appears to be in danger, services may be provided to alleviate the risk. These may be provided while the child remains in the home, if the child's safety can be assured.
- If a child cannot be maintained safely in the home, out-of-home care may be provided, generally either in the home of a relative (usually referred to as kinship care), or in a nonrelative foster

* The views expressed here are those of the authors and do not necessarily reflect positions of the Office of the Assistant Secretary for Planning and Evaluation, the U.S. Department of Health and Human Services, or the Child Welfare League of America.

family home. If the child's needs warrant it, care may be provided in a group home or other "congregate care" facility. Group care is most commonly used for emotionally troubled adolescents.

- If a child is removed from his or her parents' care, the agency must develop a permanency plan for the child, designed to ensure a swift resolution of the situation for the child and family so that the child is not left in limbo. The plan and progress toward it are reviewed periodically by the court. Services must be provided to achieve the plan, which is usually to reunite the family while keeping the child safe. Other possible plans include adoption, guardianship, or independent living (for some older children). The variety of reunification services that might be provided varies considerably from community to community, but among the most common are parenting training, individual or group counseling, and homemaker aides who teach basic household skills. Substance abuse and mental health treatment are usually provided through referral to local providers.

Figure 10.1 illustrates the child welfare system responses to child abuse and neglect reports. In 1994, nearly 2 million reports of child abuse or neglect were received and investigated by child protective services agencies. Of the reports investigated, just over one-third were either "substantiated" or "indicated" (different states use different categories), meaning that child protection investigators found evidence to indicate abuse or neglect had occurred. The largest group of these (53%) were cases of neglect; that is, the child was not being adequately cared for by the parent(s). Additionally, 25.5% were cases of physical abuse, 14% involved sexual abuse, and 2.5% were classified as medical neglect. The remainder were "other" or "unknown" (National Center on Child Abuse and Neglect, 1996).

While many people think of child welfare as synonymous with foster care, relatively few children are actually removed from their homes. Of these, most are returned to their parents' custody relatively swiftly, once the child's safety can be adequately assured. For instance, data from Illinois and Michigan indicate that of the children first investigated for abuse and neglect in 1990, approximately one-third had at least one substantiated investigation within twelve months of the first report. Of those children on whom reports were substantiated, 13.9% were placed in foster care within one year of the first investigation in Illinois; 8.5% of such children in Michigan entered foster care within a

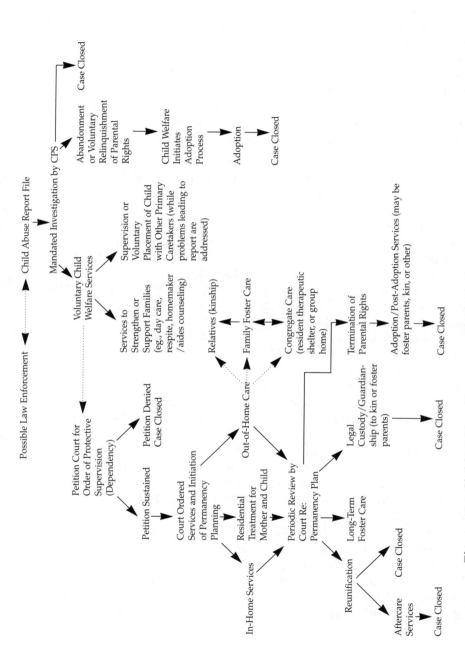

Figure 10.1 Child Welfare Responses to Child Abuse Reports

year (Goerge, Van Voorhis & Sanfilippo, 1996). Looking specifically at drug-exposed children reported to child protective services in an urban California county, one study found that 35% of children were never removed from their mothers' custody; 29% were removed on an emergency basis but were returned home within a few days; 12% were removed but returned home within 18 months; and the remaining 24% were not expected to return to their mothers' care (most of these children had been adopted or placed in guardianship arrangements with kin) (Sagatun-Edwards, Saylor, & Shifflett, 1995).

SUBSTANCE ABUSE AND CHILD SAFETY AND FAMILY STABILITY

Abuse of alcohol or other drugs affects child development and family systems. One of the most common characteristics of substance abuse or addiction is the individual's failure to fulfill major role obligations at work, school, or home. When the substance-abusing individual is a parent, impaired judgment and decision-making abilities may place his or her children in danger. Standard diagnostic criteria specifically identify "recurrent substance use resulting in . . . neglect of children" as a symptom that can be used to diagnose substance abuse disorders (American Psychiatric Association, 1994). Maltreating parents have much higher rates of alcohol and drug abuse than do other parents (Famularo, Stone, Barnum, & Wharton, 1986; Kelleher, Chaffin, Hollenberg, & Fischer, 1994). Conversely, parents with substance abuse problems show much higher rates of abusive and neglectful behavior toward their children than other parents (Kelley, 1992).

Substance abuse is among the most common family problems leading to the abuse or neglect of a child and entry into the child welfare system. Nationally, caseworkers were aware of parental substance abuse in approximately one-third of the families they served in 1994 (Westat, forthcoming); in urban centers and among families with children in foster care, the figures are even higher. A study conducted in Boston in 1988 found that 64% of substantiated child abuse and neglect allegations involved illicit drug or excessive alcohol use, and substance abuse was a factor in 89% of cases involving infants (Herskowitz, Seck, & Fogg, 1989). Of 513 children born drug-exposed at one Chicago hospital between 1985 and 1990, by the end of 1991, 20% had been the subjects of substantiated child abuse and neglect reports (Jardes, Ekwo, & van Voorhis, 1995).

Drug-exposed children in particular, and substance-abusing families generally, pose challenges to the child welfare system. Compared to other children in foster care, children from alcohol- or drug-involved families tend to enter care at a younger age and remain in care longer (Walker, Zangrillo & Smith, 1994). Substance abuse treatment appropriate for mothers with young children is often unavailable, or programs have long waiting lists. And even when mothers overcome their denial and participate in treatment programs, the potential for relapse remains a concern for child welfare caseworkers responsible for ensuring children's safety.

Child welfare involvement is neither feasible nor desirable for every family with a substance-abusing parent. An estimated 3.4 million parents with children under age 18 living in their households report using an illicit drug in the past month; 625,000 parents report past-month cocaine use (U.S. Department of Health and Human Services, 1994b). Many more are alcoholic. While many of these individuals are certainly less than ideal parents, few are so impaired that we would seriously consider child protective services intervention. Even in situations where the substance abuse is serious, it is unlikely that most or many of these children would enter foster care. There are far too many children for this to be a feasible option, even if it were desirable. What is desirable is a comprehensive, coordinated response between the child welfare and public health systems to address the difficulties faced by substance-abusing parents and their vulnerable children.

CHALLENGES WITHIN THE CHILD WELFARE SYSTEM

A combination of obstacles jeopardizes the child welfare system's ability to protect and serve at-risk children and families affected by substance abuse. There has been a rapidly increasing demand for services, coupled with too few workers who are qualified by experience and training to respond. There is too little known about how to successfully intervene with substance-abusing parents to promote recovery from chemical dependency while ensuring child safety and family stability. Assessment skills have not kept pace with the changing characteristics and needs of children and families who come to the attention of child welfare. Even with accurate assessments, we often do not have adequate service options for the child or the family.

INCREASED REFERRALS

Referrals to child protective services in recent years have increased dramatically. In 1993, 43 reports of child abuse and neglect were received for every 1,000 children under 18 in the U.S. population, up from 24 per thousand in 1983 (National Center on Child Abuse and Neglect, 1995). The number of children in foster care rose during this period from 270,000 to 445,000 (Tatara, 1993), although there are signs that the figures have leveled out somewhat recently.

Unlike other public services, the child welfare system cannot simply start a waiting list when resources fail to keep pace with growing needs. Child protective services agencies are required to investigate all reports within short time frames (generally less than a week), and must provide foster care to all children who are judged at imminent risk. The surge in CPS referrals has resulted in backlogs of uninvestigated cases, with many workers carrying caseloads in excess of 50 cases. Standards developed by the Child Welfare League of America call for caseloads of no more than 12–17 families. Parental substance abuse is often correlated with these increased referrals. In addition, making a timely investigation with a drug-using parent is more difficult, because the parent may be harder to track due to frequent moves and the chaotic lifestyle of the drug culture.

FEWER SERVICES AND HIGH STAFF TURNOVER

Increasing numbers of child abuse reports, the increasing seriousness of reports received, and higher caseloads have led the system to concentrate almost entirely on investigative activities and the provision of foster care. Little prevention or in-home service provision is being conducted. Nationally, preliminary results from a new study indicate that the number of families provided in-home services by the child welfare system dropped 62% between 1977 and 1994, from 1.3 million to 500,000 (Westat, forthcoming). This inability to respond to the children not requiring foster care placement leaves the bulk of the children in CPS caseloads at increased risk of abuse, neglect, or fatality.

Increasing pressures and frustration inevitably lead to significant staff turnover. At the height of the crack epidemic in New York City during the late 1980s, when caseloads were particularly high, staff turnover in the child welfare agency reached 50–60% per year (Sabol, 1994). Agencies in many other communities continue to face unacceptably high turnover rates, especially among direct care staff.

CHANGING CHILD CHARACTERISTICS

The characteristics of children entering the foster care system have been changing for the past decade. An increasing number of children enter the system with serious medical, emotional, and behavioral problems. Many more infants have been entering the foster care system due to drug exposure than in the past (Barth, Courtney, Berrick, & Albert, 1994). Children entering foster care as infants (under 1 year of age) are one of the most quickly growing segments of the child welfare population. In New York City, between 1984 and 1989, the number of infants entering foster care at birth quintupled (Goerge, Wulczyn, & Harden, 1995). Many of these infants are the children of addicted mothers, and have entered foster care directly from the hospital at birth or very soon afterwards. These children present particular dilemmas for child welfare professionals. Children who enter foster care as infants tend to remain in care longer than other children (Wulczyn, 1994). Data from California, New York, and Illinois indicate that only about 25% of very young children entering foster care are back home within one year (Barth et al., 1994). Many are medically fragile, HIV-positive or have other special needs. Infants, even more than other children, require consistent caregiving for proper social and emotional development, but the child welfare system is often unable to provide such consistency.

In addition to the growing number of infants in the child welfare system, there is a large number of extremely troubled adolescents. These children are also often the product of substance-abusing families. They are at significant risk of destructive alcohol and drug use themselves and are in need of substance abuse prevention and treatment programs if they are not to become the next generation of addicted parents.

ASSESSMENT SKILLS

Standardized assessments should guide case planning and service delivery. Improved assessments are needed to guide all decisions in the child welfare field. For example, current practices and tools are not adequate in assessing the risk to a child of living with a substance-abusing parent. Dore and her colleagues (Dore, Doris, & Wright, 1995) note that "many structured assessment procedures do not adequately address risks to children associated with parent/caregiver substance abuse (p. 536)" and those that "do include parental substance abuse . . .

often fail to provide workers with specific ways of identifying substance abuse in a family under investigation (p. 536)." Research is needed to better understand what factors might predict whether a child living with a substance-abusing caretaker is in danger, and to help workers assess when an abusive or neglectful caretaker is not likely to become an adequate parent and therefore, alternatives must be sought for the child. Decisions about which services to provide to attain best outcomes are not guided by accurate assessments. Too often, children and families get what is available, rather than what is needed based on a comprehensive, reliable assessment of their strengths and needs.

PLACEMENT DILEMMAS

We have known since the 1970s that children of drug abusers remain in the foster care system longer than other populations, are moved from one placement to another more frequently, and are less likely to return home to their parents. They are more difficult to plan for, in large part because of their parents' inability to participate actively in the case-planning process (Fanshel, 1975).

When a decision is made to place a child in out-of-home care, there are several options available—including family foster placement, congregate care, and placement with relatives, often referred to as kinship care. Each of these options carries risks to the child. In the case of family foster care, a shortage of foster parents has resulted in placing more children in each of the homes, in shifting children from one home to another, and in frequent separation of siblings. Between 1983 and 1992, while the number of children in foster care nationally rose by 74, the number of foster family homes available declined by 11%, from 140,000 to 125,000 (U.S. Department of Health and Human Services, 1994a).

For some children requiring placement, residential care is chosen. Congregate care is too often used, especially for young children, because more appropriate options were not available in the community. In other situations, when residential care would benefit the child, less restrictive options are chosen and children have to "fail" their way up to the more intensive services. Children are damaged by placements in settings that are more or less restrictive than their needs require.

The placement option that most challenges our thinking about permanency planning is kinship care. Increasing numbers of children in foster care are placed in the home of a relative who is reimbursed for the cost of the child's care. In some cases the relative receives reimbursements that equal those of nonrelative foster care providers; in other cases, the relative receives payment through the Aid to Families with Dependent Children Program (AFDC, or welfare) or at some other, intermediate rate. The growing use of such care has created a series of policy issues for state child welfare programs. Although figures vary considerably from state to state, several large states including California, New York and Illinois, now place between one third and one half of their foster care children with relatives (Goerge et al., 1995).

Kinship foster care has many advantages for children who must be removed from their parents' care because of abuse or neglect. These include reducing the trauma of placement for the child and maintaining family relationships. Such placements may provide additional continuity for the child who will be in a more familiar environment, with people s/he knows. But there may be disadvantages to relative placements as well. For instance, children may not be as well protected from abusive parents.

The child welfare system was designed to provide short-term substitute care for children in danger. Children placed with relatives, however, tend to stay in care for significant lengths of time, often permanently. The appropriate role of the government in such extended family relationships is unclear. For instance, in 1992, approximately 4% of children in families receiving AFDC were living with relatives other than their parents (Spar, 1993). And in approximately 10% of kinship foster care placements in 1994, the child was living with the relative before the child welfare system became involved with the family (Westat, forthcoming). It is not clear whether or not there are differences between the characteristics, circumstances, and needs of families with kinship care arrangements who are served through these systems, although the relationship between the family and the government is quite different.

PERMANENCY PLANNING ISSUES

Regardless of the placement setting, permanency planning is made more difficult when parents are substance abusers. Simply stated, permanency planning means safely reducing entrances into foster care and expediting exits from foster care via reunification, adoption, or permanent guardianship (Barth et al., 1994). The ability to achieve a permanent placement for a child in a timely manner is affected by many things. The probability of reunification is greatest immediately following a placement. The longer a child remains in care, the less likely the child will be successfully reunited with family (Courtney, 1994). Reuniting a child and family in a timely manner when the parent is addicted to substances is much more difficult due to the chronic, relapsing nature of the disease.

Adoption has been an underutilized permanency option for all children in the foster care system. Adoption is the option chosen for fewer than 10% of the children who enter foster care. In the case of infants in foster care, who never developed an attachment to their birth mothers, adoption should be a particularly feasible option. Yet even in cases where reunification is extremely unlikely, the termination of parental rights often takes 2 to 3 years or more, at which point finding an adoptive home for the child becomes more difficult. A number of states are experimenting with expedited adoption procedures designed to hasten the process. It is vital, however, that the circumstances under which expedited adoption will be considered are clearly and carefully defined (Wald, 1994). For those drug-exposed children who are adopted, recent research shows their adoption experiences are generally positive, and are quite comparable to those of other children (Barth, 1994).

Research on Effectiveness of Child Welfare Interventions

Child welfare policies, programs, and practices related to serving all children and families should be guided by research and empirical data. However, there is very little information available in the child welfare field about "what works." Even less is known about whether certain service strategies are effective with particular types of families, such as those with a substance-abusing parent.

Studies comparing the effectiveness of different approaches to dealing with families are especially lacking. New service methods are adopted primarily because the philosophies behind them appeal to an agency, but often few data are available to show that the approach yields good outcomes for children and families (or outcomes that are better than alternative approaches). In fact, outcomes for children and families often are not measured at all. Many programs, when asked how they judge their success, point to the numbers of clients served or the length of time families attend program sessions, rather than whether family functioning improved or whether children were safer, healthier, and better adjusted than they would otherwise have been.

Increasingly, there will be political pressure on social service agencies to justify their approaches with regard to outcomes for children and families, and the cost-effectiveness of delivering services. Does mandatory reporting of drug-exposed children protect children by preventing abuse or neglect, or harm children by discouraging prenatal care? Do family preservation services actually prevent foster care placements? Can family support services prevent child abuse or neglect, or, in the case of substance-abusing families, are they more likely to enable the parent's continued addiction? Do expedited adoption procedures yield better results than alternatives for certain groups of children? Over what time frames should services be maintained for families impaired by substance abuse in order to have the most impact for parent and child? Data on these and other questions of intervention effectiveness are needed to make sound decisions about the best ways to structure services to protect children and promote healthy families.

CONFLICTS AMONG PROFESSIONALS AND SYSTEMS

Not all of the challenges in serving families with substance abuse problems are confined to obstacles within one system. In some communities, the greatest difficulties involve finding common ground and overcoming conflicts between different systems and professions. Problems may arise because the child welfare and public health systems in a community may have different but equally valid goals. In the case of a family headed by a substance-abusing woman, service providers have at least two clients: the woman and her child(ren). In collaborative efforts between public health or substance abuse treatment agencies and child welfare agencies, conflicts may arise depending on who is considered the primary client.

Child welfare professionals may perceive substance abuse treatment providers as willing to overlook potentially unsafe family situations, placing children in jeopardy in order to avoid alienating the mother. Alternatively, substance abuse treatment professionals may see child welfare caseworkers as overly eager to remove children from the home or to terminate parental rights, and as unwilling to give mothers a chance to prove themselves.

Around the issue of relapse the two professions are often particularly at odds. To a substance abuse professional, relapse is a normal and expected part of the recovery process, but to a child welfare professional, relapse means potential danger for the child. Substance abuse treatment providers rightly observe that addiction is a chronic, relapsing disease and that repeated treatment attempts are often necessary before an individual achieves a stable recovery. Even so, many addicts will never recover and will ultimately die of problems related to their addictions. From the perspective of a child welfare professional, the recognition that substance abuse and addiction are chronic problems fails to address the immediate needs of a child residing in an abusive or neglectful household, or who has been removed to foster care. The child needs a stable, nurturing environment and cannot wait indefinitely for a parent to be "ready" for treatment or recovery.

An Example of Conflict: Mandatory Reporting Policies

Most children who come to the attention of the child welfare system do so because a professional working with the child or family makes a report to the local child protective services agency. Every state has a law requiring certain professionals, such as teachers and health care providers, to make such reports when abuse or neglect is suspected. Others, such as neighbors and family members, may also report suspected abuse or neglect. Laws vary considerably from state to state regarding whether perinatal drug exposure, in and of itself, requires a mandatory report. In some states, drug exposure is not mentioned specifically, leaving it to the service provider's best judgment as to whether the caregiving situation is bad enough to warrant a report. In other states, a physician is required to report the family even if there is no indication that the child may be in any danger. Further, in some jurisdictions a drug-exposed child may automatically be placed in foster care (or may not be released from the hospital) pending a full child protection investigation.

The laws requiring professionals to report all cases of drug exposure are controversial. Many public health professionals believe such reporting policies discourage pregnant substance-abusing women from obtaining prenatal care or substance abuse treatment because they may fear that admitting their substance abuse will lead to the loss of their children. Others point out that health care providers are not trained to judge child safety and are not in a position to evaluate factors in the family's home environment which may affect caregiving. Regardless of the situation in your community, hospitals and substance abuse treatment programs should have clear policies in place regarding when a child protective services report should be filed.

ISSUES ON THE HORIZON: MANAGED CARE

The current political climate and legislative agendas outside of the child welfare system are having a dramatic impact on the children and families served by child welfare and on the agencies—public and private—that serve them. The child welfare system's ability to protect children and serve at-risk families will be affected by managed care initiatives at the federal and state levels and by welfare reform.

There are two ways in which managed care systems affect child welfare. In the first instance, under Medicaid proposals, managed care organizations receive funding to deliver physical and behavioral health care services to children and families served by child welfare agencies. In the second instance, child welfare administrators at state or local levels may adopt managed care models for the funding and delivery of various child welfare services.

Managed care approaches are designed to balance costs, quality, and access to care. Managed care is attractive because it has the potential to reduce costs; improve access to care in underserved areas; improve the quality of care through standardized protocols; and increase the focus on preventive care and "wellness" rather on than crisis-driven treatment. Most managed care approaches rely on groups of providers who agree to provide specific services for defined populations at a predetermined rate for a specified period of time. Various types of risk-sharing payment arrangements allow providers more control and flexibility in determining how dollars are spent and encourage reliance on the most appropriate and cost-effective interventions. In a quality managed care system, eligible persons get the services they need, when they need them, and in the right amount, no more, and no less. However, in many managed care programs, the main focus has been on profits, or cost containment, rather than on providing quality services that meet client needs.

MANAGED HEALTH AND BEHAVIORAL HEALTH CARE FOR MEDICAID POPULATIONS

Fundamental changes in the financing and delivery of health care services for low-income populations appear inevitable. Managed care has been evolving in the United States for over 50 years, but recent developments have accelerated its growth and impact on service delivery. Dramatic reforms are under way in Medicaid, the nation's primary insurance program for low-income persons and a major funder of children's mental health services. At the federal level, the Medicaid reform debate is still in progress. Under current proposed federal reforms, states will gain greater flexibility with regard to key features of their Medicaid programs.

Many states are not waiting for federal change and are in the midst of significantly altering their Medicaid systems through the use of waivers granted by the U.S. Department of Health and Human Services via the Health Care Financing Administration. Nearly every state has applied for and/or received a Medicaid waiver to adapt primary health or behavioral health services for different Medicaid-eligible populations. All waivers include some managed care components. In 1982, only 2% of Medicaid recipients were enrolled in managed care plans. By the end of 1995, nearly 40% were enrolled in such plans.

Because the incidence of serious health and behavioral health problems among the children and youth in foster care is unusually high, current Medicaid plans will dramatically affect the physical and behavioral health of these children. In addition, because parental substance abuse is a primary reason that children enter the foster care system and remain there for prolonged periods of time, the attention of behavioral health care plans to the substance-abuse treatment needs of pregnant and parenting women will be of critical importance.

With few exceptions, current managed care approaches to the delivery and financing of physical or behavioral health care have not undergone rigorous evaluations to answer critical questions, especially related to vulnerable populations, such as children and families served by the child welfare system. Child advocates are concerned that the designers of managed care plans have only limited understanding of the special health and behavioral health needs of abused and neglected children or of their parents, and that plans will fail to allow access to the level of services required over time to ameliorate problems.

Managed Care Approaches to Child Welfare

While there is little experience available regarding managed care in the child welfare arena, child welfare administrators are attracted by the twin promises of managed care—cost containment and improved quality—and hope that managed care can improve shortcomings in the current child welfare system. In an effort to get a snapshot of important trends, perceptions, and needs of child welfare administrators, the Child Welfare League of America conducted a public agency survey in the spring of 1995. Over 80% of the respondents said they were exploring using some elements of managed care in the financing and delivery of child welfare services.

There is no one model for transferring managed care concepts and technologies designed for the medical system to social services, specifically child welfare. There is great variability among all of the managed care child welfare plans under consideration, but there are also some common features. Under many plans there is an increased emphasis on:

- More accurate initial assessments;
- The use of standardized clinical protocols;
- Better utilization management (i.e., matching clients to the most appropriate, least restrictive, most cost-effective services);
- More aggressive case management;
- A greater focus on attaining desired outcomes;
- Use of state-of-the-art management information systems technologies to drive decision making and evaluate system performance;
- The sharing of financial risks (and potential rewards) with providers; and
- Expedited permanency planning.

In the future, under a managed care child welfare system, public agencies or private behavioral health companies may serve as the system's "gatekeepers," monitoring child welfare cases through performance-based contracts. Monitoring individual cases may resemble monitoring in the health care system—looking at cost, quality, and outcomes.

A successful conversion to managed care involves start-up investments to assure the availability of a complete array of high-quality services, qualified providers, and sophisticated technology. But, in far too many instances, a managed care approach to child welfare is proposed in order to contain costs without provisions to ensure the development and testing of new technologies, the preparation of public and private providers for their new roles and responsibilities, or the availability of a full array of quality services needed to protect children and serve families. Managed care has the potential to improve child welfare service delivery, but the risks are also very real. It is so far unclear what impact these proposed plans will have on individual children and families.

THE POTENTIAL IMPACT OF WELFARE REFORM

For decades, the United States has assured that poor children and families who meet certain requirements will receive some level of cash assistance toward survival needs, no matter how many people need help. The new welfare reform law (P. L. 104-193, not yet codified) ends this commitment, providing states with almost complete flexibility regarding the design of welfare programs, and freedom to deny benefits to families who fail to follow state guidelines. States may use the new law as a tool to encourage drug-dependent women to seek substance abuse treatment, improve their parenting skills, and enhance their lives. Alternatively, they could drive families with substance abuse problems further away from intervention and place children at risk. Few features of welfare programs will be mandatory and it is likely that in the future state welfare programs will diverge significantly from one another. For this reason, the discussion that follows will focus on relatively broad themes rather than on specific programmatic features.

INCREASING THE RISK OF CHILD ABUSE AND NEGLECT

Welfare reform is predicated on the notion that too many families who could and should be supporting themselves are instead relying on public support. As a consequence of placing time limits on benefits and other policies to encourage work, some families will be at risk, even with efforts to design policies in such a way as not to hurt children. Undoubtedly, many parents will successfully enter the workforce and their families will thrive or survive one way or another. Others, however, will not. In some number of cases, the parent(s) will be unable to cope on their own and their child(ren) will be neglected, or the additional stress on families will cause some parents to abuse their children. There are no estimates of how many additional children will need child welfare system intervention as a result of the limits on cash assistance and other supports. But, undoubtedly, families headed by a drug dependent woman are particularly likely to fall into this category.

INCREASING BUDGET PRESSURES

Welfare reform proposals are being driven in part by a desire for particular policy changes, but pressures for cost containment and deficit reduction at both the federal and state levels play a major role as well. Such pressures are likely to endure and increase. With fewer funds available and potentially more children in need of protection, addressing the inadequacies of the child welfare system will be more difficult.

In order to justify their existence, programs will need to be armed with data regarding the cost-effectiveness of the services they provide.

DECREASING TOLERANCE FOR ADDRESSING SUBSTANCE ABUSE AS A HEALTH PROBLEM

Provisions of the new welfare reform law and other related legislation address substance abuse primarily as a criminal/behavioral issue rather than as a health issue. The welfare law provides that states are not prohibited by the Federal Government from testing welfare recipients for illegal drugs and from penalizing those who test positive (P.L. 104-193, section 902). Some states are already moving to deny social services to individuals testing positive for illegal drugs (Booth, 1996). Further, cash assistance and Food Stamp benefits are denied to individuals convicted after the date of enactment of drug-related felony offenses, although states may opt out of this provision or limit its scope (P.L. 104-193, section 115). The law does not mention substance abuse treatment, and treatment cannot count toward states' work participation requirements for welfare recipients. Similarly, while passed by Congress as part of a separate measure, recent amendments to the Social Security Act require the Social Security Administration to disregard alcohol and drug-related impairments in determining the disability status of applicants to two federal disability programs (the Social Security Disability Insurance Program and the Supplemental Security Income Program) (P.L. 104-121, codified as 42 U.S.C. 423(d)(2) and 42 U.S.C. 1382c(a)(3)). These measures all use denial of aid, rather than substance abuse treatment, as the preferred consequence of the detection of a substance abuse condition, and there is no consideration of the substance abuser's children who are likely to suffer from such an approach.

INCREASED PRESSURE ON KIN CAREGIVERS

In many families headed by a substance abuser, a grandparent, aunt, or other relative has stepped in to provide care for the children. Many of these kin caregivers are elderly, have health or financial difficulties themselves, or are otherwise in need of support to enable them to care for the substance abuser's children. State policies differ regarding whether such kin are eligible for foster care maintenance payments, welfare payments, or other support. Welfare reform is likely to put increased financial pressure on such caretakers, and may encourage additional parents to transfer custody of their child(ren) to relatives so that children's benefits may continue beyond time limits or if parents' benefits are cut. Work requirements and time limits on the receipt of welfare benefits do not exempt such caretaker relatives, and federal Emergency Assistance funds which many states had used in part to support kinship caregivers, are eliminated.

CONCLUSION

The primary mission of any child welfare agency is to protect children and, whenever possible, to strengthen and support families. The mission does not change when parental substance abuse is present.

The National Association of Public Child Welfare Administrators (NAPCWA) in 1991 adopted a series of "Guiding Principles for Working with Substance Abusing Families and Drug-Exposed Children." The first of these states that "[t]he mission of child welfare is to protect children and help insure their healthy development. Since children grow and develop best in families that provide safe, nurturing environments, child welfare agencies work with families in times of need to strengthen their ability to provide safe homes. When families refuse or are unable to safely care for a child, however, child protective services must and will intervene and provide a safe living environment" (NAPCWA, 1991, p. 2).

While child protection was NAPCWA's first principle, collaboration was its second: "A comprehensive child and family service system, not CPS alone, should be developed to take the lead, in collaboration with health, mental health, and substance abuse systems, in identifying and providing follow-up services for drug-dependent infants, and their siblings and parents (NAPCWA, 1991, p. 2)."

In 1992, the collaborative theme was echoed in the final report of the National Commission on Chemical Dependency and Child Welfare. The Commission called for "a comprehensive alcohol and drug and child welfare agenda [to] address service gaps, service barriers, and coordination issues that limit a community's ability to provide access to a full array of services" for families who come to the attention of child welfare. . . . The Commission also suggested that standard protocols should be developed and used in every community to assess when child welfare interventions for substance-abusing families are warranted. When child welfare services are indicated for families with substance-abuse problems, interventions should be comprehensive, community-based, and coordinated by an active case manager who provides linkage with a range of substance-abuse prevention and treatment services. Child welfare agencies and substance-abuse treatment providers must join forces to help substance-abusing parents address alcohol or other drug problems while ensuring safety of their children (Child Welfare League of America, 1992, p. 122 and p. 140).

The problems posed by alcohol and drugs require a coordinated response by multiple agencies and systems. It is imperative that child welfare and substance abuse treatment agencies overcome their differences to forge partnerships to better serve families affected by substance abuse. We must ensure the availability of an adequate array of services, objective outcome data to determine which intervention is most appropriate for which population, and continued discussion and debate within the field and between disciplines to find consensus on unresolved issues. And, finally, we must recognize that "reform" agendas and policies implemented at the federal, state, or local levels can have unforeseen and unintended consequences that jeopardize child safety and family stability in vulnerable families, especially those with substance abuse problems.

REFERENCES

American Psychiatric Association. (1994). Diagnostic and statistical manual of mental disorders (4th ed.). Washington, DC: American Psychiatric Association.

Barth, R. (1994). Adoption of drug-exposed infants. In R. Barth, J. D. Berrick, & N. Gilbert (Eds.), *Child welfare research review* (pp. 273–294) . New York: Columbia University Press.

Barth, R., Courtney, M., Berrick, J., & Albert, V. (1994). *From child abuse to permanency planning.* New York: Walter de Gruyter.

Booth, W. (1996). Florida county sets drug tests for welfare clients, *The Washington Post,* September 17, 1996, p. A3.

Courtney, M. E. (1994). Factors associated with the reunification of foster children with their families. *Social Service Review, 68,* 81–108.

The CWLA North American Commission on Chemical Dependency, (1992). *Children at the front: A different view of the war on alcohol and drugs.* Washington, DC: The Child Welfare League of America.

Dore, M. M., Doris, J., & Wright, P. (1995). Identifying substance abuse in maltreating families: A child welfare challenge. *Child Abuse and Neglect, 19,* 531–543.

Famularo, R., Stone, K., Barnum, R., & Wharton, R. (1986). Alcoholism and severe child maltreatment. *American Journal of Orthopsychiatry, 56,* 482–485.

Fanshel, D. (1975). Parental failure and consequences for children: The drug abusing mother whose children are in foster care. *American Journal of Public Health, 65,* 604–612.

Goerge, R., Van Voorhis, J., & Sanfilippo, L. (1996). *Final report of the Core Dataset Project—Child welfare service histories.* Washington, DC: U.S. Department of Health and Human Services, Office of the Assistant Secretary for Planning and Evaluation.

Goerge, R. M., Wulczyn, F. H., & Harden, A. W. (1995). *Foster care dynamics 1983–1993: An update from the multi state foster care data archive.* Chicago: The Chapin Hall Center for Children.

Herskowitz, J., Seck, M., & Fogg, C. (1989). *Substance abuse and family violence.* Boston: Massachusetts Department of Social Services.

Jaudes, P. K., Ekwo, E., & Van Voorhis, J. (1995). Association of drug abuse and child abuse. *Child Abuse and Neglect, 19,* 1065–1075.

Kelleher, K., Chaffin, M., Hollenberg, J., & Fischer, E. (1994). Alcohol and drug disorders among physically abusive and neglectful parents in a community-based sample. *American Journal of Public Health, 84*(10), 1586–1590.

Kelley, S. J. (1992). Parenting stress and child maltreatment in drug-exposed children. *Child Abuse and Neglect, 16,* 317–328.

McCullough, C. (1991). The child welfare response. *The future of children: Drug exposed infants,* (1), 61–71.

National Association of Public Child Welfare Administrators (1991). *Guiding principles for working with substance-abusing families and drug-exposed children: The child welfare response.* Washington, DC: The American Public Welfare Association.

National Center on Child Abuse and Neglect (1996). *Child maltreatment 1994.* Washington, DC: U.S. Government Printing Office.

Sabol, B. (1994). The call on agency resources. In D. Besharov (Ed.), *When drug addicts have children.* Washington, DC: The Child Welfare League of America and the American Enterprise Institute (pp. 125–144).

Sagatun-Edwards, I. J., Saylor, C., & Shifflett, B. (1995). Drug exposed infants in the social welfare system and juvenile court. *Child Abuse and Neglect, 19*(1), 83–91.

Spar, K. (1993). *Kinship foster care: An emerging federal issue.* Washington, DC: Congressional Research Service.

Tatara, T. (1993). *Characteristics of children in substitute and adoptive care: A statistical summary of the VCIS National Child Welfare Data Base.* Washington, DC: American Public Welfare Association.

U.S. Department of Health and Human Services. (1994a). *Respite care services for foster parents.* Washington, DC: HHS Office of Inspector General.

U.S. Department of Health and Human Services. (1994b). *Substance abuse among women and parents.* Washington, DC: HHS Office of the Assistant Secretary for Planning and Evaluation.

U.S. General Accounting Office, (1995). *Foster care: Health needs of many young children are unknown and unmet.* Washington, DC: U.S. General Accounting Office.

Wald, M. (1994). Termination of parental rights. In D. Besharov (Ed.), *When drug addicts have children* (pp. 195–210). Washington, DC: The Child Welfare League of America and the American Enterprise Institute.

Walker, C. D., Zangrillo, P., & Smith, J. M. (1994). Parental drug abuse and African American children in foster care. In R. Barth, J. D. Berrick, & N. Gilbert (Eds.), *Child welfare research review* (pp. 109–122). New York: Columbia University Press.

Westat, Inc. (forthcoming). *National study of preventive, protective, and reunification services delivered to children and their families.* Washington, DC: U.S. Department of Health and Human Services, Children's Bureau.

Wulczyn, F. (1994). Status at birth and infant foster care placement in New York City. In R. Barth, J. D. Berrick, & N. Gilbert (Eds.) *Child welfare research review* (pp. 146–184). New York: Columbia University Press.

11

Training Teachers to Educate Drug-Affected Children

Ted Lardner, Ph.D.

I have been working for five years with high school teachers from a variety of districts in the greater Cleveland area in an ongoing staff-development project focused on the teaching of writing. Our model is collaborative and it emphasizes dialogue. We from the university do not arrive at a school site and lecture to teachers, because we do not know and cannot know for each teacher what to do and how to do it in her or his classroom. With teachers, we establish principles which may guide practice, and our work together is guided by focused agendas aimed at solving problems which teachers are facing. Naturally, as we move toward resolution on some problems, other questions and problems arise. There are so many variables that affect what happens in a classroom, it seems sometimes that we are barely able to grasp the true outlines of a single problem, let alone to navigate toward its practical solution.

As a result of being immersed in this process with these teachers, I have managed to gain a sense of how they think and talk about what they do and what they would like to do. It may be that the most significant fact about the practical world in which these teachers operate is that it is deformed by a kind of structural contradiction which plays itself out materially and conceptually. The contradiction is this: On the one hand, individual teachers are charged with responsibility for student performance (achievement and behavior) in a classroom. On the other hand, teachers have almost zero control over most of the factors relative to student performance. Materially, the structure of the class "hour" and the classroom serves to limit the degree and kind of interaction through which teachers may influence students. This structure also isolates teachers from other potential partners in the educational system: other teachers, parents and caregivers, administrators. Conceptually, teachers must try to solve problems, evident in their classrooms, about which they often have too little information. The conversation of the teachers with whom I work is filled with second-hand information and rumors.

This is not a knock against the professionalism nor the dedication of these teachers. It is a description of a working reality in which well-meaning individuals do their best to make sense, by every practical means at their disposal, of a contradictory, conflicted situation.

Last spring I was doing a workshop with English teachers at a sub-urban high school. This high school is a changing place in terms of its history and the living memory of most of the teaching staff there. The demographics of the district are changing, which means that the faculty does not work nearly as much anymore with its accustomed middle-class college-bound student body. Like other districts across the United States, this district has been visited by the effects that social and economic upheaval have had on families. The teachers are seeing more students who are "at risk" by several definitions. This topic of the changing student population is (properly) a recurring theme at our workshops in this school, and we were visiting the subject again when one teacher spoke up to say, "And you know what's coming, don't you? The crack kids. They're in middle school now, and we're going to get them." This comment ended the exchange the group had been having; it acted as a sort of trump, an expression of the ultimate barrier against which a teacher's effort and thinking might spend itself for nothing. There was a moment of silence. Then a sigh. We moved on.

The moment illuminates what seem to be the most salient issues relating to the response of the educational system to drug-exposed children. Whatever type of education interventions would benefit the children, the only way to make sense of the construct, "the educational system," is to recognize the practitioners, the teachers, who constitute the most important element of its operation. The implication is that teachers are the ones in whose hands the real work of developing effective responses rests. What follows from this is the requirement to understand what it is that teachers lack that prevents them from responding effectively. Obviously, teachers need information of precisely the kind included in this book. Information is important because it can lead to changed attitudes and changed attitudes can lead to changed behavior. However, information is only one part of the picture. Teachers also need the power to change the structures within which they presently work, including the organization of time and space in schools and classrooms, and the less tangible but equally significant structure of interaction among students, teachers, and other partners in the educational system.

The teachers I am referring to in this anecdote are almost without exception hard-working, deeply committed professionals who struggle to make sense of their circumstances. The label, "crack kids," comes to them as a ready-made device which, for better or worse, but generally worse, helps define their terrain. If the response of the teachers at this high school evinces hopelessness, these teachers are not despairing. Mainly, these teachers are busy, nearly to the point of distraction, and their hopelessness, if that is what it is, is the abrupt end of a conversation, a sigh, then the next thing.

Educational responses play an enormous role in the development of all children. The response of the education system to children exposed to crack cocaine may usefully be thought of in terms of teacher knowledge and practice on the one hand, and institutional structure and practice on the other. To find the best educational response, in other words, we need to think through what happens inside the classroom, and also what happens between the classroom, the family, and the community.

There are two issues related to the topic of teacher knowledge and practice in the classroom. The first is the need for further research to illuminate the multiple causal relationships linking prenatal exposure to crack cocaine with school achievement. The research to date suggests a complicated picture:

> [I]t is not clear whether the characteristics seen in cocaine-exposed children are actually caused by the cocaine itself, or by other factors associated with poverty such as other drug use, violent/disruptive environments, homelessness, or a combination of these factors. (National Health/Education Consortium, 1992, p. 8)

The second is the issue of labeling in conjunction with teacher attitudes, expectations, and student achievements. Since Rosenthal and Jacobson's groundbreaking "Pygmalion" study in 1968, hundreds of studies have documented the existence of the self-fulfilling prophesy phenomena of teachers' expectations and student achievements (Rosenthal 1987). Though to date we lack empirical evidence in the specific case of drug-exposed children, it seems reasonable to suggest that children who are identified as "crack babies" in school are likely to suffer the negative consequences of labeling. Good (1982), noting that the original *Pygmalion* study lacked direct classroom-observational data, offers a five-point model relating teacher expectations for student achievement, the behavior toward students through which these expectations are communicated, and the responsive changes in students' motivation, behavior, and achievement. While Good suggests that more observational research is necessary to better understand students' responses to teachers' different expectations and behaviors, research on the subject of Special Education labeling and tracking points to lower teacher expectations (Dupuis & Badiali, 1988; Parish, Menvey, & Knowles, 1993) and reduced educational achievement (Gama & de Jesus, 1986; Juliebo & Elliott, 1984). Fogel and Nelson (1983) report that Special Education labeling negatively biased teachers' global evaluations of children, though it did not influence the grading of student work, nor teachers' behavioral observations of students. Finally, much of the research relating teacher expectations and student achievements has looked specifically at expectations regarding *academic* ability and achievement. Crano and Mellon's study (1978), on the other hand, reports that

> [T]eachers' expectations and evaluations of children's social development . . . appeared to exert a greater influence on later academic performance than those expectations concerned specifically with academic potential. (p. 47)

The research documenting the interrelationship of labeling, teachers' attitudes and expectations, and student achievement is extensive. Student labeling and tracking influences attitudes and expectations of educators. While Labov (1983) has argued (in the context of dialect-variation and teachers' language attitudes) that "negative attitudes can be changed by providing people with scientific evidence" (p. 32), other evidence suggests that teacher attitudes maybe somewhat less malleable through the application of information. Sachs and Smith write that:

> Forms of consciousness, knowledge, sentiments and values that teachers use as part of their cultural repertoires in schools are the result of social constitution. The "social" is composed of a number of overlapping discourses that are characteristic of schools everywhere. (p. 423)

Educational research has traditionally relied on scientific methodology like controlled experiments, presuming an "objectivity" always unavailable to the classroom teacher who is a participant in the scene being studied. The conventional narrative frame which guides our thinking about teacher knowledge and practice holds that the application of research findings can result in teacher practice coming closer and closer to some ideal. The model is top-down and one-directional, and therefore problematic. It often supposes single-factor explanations of phenomena. It perhaps misrepresents the connection between teacher knowledge, attitudes, and practice. Results of an inservice program aimed at remediating K-6 teachers' attitudes and practice in relation to Black English Vernacular showed that while teachers had a better understanding of the facts of social variation in language, they were less confident of the pedagogical application of this information (Howard, Hanson, & Pietras, 1980).

SCHOOL, FAMILY, AND COMMUNITY

Many have pointed out that cries of educational crisis often reflect social displacements and economic changes which produce anxiety among those threatened by displacement and change. In the United States, such social anxieties have continued to resurface periodically since World War II (Heath & McLaughlin, 1987) as seen in *Newsweek*'s memorable "Why Johnny Can't Write," published in 1975, and, in 1983, the National Commission on Excellence in Education's *A Nation at Risk*. The responses have varied over the decades. According to Heath and McLaughlin (1987), education initiatives focused on new teaching methods and technologies in the 1950s, while remediating societal problems such as urban blight and rural poverty were seen as the key to solving the problems of education in the 1960s. In the 1970s, school improvement efforts targeted teacher accountability, while in the 1980s, the roles played by the family and the workplace in education were critical: "[E]ducation for the 21st century could not be limited to a single institution and . . . piecemeal approaches to reform that ignored the interdependent nature of the workplace, families, schools, and community institutions were doomed" (Heath and McLaughlin, p. 577). In particular, these latest initiatives have singled out the role of parents "as extensions of the schools' business—supporters of homework, monitors of activities, and reinforcers of school values" (Heath & McLaughlin, p. 577).

Heath and McLaughlin call for "moving beyond" dependence on the school and the family, reframing educational policy for the 21st century in local terms which take into account the variety of potential support systems available to children. "[S]chool becomes the nexus for community, business, and family collaboration" (1987, p. 580). Their call for radically rethinking the structure and relationships among educators, business people, families, and the community has much in common with emerging school-based and community-based educational responses to the needs of cocaine-exposed children.

Reports of school-based programs developed to serve the needs of drug-exposed children shed light on the needs which drug-exposed children pose to schools and teachers, and the directions teachers and school policymakers need to go in order to meet them. Three themes are evident in reports from two different sites, one, a day-care program housed in the Ravenswood School District in East Palo Alto, California, the other, Project DAISY, a program consisting of team-taught, limited-enrollment classrooms established in four Washington, DC, public elementary schools. Testifying before the Congressional Black Caucus in 1991, Dr. Charlie M. Knight, Superintendent of the Ravenswood City Schools, and Dr. Diane E. Powell, Director of Project DAISY in Washington, DC, identified the strong connection between teacher training in cultural sensitivity and the teaching of drug-exposed children. Second is the need to recognize the role of the teacher, and the school more generally, as members of a team, that is, as part of a network of interconnecting support services. Third is a need to reconceive the traditional, individual-oriented focus of instruction by recognizing and including the family—particularly the mother and/or the primary caregiver—in the work of the school.

But both Dr. Knight and Dr. Powell place their reports in contexts provided by larger public concerns and perceptions of "at risk" students and schools, suggesting that as educators and policymakers consider the role of the educational system in responding to drug-exposed children, the scope of inquiry needs to be widened; to imagine "what works in the classroom," it becomes necessary to account for the social and economic contexts in which classroom work takes place. In thinking through the role of schools, therefore, it is important to recognize contexts conventionally thought of as external to the process of schooling itself. And in her statement, Dr. Knight (1991) places the effort of the Ravenswood Schools in the context of diminished opportunities for mainstream success available to the low-socioeconomic-status Black youth in East Palo Alto. Noting a 500% increase in spending by California on incarceration, Dr. Knight states that by around 1990, one in three young Black men in California were either on parole, on probation, or in jail (pp. 27–28). At the same time, education policymakers were recognizing that disproportionate numbers of Black male children were being placed in Special Education Programs. Dr. Knight links these observations to the fact that for many youngsters in the community, the alternative to school success is grim: drug use, pregnancy, and prison.

Experiences in the first 2 years of the day-care program suggest that many children prenatally exposed to crack cocaine, by perhaps age 2 behaved "so similarly to nonexposed children as to be indistinguishable" (Knight, 1991, p. 29). Visiting the day-care center several times each week, mothers are offered "drug and family counseling, parent training, preventive health care, and continuing education" (p. 29). Based on experience with this day-care program, Dr. Knight concluded that when public schools in a poor community are the last credible governmental institutions, they should become the focal point for the necessary multi-agency outreach efforts serving drug-exposed children and their mothers. Dr. Knight pointed out the need for improved teacher training, because too often, teachers seemed to "lack both the belief that these children can learn and the skills to effectively serve them" (p. 34). At the same time, the issue of teacher preparation is layered; new teachers continue to be ill-prepared to teach effectively in culturally diverse classrooms. Dr. Knight argued that effective teacher education programs would "require direct experience in urban schools, and must require teacher candidates to participate in both cultural orientations and class work in dealing with disabilities" (p. 35).

The themes sounded in Dr. Knight's testimony recur in the statement of Dr. Diane E. Powell, Director of Project DAISY in Washington, DC: As of 1991, Project DAISY was located in four schools in Washington, DC. Children served by the mixed-age classrooms ranged from 3- to 5-years-old. A teacher and a teacher's aide staffed each class. Enrollment was limited to fifteen students, five of whom were prenatally exposed to drugs. The classroom staff was supported by a project team which included a clinical psychologist, a clinical social worker, and a speech language pathologist. Work in this project suggests the following areas of concern: the need to offer support and to be culturally sensitive to the community which these schools serve; and the need for cultural sensitivity when reaching out to the primary caregiver, who is nearly always female and often a senior citizen. In other words, teachers need to learn how to go to a grandmother's house and to show a grandmother how to help her grandchild do her homework. Staff observations suggest that while many of the children in Project DAISY seemed to have "deficits in language" (Powell, 1991, p. 40), this seemed to result from the fact that "when these children were young they didn't have that initial bonding experience with a significant other, so they didn't have a lot of exposure to language models" (p. 40). Further research on this point is in order, since concern over the "language deficits" of "underprivileged" African-American children has a long history in education.

In addition to collaboration among support agencies, the need for home-based assistance and parent support groups, Dr. Powell calls for integrating these children in relatively small classrooms staffed with two adults. Educators require new training as well, to prepare them to act as members of interagency collaborative teams, and to work closely with families in community-based programs (Powell, 1991, 44–45). Dr. Powell contextualizes her report of Project DAISY by drawing attention to the language with which the conversation about these children has been fashioned. Those whom Project DAISY serves, Dr. Powell states, are "children first. . . .

> They're not a biogenic underclass. They're not shadow children. They're not crack babies. They're not those children. They're children. They have names. They have parents. They have grandparents. They have a father. They came from somewhere, and there's a place for them to go. (p. 37)

Werner (1994) tips off educators to the implications of Dr. Powell's statement. Describing resilience research, Dr. Werner states that "[s]upport from . . . an informal network of kin and neighbors and 'ordinary' members of the community was more often sought and more highly valued . . . than the services of community organizers, mental health professionals, and social workers" (pp. 6–7). Playing their roles most effectively in responding to the needs of these special children will require schools and teachers to remake themselves as able partners in these support networks. That will require of many teachers and administrators a radical rethinking of their professional, and, perhaps, personal identities and commitments. We need models to show the way.

REFERENCES

Crano, W. D., & Mellon, P. M. (1978). Causal influence of teachers' expectations on children's academic performance: A cross-lagged panel analysis.

Journal of Educational Psychology, 70(1), 39–49.

Dupuis, V. L., & Badiali, B. J. (1988). Classroom climate and teacher expectations in homogeneously grouped, secondary schools. *Journal of Classroom Interaction, 23*, 28–33.

Fogel, L. S., & Nelson, R. O. (1983). The effects of special education labels on teachers' behavioral observations, checklist scores, and grading of academic work. *Journal of School Psychology, 21*, 241–51.

Gama, E. M. P., & de Jesus, D. M. (1986, April). *Teachers' expectations and causal attributions for students' academic achievement,* Annual Meeting of the American Educational Research Association, San Francisco, CA.

Good, T. L. (1982). How teachers' expectations affect results. *American Education, 18*, 25–32.

Heath, S. B., & McLaughlin, W. (1987). A child resource policy: Moving beyond dependence on school and family. *Phi Delta Kappan, 68*, 576–580.

Howard, H., Hanson, L., & Pietras, T. (1980). *Final evaluation: King Elementary School Vernacular Black English Inservice Program.* Ann Arbor, MI: Ann Arbor Public Schools.

Juliebo, M. F., & Elliott, J. (1984). *The child fits the label.* Edmonton, Alberta: University of Alberta. 1984. ERIC number ED 285143.

Knight, C. M. (1991, September 13). *Statement of Charlie M. Knight Hearing before the Select Committee on Narcotics Abuse and Control* (pp. 25–36). Washington, DC: U.S. Government Printing Office.

Labov, W. (1983). Recognizing black English in the classroom. In J. W. Chambers (Ed.), *Black English educational equity and the law* (pp. 29–55). Ann Arbor: Karoma.

National Commission on Excellence in Education. *A nation at risk: The imperative for educational reform.* Washington, DC: U.S. Department of Education, 1983.

National Health/Education Consortium. (1992). *Cocaine-exposed children: a growing health/education issue.* Washington, DC: Author.

Parish, T. S., Menvey, M. D., & Knowles, W. C. (1993). An investigation of teachers' attitudes toward gifted and handicapped students. *Reading Improvement, 30*, 250–51.

Powell, D. E. (1991, September 13). Statement of Diane E. Powell. *Hearing before the Select Committee on Narcotics Abuse and Control* (pp. 37–46). Washington, DC: U. S. Government Printing Office.

Rosenthal, R. (1987). "Pygmalion" effects: Existence, magnitude, and social importance. *Educational Researcher, 16*, 37–41.

Rosenthal, R., & Jacobson, L. (1968). *Pygmalion in the classroom.* New York, NY: Holt, Rinehart & Winston.

Sachs, J., & Smith, R. (1988). Constructing teacher culture. *British Journal of*

Sociology of Education, 9, 423–436.

Select Committee on Narcotics Abuse and Control (1991). *Drug-exposed kids: A crisis in America's schools.* Washington, DC: U.S. Government Printing Office.

Sheils, M. (1975, Dec. 8). Why Johnny can't write. *Newsweek,* pp. 58–65.

Werner, E. E. (1994, December). *Applications of resilience: Possibilities and promise.* Paper presented at Conference on the Role of Resilience in Drug Abuse, Alcohol Abuse and Mental Illness, Washington, DC.

PART III

Contrasts and Conclusions

12

Bridging the Public Policy/ Public Health Gap: Organizing Multiple Agencies to Deliver Coordinated Services

Leslie L. Jordon

S everal years ago, in an effort to significantly improve the availability and quality of community services and access to them, the Missouri Department of Mental Health, in conjunction with a number of its community stakeholders, undertook several major initiatives to develop mechanisms for more comprehensive mental health service systems.

One of the most far-reaching of Missouri's community initiatives was the design and development of a new alcohol and drug treatment model: The Comprehensive Substance Treatment and Rehabilitation program, more commonly referred to as CSTAR. CSTAR was designed to provide holistic treatment and support to individuals and their families, in the community. Outcome evaluations indicate the model is successful in terms of recovery rates, also in client satisfaction.

The success is due in large part to: case management, the use of multidisciplinary teams, and the emphasis on long-term treatment which is individualized. The design and implementation presented serious challenges and controversy over policy. These were overcome in large part by the underlying commitment on the part of the design work group to certain guiding principles.

THE WORK GROUP

The CSTAR model was designed by a work group formed in 1990 that included representation from alcohol and drug programs (ranging from hospital-based to outpatient), maternal and child health specialists from the Missouri Department of Health, consumers, and family members. The work group, with the assistance of staff from the Missouri Division of Alcohol and Drug Abuse, created a new, statewide model that offered individualized treatment from a menu of services, emphasized community and family, and either offered or arranged the necessary support services clients needed to succeed in long-term recovery.

As a result of monies that had been appropriated during the previous state legislative session, the original focus was to develop a treatment program for crack-addicted, pregnant women. This was also a time when national interest was high and media attention was being paid to the dramatic rise in the number of "crack babies." The work group, however, expanded the vision to take a much broader look at the needs of all drug-addicted, high-risk populations. Women and their children became a major component of the model, with the focus being on the family unit as a whole.

THE PROGRAM DESIGN

The work group developed the following major bottom-line criteria (principles and policies) that subsequently shaped (and impacted) the design of the CSTAR program:

- Treatment should be based on the individual's assessed need, and services offered within the least restrictive environment.
- Treatment programs must utilize a cooperative interdisciplinary team approach. This interdisciplinary team shall consist of, at a minimum, an alcohol and drug counselor, a physician, and a case manager.
- Individuals and their families should (whenever possible) be able to receive treatment in the community where they live.
- Family members should be able to continue in treatment even if the primary abuser refuses treatment. Extensive family involvement in the treatment process is critical to successful recovery.
- CSTAR will contain Medicaid-eligible services; thus the program design will need to meet specific Medicaid requirements.

- In addition to being covered by Medicaid, CSTAR will have several other major funding services, such as federal block grant dollars and state general revenue. The funding should not determine who is eligible to enter the CSTAR program
- Many of the CSTAR clients, especially those clients with multiple needs, should be offered the structure and support of supervised, chemical-free housing if they are to succeed in treatment. Monies should be available to assist with rent for up to one year.
- Children should be able to accompany their mother (parent) to treatment. CSTAR programs across the state shall have monies to fund local 16-bed, supervised residential sites for families. Programs shall be required to accommodate large families and not limit the number of children who can accompany their parent to treatment.
- Treatment and recovery services should be available and accessible on a long-term basis or for at least two (2) years. Ideally, treatment and support shall continue as long as clinically indicated.
- To assure accessibility, transportation shall be a required component of all CSTAR programs.
- Clients, especially women and children, should be given assistance in finding permanent housing, and this service should be a major component of case management. The state shall also assist by applying for Shelter Plus HUD monies specifically for CSTAR families in recovery (Missouri did apply and did receive HUD monies for several of its metropolitan areas).

THE CORE SERVICES

Comprehensive standards and regulations were developed by the work group over a 12-month period. To become a provider of CSTAR services in Missouri, the standards must be met as determined by a certification survey conducted by Missouri Division of Alcohol and Drug Abuse staff. All CSTAR programs must deliver the following core components or services:

- *Intake Screening.* The process of gathering and evaluating relevant information about a client to determine initial admission for CSTAR services and to develop the initial service plan.
- *Assessment and Treatment Planning.* A comprehensive assessment that addresses substance use history; prior treatment; social, family, educational, and vocational history; and, current use of com-

munity resources. A psychologist or physician with one year of experience in the treatment of substance abuse develops the diagnosis. Based on the assessment and diagnosis, the interdisciplinary team, in cooperation with the client, develops a treatment plan.

- *Day Treatment.* A structured package of therapeutic activities offered 7 days a week (10 hours a day) for a prescribed period of time. Day treatment includes individual and group counseling, group education, family therapy, recreational activities, study sessions, orientation to self-help groups, events involving family members and, as needed, case management. Clients participate in day treatment for an average of 60–90 days. Once this intense level is completed, the client receives a more individualized continuum of services.
- *Individual Counseling.* A goal-oriented therapeutic process in which the individual interacts with a counselor to promote recovery from substance abuse and a resolution to related problems that interfere with the client's functioning.
- *Group Counseling.* Goal-oriented, therapeutic interaction between a counselor and two or more clients to promote the client's self-understanding, self-esteem, and resolution of problems through personal disclosure and interpersonal interaction among group members.
- *Group Education.* Presentation of information and application of the information to participants through group discussion designed to promote recovery and enhance social functioning.
- *Family Therapy.* Goal-oriented, therapeutic interaction of a family therapist with the client and/or one or more members of the client's family to address and resolve the family system's dysfunction, particularly as it relates to the substance abuse problem. Family therapy shall be available both in an office setting and in the community at locations convenient to the family. (A higher reimbursement rate was established for therapy that takes place outside the office.)
- *Codependency Counseling.* Goal-oriented, therapeutic interaction with an individual or a group to address dysfunctional behaviors and life patterns associated with being a member of a family in which there is a substance abuse problem.
- *Case Management.* Specific activities with or on behalf of a particular client or their family in accord with the individual's rehabilitation plan to maximize adjustment and functioning with the community.

ADDITIONAL CORE SERVICES FOR WOMEN
AND CHILDREN

As noted earlier, a major feature of the CSTAR program was the development of a statewide treatment system specifically for women and their children. Currently, Missouri has nine programs across the state for women with their children, with the capacity to serve approximately 2,000 women and 6,000 to 7,000 children annually. The following services, in addition to the core services, are provided:

- *Residential Support.* Twenty-four-hour staff coverage (including nursing staff) for both a mother and her children (up to age 13). The average length of stay is 60 days; stays of 90 days or longer are permissible with prior approval from the Division of Alcohol and Drug Abuse. During the days and early evenings, the mother receives CSTAR day treatment services. (In order to receive Medicaid funds, the residence size is limited to 16 women at any one time.)
- *Child Care.* Each women's CSTAR program is required to provide a child care and development program for the children of women who are concurrently receiving treatment. Each center must design appropriate services that address the following goals: 1) building self-esteem; 2) learning to identify and express feelings; 3) building a positive family relationship; 4) developing decision-making skills; 5) understanding chemical dependency as a family illness; and 6) learning and practicing nonviolent ways to resolve conflict.
- *Supported Housing* (rent subsidy). The Division provides a housing allowance to pay for safe and appropriate housing (for up to 1 year) for women and their children who are financially unable to purchase such housing and who need housing in order to benefit from treatment and continue in recovery.

PROGRAM POLICY DESIGN ISSUES

During the design of the CSTAR program, the work group often had to examine and discuss not only differing philosophies among the members but also (revisit) the originating principles. The work group needed to reassure themselves that they were creating a model that would address the gaps in alcohol and drug treatment based on the group's collective experiences. The group had permission from the state's leaders to be bold with the model design and build in the necessary program flexibility so the model could change as experience dictated. Perhaps the most unique aspect during the design of the CSTAR program was the almost total commitment of the work group to concentrate on what the consumer needed, *not* what was convenient for the program or its staff.

The following are examples of some of the larger issues the work group faced. These issues are not necessarily unique to the development of alcohol and drug programs for women. However, they go to the core of issues facing the treatment community as its programs become more comprehensive and better integrated with other community agencies.

INTERDISCIPLINARY TEAMS

The concept of using interdisciplinary teams was not, in itself, controversial. However, defining the team members, their credentials, and the requirement that teams truly function as teams with meaningful input into and oversight of each client's treatment and recovery process was extremely controversial.

The interdisciplinary team eventually became defined as a group of professional staff members within the CSTAR program that consists (at least) of a case manager, a qualified alcohol and drug counselor, and a diagnostician (licensed psychologist or physician).

The treatment team, a component of the interdisciplinary team, is comprised (at least) of the qualified alcohol and drug counselor and a case manager.

The requirement that a licensed psychologist, board-certified psychiatrist, or a licensed physician with at least 1 year's experience in treating persons with substance disorders, perform a complete diagnostic formulation with all five (5) axes (including diagnosis, degree of severity for dependency, and review of patterns) was new to the state alcohol and drug treatment agency and its provider system. The majority of the work group felt that the involvement of a qualified diagnostician and ongoing diagnostic assessment, both for mental health problems and alcohol and drug addiction, was critical if we were to address all the underlying factors causing a person's addiction.

Major concerns were affordability, and availability of qualified physicians/psychologists. Adequate reimbursement rates were set to address the affordability concern, and as a result, availability was no longer an issue. To further emphasize the importance of the diagnosis, standards were written that required that it be based on an interview and that the physician/psychologist participate in regular team meetings.

The introduction of a case manager, who is charged with specific responsibilities and goals pertaining to a client's treatment and recovery, was perhaps the most difficult issue faced by the work group. Every client in CSTAR has an assigned treatment team consisting of the counselor *and* the case manager. There was tremendous discussion and concern raised, not only over the "introduction" of "enabling social work types to alcohol and drug treatment programs," but also the question of who would supervise and direct the case manager's activities; should it be the counselor or a separate individual specifically qualified to supervise a case management section? The deciding argument came from an unexpected source: work group members who had long-term and well-established connections with the AA community in Missouri. It was argued that a separate staff person to help not only clients broker services in the community, but to also negotiate the services within the treatment program, would be a valuable advocate and should be viewed as an equal member of the treatment team, not a subordinate to the alcohol and drug counselor. Concerns over "enabling," "manipulation," and "control" should be addressed with training. The group concluded that the use of treatment teams would add more expertise, experience, and objectivity to the treatment and recovery process.

Residential versus Outpatient Treatment

Prior to CSTAR, treatment in Missouri was almost exclusively residentially based. A client went away to a program, not necessarily in his or her community, received 30–60 days of treatment and was discharged to the community with little or no aftercare. For programs with aftercare, there was no outreach attempt to follow the client on an outpatient basis. CSTAR takes a different approach and attempts to separate treatment needs from the need for safe or supervised housing. The client is assessed both upon admission and throughout treatment as to the level of supervision and structure needed during the evenings, nights, and weekends. Programs should have the flexibility of offering structured overnight supervision, monies to pay for up to 1 year's rent in an apartment, or other safe housing. This flexibility in living arrangements was considered essential if we were to offer long-term habilitation and not just short-term treatment.

Two main issues were raised by separating housing needs from treatment needs. One: from a provider's viewpoint, this "flexibility" appeared to present a nightmare for administering multiple services as well as for monitoring clients. Two: there was fear that with the decreased emphasis on the traditional model of 30-day residential treatment, and the placement of treatment *in* the community (including the home, schools, etc.), new residential beds would no longer be funded and existing programs might be forced to convert to the CSTAR model.

DIVERSION OF HOSPITAL INPATIENT FUNDS

During the development of the model design, the work group had to be sensitive to program model costs and availability of necessary monies to fund the program. The work group was united in pursuing Medicaid funding, although not without fear and trepidation. There was a problem, however, with starting a statewide, comprehensive outpatient treatment model funded by Medicaid when Medicaid inpatient costs for alcohol and drug abuse treatment were skyrocketing.

In 1989 and 1990, when CSTAR was in the initial stages of development, the prevailing policy and funding issues included an increase in Medicaid hospital inpatient utilization and in recidivism. Medicaid hospital costs for primary alcohol and drug inpatient care alone rose 30% from FY 1988 to FY 1989. At the same time, there was a growing recognition that inpatient, or acute care, settings should no longer be the first or only choice for alcohol and drug treatment. In addition, many of the persons receiving inpatient alcohol and drug treatment were AFDC mothers whose children were placed in foster care while the mother received treatment. Services for the family members of the addicted Medicaid-eligible persons were nonexistent.

A decision was made by the Department of Mental Health and the state Medicaid agency to restrict inpatient alcohol and drug treatment hospital utilization to purposes of medical detoxification only and divert a percentage of the dollars used in the inpatient hospital program to the new CSTAR program. The decision to stop reimbursement for Medicaid hospital inpatient treatment put tremendous pressure on the CSTAR work group to have the model operating statewide, prior to the cutoff of inpatient treatment funds.

Meetings were held with the Missouri Hospital Association to obtain their support of the CSTAR model and to encourage their members with inpatient alcohol and drug treatment units to convert to the

CSTAR model and become CSTAR providers. The decision to encourage hospitals to become CSTAR providers was controversial within the alcohol and drug community and the state's alcohol and drug division. Prior to using Medicaid funding, the state's alcohol and drug division had control over who received contracts. It also had control over the amount of dollars awarded in a contract, and thus total control over expenditures. In the Medicaid program, any provider who is surveyed and meets standards is eligible to become a provider. There was concern over runaway costs and unwanted growth. Hospitals *did* become CSTAR providers, but not in the large numbers that was feared. They also demonstrated they could successfully provide a comprehensive, community-based model, and indeed, several have very successful CSTAR programs.

A positive benefit to new providers entering the publicly funded system—for example, schools, hospitals, women's shelters, and mental health centers—is better integration with other agencies in the community, and most important, greater access to treatment.

The Use of Medically Trained Staff

The CSTAR work group was also divided over whether the program standards should require the use of medically trained staff, specifically nurses. Traditionally, the state-funded treatment programs did not require medically trained staff in treatment other than for social setting detoxification programs. Members of the work group argued (and especially those with maternal and child health backgrounds) that a medical component was vital in a holistic model and imperative in a women and children's program. The final decision was that all the women and children's programs would be required to have full time RNs and LPN staff scheduled throughout the day and evenings. As true with many publicly funded programs, once money is allocated for certain services, it is hard to receive more money to expand the service in the future. As a result, general adult and adolescent CSTAR programs do not have a medical component and are unlikely to ever have this service added.

Strengths-Based Case Management

The introduction of case managers as a regular resource within the alcohol and drug treatment community has been late in coming. Early in the development of the CSTAR model it was decided that the case manager would play a vital role in the model and would act as the "navigator" who directed the many and diverse needs of the clients through a system of services that could address the needs, and also provided long-term support for the client during recovery.

Missouri was fortunate to have access to an individual who had worked previously with Missouri's Department of Mental Health in implementing case management models. Dr. Pat Sullivan, at that time a Professor of Social Work at Southwest Missouri State University, was contracted by the state to develop the case management model, prepare a case manager training manual, and conduct periodic training for CSTAR program staff.

The case management model, as taught by Dr. Sullivan, is called "strengths-based case management." Case management from a strengths-based perspective is intended to encourage health through the emphasis of positive interactions between the client and his or her environment, and individual strengths versus pathology. This perspective does not deny the importance of the addiction, but rather demonstrates the equal importance of positive goals that focus on the healthy strengths of a person, rather than just the weaknesses. The Division of Alcohol and Drug Abuse's Case Management Manual (Sullivan, 1991) lists as the goal of case management services:

> To promote stability in the daily life of clients as indicated by increased employment levels, family stability, and satisfactory, reduced substance usage, improved health, and enhanced overall life satisfaction. (p. 58)
>
> The relationship between a case manager and a client, particularly as advocated in this model, is an intense one. Done well, case management from this perspective requires that a great deal of time and energy is devoted to each client served. Indeed, when case management is operationalized, as intended, caseloads should rarely exceed 25 clients (p. 60).

Implementing this model requires the case manager to be active with the client in the community. The case manager offers support and instruction to clients as they struggle with daily activities, learn new skills, and strive to attain their individual goals. To the greatest degree possible the clients should direct the process of helping.

It is recognized that those in treatment for substance abuse often have long track records of unreliability and manipulative behavior.

These traits create many of the problems the recovering person faces when trying to relate positively as a sober individual. If these are the traits that are the core of the client's problems, then addressing them should be at the core of recovery.

> Case managers are in a prime position to encounter these longstanding personality patterns. It is not, at times, an enviable position. Furthermore, by virtue of the focus on resource acquisition and community integration, the case manager works to help the client secure resources from other community vendors, obtain housing and employment and work towards other life goals, the more there is potential for manipulation and deceit. Framed positively, these crises are the basis for change to occur. The case manager who establishes a solid, helping relationship can use incidences of manipulation and deceitfulness as examples of negative patterns of behavior. Job failure, evictions, and broken relationships are all examples of negative consequences of unhealthy behavior. In short, those characteristics and patterns of behavior that may cause some professionals to pause when considering the value of case management, are precisely the pivots for positive change. (Sullivan, 1991, p. 62)

The concept of a Counselor/Case manager team, where the two individuals can work on their respective goals with the clients and complement each other's expertise is sound clinical practice in working with (multiple needs) clients.

The introduction and integration of a strength-based case management system into alcohol and drug treatment programs proved to be difficult and time-consuming. In anticipation of this, the Missouri Division of Alcohol and Drug Abuse provided a very ambitious training program not only to start the case management service, but also to provide ongoing consultation with individual CSTAR programs. More than 500 individuals were trained during the first year of CSTAR program implementation. The CSTAR program directors were trained first, then clinical supervisors, counselors, and on a continuous basis *all* staff hired as case managers.

The time involved in developing a case management system that is both accepted within the alcohol and drug treatment program and is successful at crafting comprehensive solutions to complex problems cannot be underestimated. This is especially true with family and children's services agencies that have pronounced dissimilarities in professional orientation from the alcohol and drug treatment staff. The most successful CSTAR programs have formed strong relationships, and in some instances, collaborations with the myriad of public and private sector community-based agencies that are essential components of a particular client's long-term recovery.

During the first 2 years of CSTAR implementation, the following problems were often noted during consultation and certification visits with various programs:

- Lack of an understanding and acceptance by treatment staff, especially the counselors, of the case manager's role and the key principles of a strengths-based case management model.
- Resistance to a counselor/case manager "team" approach where the two professional disciplines are equal. Serious problems of control, authority, and boundaries were often noted among team members.
- If the CSTAR program administration was not comfortable with the role of the case manager or had a particular bias against it, case management services were never implemented properly and the case manager was often delegated jobs no one else in the agency wanted.
- Timing of and decisions about which life areas the case manager works on with the client are highly individualized, and the hours spent per client can and should vary. Teams that did not communicate frequently were unable to exercise the necessary flexibility to successfully prioritize items in a client's individualized treatment plan. For example, when a client (in this case, a woman with a child) first enters the CSTAR program, it might be assumed that the major focus would be on treatment and starting the recovery process; this is true if all the other life areas are under control and not negatively impacting the client. If, however, the client is having a housing crisis, is about to lose her public assistance or is facing a court hearing where she may lose her child, treatment, *at best,* will only aggravate the stress. Some of these areas need to be worked on aggressively before treatment can effectively be started. A functional team will plan through this and feel confident with each other's ability to address their respective responsibilities and roles with the client. All the skills necessary in an interagency collaboration come into play here. Once collaboration is developed in the team, these skills readily transfer outside the agency to the community.

Interestingly, the one area that was originally voiced as a major concern during program design about alcohol and drug treatment staff "enabling" turned out to be a nonissue once the model was in operation. Case management training helped significantly, but it also became apparent that most of the case managers were social workers by training, and understood the difference between "enabling" in the sense of alcohol and drug addiction and "enabling" someone in assisting them to make positive changes.

INTERAGENCY CASE COORDINATION

There are several key services that the majority of CSTAR clients, especially women with children, are either already receiving or need access to when entering treatment. It is not uncommon for clients to have several case managers across several agencies. It is the responsibility of the CSTAR case manager to assist in accessing services and to coordinate with existing service agencies and other case managers while the client is in treatment. Case coordination with outside agencies requires considerable skills in the art of communication, consensus- building, and compromise. This is especially true of the agencies that may have very different professional orientations from the alcohol and drug treatment community.

Perhaps the most common difference noted was between child protection agency staff and the client's alcohol and drug treatment staff. The children's services workers' primary concern is protection of the child, and they may have little or no patience for the mother's need for a *long*-term treatment program and even less tolerance for the parent's relapses. The coming together of these different professionals to work on a joint plan for the family is critical and is one very positive outcome of successful CSTAR programs.

At a minimum, successful CSTAR programs are required to form strong working relationships with the following agencies within their community that provide:

- Health care
- Housing
- Child care
- Social services
- Public assistance (Welfare & Food stamps)
- Family support (i.e., family preservation, respite, and other services necessary for "at risk" families)

- Mental health, and
- Criminal justice

Part of the CSTAR program provider certification process involves interviews, by surveyors, of these various agencies in the community. Discussed are such topics as: any knowledge of the existence of the local CSTAR program; the amount, if any, of contact with the program; the ability and willingness of the CSTAR program to coordinate and problem solve; the willingness on the part of the agency to be an educator for agency staff in the area of alcohol and drug abuse; and the willingness to share resources to meet common goals for the client.

FUTURE DIRECTIONS

The CSTAR program was designed and implemented in Missouri during a time when the state's leaders were emphasizing the development of comprehensive, community-based treatment models. Their leadership has proved successful; the ongoing evaluation of the CSTAR program, and an analysis specifically of the CSTAR women's and children's programs, has been very positive.

The individuals who were responsible for empowering the work group to design and implement the CSTAR model are gone. Much of the future impetus for change or growth of the CSTAR model, therefore, will need to come from the providers of CSTAR services and the communities where they are located. Simultaneously, there are significant changes occurring in Missouri, like the rest of the country, in the area of health care and human services delivery systems that will have a major impact on comprehensive treatment programs.

MANAGED CARE

Managed care is becoming increasingly the system of choice for the delivery of health care services. In Missouri, the Medicaid agency is in the process of implementing managed care for the welfare population in all of the state's major metropolitan areas. Managed care plans will be required to provide a behavioral health benefit package (comprised of both mental health and alcohol and drug treatment) that is the "equivalent" of 30 days inpatient and 20 days outpatient care. The Department of Mental Health, however, still administers and receives Medicaid funding for the CSTAR programs. Clients enrolled in managed care plans will be required to "exhaust" their behavioral health benefits before entering a fee-for-service Medicaid program i.e., the CSTAR program, for further treatment. This policy is wrought with problems, and has been opposed by both the Department of Mental Health and the mental health community. The health plans have not yet been implemented, so it is too soon to tell if the community agencies will work out a system locally which prevents clients from being dumped from one treatment to another.

Managed care, in general, poses many questions for the behavioral health field, and how long the CSTAR program will continue to exist outside the managed care system is unknown. As more healthcare-system decisions are being made based on cost containment, long-term comprehensive treatment models that mandate delivery of essential support services, i.e., housing, childcare, and transportation, could be lost.

COMMUNITY COLLABORATION

CSTAR programs are in the initial stages of collaboration with other community agencies and services. It took tremendous collaboration *within* the state agency to develop and implement the CSTAR model, and that collaboration came only after a considerable time of building trust.

There is some level of coordination between the CSTAR treatment programs and other community agencies. Coordination between CSTAR program staff and criminal justice staff and health service professionals is strong, partly based on past relationships. Good coordination with family and children service agencies is still tentative. There is an opportunity for improvement, however, by a movement within the Missouri Department of Social Services (which houses the family and children's services divisions) to create neighborhood-based family resource and service centers in connection with extensive school-based services.

FAMILY CENTERS

Missouri is currently opening family centers in low-income, high-risk neighborhoods. Necessary services are located at one physical location ("one-stop-shopping"). However, the centers are more than a group of agencies sharing space. Each center has a governing board that establishes policies and guidelines for the various agencies not only to interact, but also to collaborate on needed services. Mental health and alcohol and drug treatment services have been a part of the centers since their inception. The CSTAR program, with its emphasis on holistic treatment and support services, parallels the mission of the family centers. The colocation of family and children's services staff in the same building as the CSTAR program and the children's day care center allows for, and encourages, a problem-solving partnership among practitioners and clients. This "marriage" of the CSTAR programs into family centers brings hope for future collaboration.

Integrating women and children's alcohol and drug treatment programs into a community system recognizes that early, accessible, and comprehensive interventions for drug-abusing women are critical for healthy neighborhoods.

REFERENCE

Sullivan, W. P. (1991, July). *Case management in alcohol and drug treatment.* Southwest Missouri State University Center for Social Research.

Afterword

The Integration of Basic, Clinical and Policy Research

Roger E. Meyer, M.D.

Adam's mother . . . died of alcohol poisoning. . . . I'd feel sorrier for her, if we didn't have Adam. As it is, I only hope that she died before she had a chance to produce another child with his problems. I can't help but wish, too, that during her pregnancy, if she couldn't be counseled or helped, she had been forced to abstain for those crucial 9 months. On some American Indian reservations, the situation has grown so desperate that a jail internment during pregnancy has been the only answer possible in some cases. Some people . . . have taken more drastic stands and even called for the forced sterilization of women who, after having previously blunted the lives of several children like Adam, refused to stop drinking while they are pregnant. This will outrage some women, and men, good people who believe that it is the right of individuals to put themselves in harm's way, that drinking is a choice we make, that a person's liberty to court either happiness or despair is sacrosanct. I believe this, too, and yet the poignancy and frustration of Adam's life has fed my doubts, has convinced me that some of my principles were smug, untested. . . . Where, exactly, is the demarcation between self-harm and child abuse? . . . . Where do we draw the line? (Erdrich, 1989, p. xvii)

In the best of worlds, the common focus of concern of clinicians, clinical investigators, basic scientists, and policy researchers is a concern about the welfare of real human beings. The words (above) of the novelist and adoptive mother, Louise Erdrich, from the foreword to her husband's book, "The Broken Cord," should serve as a valuable counterpoint to the chapters in this text. Dorris' book presents the real life tragedy of an alcohol-exposed child and his adoptive family. There are no simple answers to the issues that are raised in his text, and in this one; indeed, the problems are larger than any single field of inquiry can comprehend.

The potentially damaging effects upon the unborn child of alcohol drinking in the mother have been known for millennia. The Old Testament refers to the advice that an angel gave to Samson's mother to drink no wine or strong drink because she was about to become pregnant. Newly married Spartan couples were prohibited from consuming alcohol on their wedding night. In the mid-1800s, the British House of Commons prohibited the sale of alcohol to pregnant women. While there are references in the clinical literature dating back to the last century, the "Fetal Alcohol Syndrome" was initially named and described by Jones, Smith, Ulleland, and Streissguth in 1973, pp. 144–145.

The literature supports the existence of a continuum of effects of prenatal alcohol exposure that range from the morphological abnormalities described in the Pagliarios' chapter (Chapter Two) to more subtle cognitive and behavioral abnormalities. The term "Fetal Alcohol Effects" has been applied to those children who exhibit some abnormalities consequent to neonatal alcohol exposure, but do not fulfill the criteria for a full-fledged diagnosis of FAS. The Pagliarios argue against this new term, preferring to consider the continuum of severity as being one syndrome. The Pagliarios also emphasize the long-term sequelae associated with the FAS, including growth retardation, developmental deficits in cognitive skills, development deficits in motor skills, and mental disorders.

The educational and social service systems are both challenged in caring for prenatally alcohol- and drug-exposed children. Because "the academic functioning of FAS/FAE patients appears to peak at around age 12 to 15," and because "the majority of these patients have received many years of special education services without alleviation of the basic deficits" (Dorris, 1989, p. 240), a more constructive focus would be on teaching vocational, survival, and daily living skills. Unfortunately, these children with learning deficits grow up to be disabled adults.

Fetal Alcohol Syndrome is one of the leading known causes of mental retardation in the United States (Abel & Sokol, 1986). The treatment costs alone for this syndrome have been estimated at nearly one-third of a billion dollars per year in the currency value of the late 1980s (Abel & Sokol, 1987). Abel and Sokol estimated the world-wide incidence to be 1.9 cases per thousand live births. The incidence rate is higher in heavy drinking communities.

Since the report by Jones et al. in 1973, the clinical research and epidemiological literature has pointed to the complexity of the phenomenon. It is now believed that the adverse effects of prenatal alcohol exposure exist on a continuum, so that the best advice to "adolescent girls and women who are pregnant or planning to become pregnant" should be to "abstain from alcohol consumption (Erdrich, 1989). This recommendation is based on the observations that: 1) no safe level of alcohol use has been demonstrated; and 2) there is no known cure for the FAS."

There is much that remains uncertain. Fetal alcohol effects have only been found variably among children born to alcohol-abusing women (Streissguth, Barr, Martin & Herman, 1980). Genetic differences and critical periods of organ development would appear to be critical variables. Because of the difficulty in quantifying alcohol consumption in association with critical periods of organ development, as well as dose, duration and genetic factors, research in animal models has proven to be invaluable. Indeed, this area of research on fetal alcohol effects has brought striking confirmation that alcohol is indeed a teratogen, and a behavioral teratogen, with effects that include abnormal stress response in adult offspring exposed in utero (Randall,1987).

As of this writing, it is unclear how alcohol acts as a teratogen on the developing brain and other organs. Knowledge gained through research can be reassuring, even if it does not offer solutions to intractable problems.

The consequences of Fetal Alcohol Syndrome involve the broad array of societal agencies and services ranging from the courts, child protective services, and the legislatures. The teratogenic effects of prenatal alcohol or other drug exposure are compounded by the lack of adequate parenting in families where parents are regularly intoxicated. The issues are not simple, and they will defy simple answers. The problem of drinking in young women and adolescent girls also increases the possibility of unintended pregnancies, rape, and incest. Senator Ted Stevens of Alaska (personal communication, 1989) has described isolated communities in his state in which it is difficult to find an 18-year-old girl who has *not* been sexually violated by a member of her own family. Senator Stevens links the incest to the problem of alcohol use in the family. While the existing welfare system has not helped to reduce the problem of FAS, it at least offered a framework for policy research-driven changes that might impact upon the problem or its consequences. As the federal government and individual states pull back substantially from supporting these programs, policymakers and researchers will face the most complex challenges in trying to address the problem of fetal alcohol exposure and its consequences.

OTHER DRUGS

The literature on FAS is much clearer than for the consequences of other types of *in utero* drug exposure. While heroin addiction results in opiate withdrawal in the neonate, there is no evidence that opiates cause teratogenic effects. The literature on cocaine is less clear on this subject, with more data needed on the developmental histories of children who have been exposed to cocaine *in utero*. The children of cocaine-exposed mothers born in the 1980s are now in school. There is a critical need for adequate developmental follow-up on these children. The same issues apply to other drugs of abuse. Nicotine, which is a known teratogen, compounds the challenge to researchers in this field because most of the women who abuse illicit drugs also smoke cigarettes. Many also abuse alcohol. Moreover, the problem of illicit use in the mother does not only relate to possible teratogenic effects. Maternal neglect, family violence, spousal abuse, child abuse, and a variety of subtle and overt forms of deprivation present major problems for children growing up in these environments. On the other hand, the birth of a child can be the point at which a new mother is responsive to referrals for treatment and social services. R. J. Sokol (personal communication, 1990) has pointed out that pregnancy should offer a physiological rationale for a woman to decrease alcohol intake. Non-alcohol-abusing pregnant women find drinking less pleasurable.

Where poverty and addiction coexist in the same individual, the severity of social consequences of the addiction is often substantially greater. It is not that poverty causes addiction; it is true that poverty is a risk factor for the severity of consequences of addiction. One of those consequences is the effect on children in the home. This is a field that needs to bring together clinical, educational, and policy researchers to develop programs that will work for parents and children. The challenges have been developed clearly throughout this volume. The challenge to society is to make the problems of drug- and alcohol-exposed children and their families real enough to care about.

REFERENCES

Abel, E. L., & Sokol, R. J. (1986). Fetal alcohol syndrome is now the leading cause of mental retardation. *The Lancet, ii,* 12–22.

Abel, E. L., & Sokol, R. J. (1987). Incidence of Fetal Alcohol Syndrome and economic impact of FAS-related anomalies. *Drug and Alcohol Dependence, 19,* 51–70.

Erdrich, L. (1989). Foreword. In M. Dorris, *The broken cord,* p. xvii. New York, NY: Harper and Row.

Jones, K. L., Smith, D. W., Ulleland, C. N., & Streissguth, P. (1973). Pattern of malformation of offspring of chronic alcoholic mothers. *The Lancet, 1,* 1267–1271.

Randall, C. L. (1987). Alcohol as a teratogen: A decade of research and review. *Journal of Studies on Alcohol, 1,* 125–132.

Streissguth, A. P., Barr, H. M., Martin, D. C., & Herman, C. (1980). Effects of maternal alcohol, nicotine, and caffeine use during pregnancy on infant development at eight months. *Alcoholism: Clinical and Experimental Research, 41,* 152–164.

PART IV
Appendixes

A

Policy Statements of National Medical, Nursing, Legal, and Social Service Organizations

THE AMERICAN SOCIETY OF ADDICTION MEDICINE PUBLIC POLICY STATEMENT ON CHEMICALLY DEPENDENT WOMEN AND PREGNANCY

BACKGROUND

Because of the adverse effects on fetal development of alcohol and certain other drugs (including nicotine, cocaine, marijuana, and opiates) the chemically dependent woman who is pregnant or may become pregnant is an especially important candidate for intervention and treatment. Similarly, prevention programs should target all women of childbearing age.

Recently, public concern for preventing fetal harm has resulted in punitive measures against pregnant women or women in the postpartum period. These measures have included incarcerating pregnant women in jails to keep them abstinent and the criminal prosecution of mothers for taking drugs while pregnant and thereby passing these substances to the fetus or newborn through the placenta.

The American Society of Addiction Medicine is deeply committed to the prevention of alcohol and other drug-related harm to the health and well-being of children. The most human and effective way to achieve this end is through education, intervention, and treatment. The imposition of criminal penalties solely because a person suffers from an illness is inappropriate and counterproductive. Criminal prosecution of chemically dependent women will have the overall result of deterring such women from seeking both prenatal care and chemical dependency treatment, thereby increasing, rather than preventing, harm to children and to society as a whole.

POLICY RECOMMENDATIONS

The American Society of Addiction Medicine supports the following policies:

1. Prevention programs to educate all members of the public about the dangers of alcohol and other drug use during pregnancy and lactation. These should include:

   - Age-appropriate school-based education throughout the school curriculum.
   - Public education about alcohol and other drug use in pregnancy and lactation, including health warning labels and posters as well as radio and television messages, educational programs and written materials.
   - Prenatal education about alcohol and other drugs for all pregnant women and significant others, as part of adequate prenatal care.
   - Professional education for all health care professionals, including education of obstetricians and pediatricians in the care of chemically dependent women and their offspring.

2. Early intervention, consultation, and case-finding programs specifically designed to reach chemically dependent women:

   - Screening for alcohol and other drug problems in all obstetric care services, as well as in all medical settings.
   - Adequate case finding, intervention, and referral services for women identified as suffering from chemical dependency.

3. Treatment services able to meet the needs of chemically dependent women:

   - Appropriate and accessible chemical dependency treatment services for pregnant women and women of childbearing age and their families, including inpatient and residential treatment. Services to care for the children and newborns of these patients should be provided. Without adequate child care arrangements, chemically dependent women are often unable to engage in the treatment they need.

- Adequate facilities for the outpatient and aftercare phases of treatment for chemically dependent women.
- Adequate prenatal care for chemically dependent women in treatment, sensitive to their special needs.
- Adequate child protection services to provide alternative placement for infants or children of persons suffering from chemical dependency who are unable to function as parents, in the absence of others able to fulfill the parent role.

4. Research:

- Basic and clinical research on the effects of alcohol and other drugs used during pregnancy.
- Model programs, with evaluation component, for case-finding intervention and treatment of chemically dependent pregnant women, and for case finding, intervention, and treatment of infants and children affected by maternal alcohol and/or other drug use.

5. Law enforcement:

- State and local governments should avoid any measures defining alcohol or other drug use during pregnancy as "prenatal child abuse," and should avoid prosecution, jail, or other punitive measures as a substitute for providing effective health services for these women.

6. Preservation of patient confidentiality:

- No law or regulation should require physicians to violate confidentiality by reporting their pregnant patients to state or local authorities for "prenatal child abuse."

Adopted By ASAM Board of Directors 9/25/89
American Society of Addiction Medicine, Inc.
5225 Wisconsin Avenue, N.W. Suite 409
Washington, DC 20015
(202) 244-8948
May 1994

STATEMENT BY RICHARD H. SCHWARZ, M.D.

President
The American College of Obstetricians and Gynecologists
February 27, 1992
at the 1992
Secretarial Conference to
Link Primary Care, HIV, Alcohol,
and Drug Abuse Treatment
Washington, DC

Chemically dependent women of child-bearing age are a critical population in their own right, but often fit into other poorly served groups as well. My fellow panelists are speaking about barriers and problems specific to some of these other critical populations. I ask you to keep in mind as we speak the multiple obstacles for women within these groups.

While attention is justifiably most often focused on the inner city, poor, young, minority population, substance abuse does occur among more affluent women as well. In 1989 the Rhode Island Section of the American College of Obstetricians and Gynecologists collaborated with the state medical society and state health department to do anonymous prevalence testing for a limited number of illicit drugs in the urine of women admitted in active labor. The sample was representative of all births occurring in the state, and included more than 65% of the women giving birth in the state during the study period. Of the 465 women tested, 7.5% were positive for at least one drug. In this study poverty and race other than White did correlate positively with the use of certain drugs. However, fully 6.6% of women who were not poor, and 7% of White women also tested positive for at least one drug.

For those who use drugs, some of the barriers faced by disadvantaged women and by their more fortunate sisters are the same; some are different. Both groups have been let down, not only by society, but also—and this is the point of this conference—by our health care system. The suburban housewife who is pregnant and regularly snorts cocaine may be seeing an obstetrician-gynecologist for prenatal care right on schedule and yet the drug use is unrecognized by the physician. The barriers for this woman include physician attitudes about who may be at risk, and the lack of training to detect the problem and intervene. On the other hand, the pregnant crack-smoking teenager in the inner city often reaches maternity care only when she is in premature labor with hemorrhage from a placental separation. This may occur because the substance abuse professionals working with the young woman have not focused on the pregnancy or have not been able to get the patient into the prenatal care system. For both women, there are significant barriers to proper and effective care and for both, our health care system and society have failed to provide a means to overcome the problems.

Our drug abuse treatment system is male oriented. The perception has been that drug abusers are mostly men. For this reason, prevention and treatment programs have been developed for men. To whatever degree causes and effects of chemical dependence have been studied, or the effectiveness of programs has been validated, the preponderance of the research has involved men. The "war on drugs" has seen criminally violent males as the enemy to be neutralized primarily through law enforcement.

Why should we be surprised, then, to find that the parsimonious allocation of resources in this country to prevention and treatment for drug abuse leaves women behind in an already inadequate system? In New York City, licensed treatment is available for only about 49,000 of the estimated 500,000 to 600,000 substance abusers. Programs attempting to provide enhanced services for women can accommodate only about 4,000. Yet it is expected that approximately 12,000 addicted women will give birth in New York City this year. Furthermore, most substance abuse treatment programs provide only outpatient care, leaving these vulnerable women to return at night, in one scenario to the streets, in another, perhaps to the sheltering facade of their suburban homes with their crack-smoking upwardly mobile husbands. The situation in New York City may be more extreme, but it reflects the general situation throughout the country.

The problem goes beyond the quantity of care. Women's needs are different. Some differences are subtle and need research. Others are painfully obvious: Women often have small children in tow. They may be pregnant. To care for these women effectively, a residential facility must have room and staff for child care, and meet an additional layer of licensure requirements beyond those needed as a drug treatment facility. If pregnant women are cared for, the facility may have additional liability concerns, real or perceived. Providing or interacting with obstetric care resources is not easy. Many physicians and hospitals do give generously of their services: many other shy away, not sure of their skills in the face of unfamiliar complications caused by drug abuse. Women must be treated differently than men. A woman who is pregnant is herself more vulnerable to the effects of substance abuse than one who is not, quite apart from the effect on the fetus. Treatment for drug abuse must be undertaken differently. Physicians see the woman's addiction as hopeless and untreatable. They see any positive effect of medical care being wiped out by lack of self-care. Reimbursement is uncertain, usually low, and bound up in red tape. Worries about physician liability surrounding these high-risk patients are inevitably in the minds of my colleagues. We have a major job to do in reducing the reluctance of many in the health care system so that the important medical needs of women beyond treatment for their chemical dependency are met.

I mentioned before that criminal justice has focused on men and crimes of violence. However, a newer and more ominous trend is for punitive measures to be applied more rigorously to women than to men for substance abuse. It almost seems women are being penalized more for the "crime" of having children or being of child-bearing age than for the drug violation itself. Men are not subjected at the birth of their babies to drug screens reportable to the state with the threat of losing child custody. Nor are they "sentenced" to surgically implanted long-acting contraception. Pamela Rae Stewart's male partner was not jailed for his role in her ingestion of street drugs and having sex with her against the doctor's advice in the final hours of her ill-fated pregnancy. Primary care physicians must not be turned into policemen and detectives against their patients. This will drive women away, not bring them into care.

Finally, the patterns of care for the diagnosis and treatment of HIV are also male oriented in many cases. In my own institution, two percent of women delivering are now HIV positive. Because of this high prevalence we have developed many special skills and programs there. We continue to undergird our efforts with analyses of the clinical research emerging from ours and similar services. But on a national basis, the experience with HIV began with, and has primarily addressed, White males. Clinical manifestations in women are different, and in pregnant women, they differ yet again. We now know that recurrent vaginitis is sometimes an early symptom of HIV in women. Concurrent disease processes are different; there is mounting evidence that susceptibility to and the progression of cervical cancer are exacerbated by HIV infection. Nationally, HIV infection in women is largely drug related, nearly half to their own drug use and almost another quarter to sexual contact with a drug-using man. In New York City, those figures are closer to 60% and 30%. The women most at risk are women of color, and those without money, education, and social supports.

Between 1989 and 1990, the number of women in this country with AIDS increased by 34%, compared with a 22% increase among men. For 1991, it was projected that AIDS would be one of the five leading causes of death among U.S. women between the ages of 15 and 44 years. Furthermore, infants born to HIV positive women are at approximately a 30% risk of being infected. We must do our best to prevent prenatal HIV infection, and to care for affected infants. But we must get beyond viewing women as disease vectors—to their infants and to sexual partners. A man is more likely to transmit HIV to a woman than to acquire it from her, in any case. Programs of research, prevention, and care must be directed specifically to women and their needs.

The regional workshops leading to this conference have identified barriers experience by women and other critical populations. Surely the recommendations offered can make the system more responsive to women. Increasing the representation of women and minorities among health care professionals, developing community participation, providing cultural diversity training for health professionals, and creating social support structures are all essentials to a successful effort. The system must become more sensitive to the critical populations it serves. Public education and prevention programs are of course the ultimate answer but I would like to suggest that given the magnitude of the problem at hand for women, interdisciplinary communication and collaboration along with professional education are key elements for us.

The obstetrician-gynecologist is often in an optimal position to recognize drug abuse and direct the patient toward treatment. This may occur when providing family planning, preconceptional, or maternity care, treatment for sexually transmitted diseases, or general reproductive health care and cancer screening. In fact the obstetrician-gynecologist often is the only health care professional in contact with the patient. Unfortunately, the obstetrician-gynecologist is not always well prepared to recognize the problem or even to ask the appropriate questions. This is especially true in practice settings where substance abuse and HIV are perceived to be uncommon—and unmentionable—but in fact are not so. The American College of Obstetricians and Gynecologists (ACOG) is facing up to the same needs for professional awareness of family violence; my successor as president is about to launch an initiative to help obstetrician-gynecologists confront battering as a serious issue in women's health. Whether it is drug abuse, violence, or another of the social pathologies, as physicians for women, we cannot opt out. Many of the solutions require physician education and the responsibility rests squarely on the medical schools and residency training programs, and on the continuing education of practicing physicians. The latter is the province of my own organization, ACOG, which represents over 31,000 specialists in reproductive health care. We must do better in that regard and I promise we will.

We as physicians must improve our attitudes about poor and minority patients, but also we must eliminate our blind spots to dangerous personal behavior by patients who seem "just like us." We must give our colleagues workable tools for identifying problems of a sensitive nature that go beyond the comfortable sphere of anatomy, physiology, and the disease process. Physicians need to hear that these patients are worth caring for, that chronic conditions require patience, and that treatment works. We must teach them how to locate and collaborate with substance abuse and HIV treatment systems and community resources. We must acknowledge that our responsibility for improving women's health care cannot stop at some neat boundary that excludes the life each woman leads with her family and significant others, and in her work and community environment.

But suppose we do all this? Suppose obstetrician-gynecologists become aware, develop skills, communicate with specialists in treating the problems beyond their training? Will there be places to refer women for appropriate care?

I have alluded to failings in the drug treatment programs in dealing with women patients. Focused as these services are on the difficult drug problem, reproductive health care often falls by the wayside. Screening for sexually transmitted diseases, especially HIV and syphilis, is critical, as is contraceptive counseling, yet these services are often not provided in these settings. Early recognition of pregnancy is essential to providing women with all their reproductive options as well as to optimal pregnancy outcome. This may not occur in a substance abuse clinic with a staff not experienced in this area and often not equipped for the appropriate examinations.

Once again the answer lies in communication and education. Perhaps the easiest solution, if the patient volume warrants, is a collaborative venture in which a prepared and willing obstetrician-gynecologist is available in the substance abuse clinic or the reverse in which, for example, there is a special prenatal clinic for drug-using patients, which is staffed by appropriate members of both teams. In fact, in the ideal situation for the pregnant patient, programs incorporate treatment for her significant other, parenting education, child care, nutritional services, and vocational guidance, and related services into the medical care and substance abuse treatment for the woman. This approach can facilitate the social reentry of the woman after delivery. A few comprehensive programs like this do exist, but they demand tremendous dedication and a commitment to pay now, rather than later, for the societal cost of drug abuse.

Just as communication and collaboration among providers are the keys to the successful management of patients, it is essential, I believe, that there be better communication among the numerous federal, state, and local agencies which provide the major share of resources and regulate and shape both public and private care. Too often failures in this are result in either gaps or redundancies in a system which is already less than adequate to meet the needs. The suggestion that there be a commission to advise Secretary Sullivan might well be a first step toward coordination at the national level. But it will be effective only if duplicated at the local level.

Drug abuse in women has not received the attention it deserves. When anyone abuses drugs it becomes a family problem. Drug use during pregnancy impacts on the fetus, and the high prevalence of HIV infection in substance abusers places the next generation in jeopardy of this infection as well. While we must focus attention for the long term on prevention, for the present, we must deal with the problem at hand and we must do so more effectively than we are now.

I said drug abuse in women has not received the attention it deserves. That is true. On the contrary, **it has received all too much attention,** by a frightened and misinformed public and by segments of the media and politicians who seek their own kind of gain from the sensational and from laying blame on others, including far more than a fair share on women whose personal circumstances they cannot possibly assess. The problems challenge the best of our scientific acumen, the most creative efforts of our public health system, a societal will to address root causes, and the utmost in compassion from all of us.

American College of Obstetricians and Gynecologist
409 12th St., SW
Washington, DC 20024-2188
(202) 638-5577

AMERICAN NURSES ASSOCIATION
APRIL 5, 1991 POSITION STATEMENT
ON
Opposition to Criminal Prosecution of Women for Use of Drugs
While Pregnant and Support for Treatment Services for Alcohol and
Drug Dependent Women of Childbearing Age

Summary: Perinatal alcohol and other drug abuse has serious consequences for mothers and children. ANA supports treatment services for women of childbearing age that are alcohol and drug-dependent and is in opposition to criminal prosecution and punishment of these women.

Perinatal alcohol and other drug abuse is a major societal problem with serious consequences for the nation's mothers and children. Addiction is a primary disease requiring specialized treatment to achieve a process of long-term behavior change known as recovery. ANA is also opposed to the application of current laws for criminal prosecution of alcohol and drug dependent women solely because they were pregnant when they used alcohol or other drugs and opposes any legislation that focuses on the criminal punishment of the mothers of drug-exposed infants. ANA recognizes alcohol and other drug problems as treatable illnesses. The threat of criminal prosecution is counterproductive in that it prevents many women from seeking prenatal care and treatment for their alcohol and other drug problems. There are presently few alcohol and other drug abuse treatment services available for pregnant women and few programs designed specifically for women of childbearing age, and due to perceived risk of liabilities of care for the unborn child and/or regulations at state levels of care. ANA supports a marked increase in funding at federal, state and local levels for development and expansion of alcohol and other drug abuse treatment services tailored to meet the special needs of women of childbearing age.

ANA is committed to prevention and treatment as primary solutions to perinatal substance abuse and addiction. There is an urgent need for nursing and other research designed to improve the knowledge base upon which prevention and treatment efforts are based and to test innovative interventions tailored to women of childbearing age.

The Coalition on Alcohol and Drug Dependent Women and Their Children reports that an increasing number of women are being arrested and prosecuted solely because they used drugs while they were pregnant. Laws are being applied that were never intended to pertain to the behavior of pregnant women. Pregnant women also find themselves receiving stiffer sentences than those being imposed on men and women who are not pregnant. Some states are considering new laws to make drug use during pregnancy a felony subject to a punishment of imprisonment. ANA joins the Coalition on Alcohol and Drug Dependent Women and their Children in opposing these trends toward criminalization of drug use during pregnancy as constituting extreme, inappropriate, and ineffective responses to health problems. In order for pregnant women to receive health care that is sensitive to potential or existing drug problems, women must feel that they can seek care and give information regarding their drug use or other problematic behavior without fear or punishment.

American Nurses Association
600 Maryland Avenue, S.W.
Washington, DC 20024
(202) 554-4444

NATIONAL COMMISSION ON CORRECTIONAL
HEALTH CARE POSITION PAPER

WOMEN'S HEALTH CARE IN CORRECTIONAL SETTINGS

Background

The number of women under the jurisdiction of state and federal prison authorities at the end of 1989 reached a record 40,556. While this number represents a relatively small percentage of the overall prison population (5.7%), the rate of growth for female inmates has exceeded that for males each year since 1981 (Greenfeld and Minor-Harper, 1990). An additional 37,383 women were held in local jails in 1989, which represents 9.5% of all jail inmates. Between 1983 and 1989, the rate of growth for female jail inmates was 138%, which was almost twice that for males (Snell, 1992).

Studies show that incarcerated women utilize health care services much more than men and the reasons for this increased utilization include a woman's more complicated reproductive system, sexually transmitted diseases, and pregnancies. Upon entry into corrections, women report problems with alcohol abuse, headaches, fatigue, drug abuse, and sexually transmitted diseases. Further it has been estimated that 10 percent of women entering correctional facilities are noted to have psychiatric problems with depression being the most common diagnostic category (*CorHealth—The Newsletter of the American Correctional Health Services Association,* Summer 1993).

Entering a correctional facility is very stressful, but for women this issue is even more intense because of separation from their children; studies across the country show that approximately 75 to 85 percent of incarcerated women have children, most of them coming from single-parent households. It has been reported that two-thirds of female prison and jail inmates had children under 18 (Greenfeld and Minor-Harper, 1990; Snell, 1992). Another study noted that between 50 and 70% of incarcerated women had one or more dependent children who were living with them prior to their imprisonment (Baunach, 1985). Thus, appropriate services for female inmates should include parenting and child custody issues.

From 40 to 60 percent of the women in prisons and jails have reported that they had been previously sexually or physically abused (Greenfeld and Minor-Harper, 1990; Snell, 1992; *CorHealth—The Newsletter of the American Correctional Health Services Association,* Summer

1993). Such experiences can lead to life long psychological problems ranging from depressive disorders, stress disorders, anxiety disorders, substance abuse (with its attendant physical health problems), behavioral disorders of violence and impassivity, and learning problems. Further, being victimized can have serious consequences on women's ability to parent their children. Unfortunately, health care professionals have not been trained to take the experience of victimization into account when they treat patients and this shortcoming limits the quality of health care they are able to deliver to women. For example, it has been suggested that having been sexually assaulted discourages women from obtaining regular Pap smears.

A history of problems with alcohol and/or other drugs is another common complaint of women entering correctional facilities and because of this abuse, many of these women are at much greater risk of becoming HIV+ from having had unprotected sex or having used dirty needles. An estimated 72 percent of the women in state prisons in 1989 had used drugs at some time in their lives prior to their incarceration. A third of all female prison inmates reported they were under the influence of a drug at the time of their offense, and 39 percent reported that they were using drugs daily in the month before their offense with 24% reporting daily use of a major drug (cocaine, heroin, methadone, LSD, or PCP) in that month (Greenfeld and Minor-Harper, 1990). That same year, almost 84 percent of convicted female jail inmates said that they had used drugs, and 37.5 percent were under the influence at the time of arrest (Snell, 1992). By 1991, 79.5 percent of the women in state prisons said they had ever used drugs and 53.9 percent said they had used drugs in the month before their current offense (Snell and Morton, 1994).

Research regarding the provision of gynecological services for women in correctional settings has been limited, but it consistently has indicated that such services are inadequate. Annual gynecological exams are not done routinely in either jails or prisons, nor are they regularly performed upon admission. Appropriate initial screening questions about a woman's gynecologic history may not be asked, and in many correctional facilities, there are no physicians who are trained in obstetrics and gynecology leading to inadequate and inappropriate gynecologic care. As a result, women in jails and prisons are at risk for the lack of detection of some diseases such as breast cancer, ovarian cancer, and abnormal Pap smears. In addition, because of past medical histories of many incarcerated women, their pregnancies tend to be more complicated. Further, many women enter jails and prisons while pregnant and they need adequate prenatal care and reproductive counseling such as family planning and birth control. In addition, postpartum screening for physical and psychiatric complications are needed.

The circumstances of women's incarceration are unique. It has been estimated that a third of the female state prison inmates in 1991 were there for violent crimes, with a third of that number serving time for a homicide. Nearly two-thirds of all female inmates serving time for a violent crime had victimized someone they knew, and among these offenders, half had victimized either an intimate or a family member such as a parent, sibling, or even their own child (Snell and Morton, 1994). More than a fourth of the women in prison for violence were convicted of the homicide of a family member, ex-spouse or, another intimate. Women incarcerated for a violent offense were the most likely to report previously having experienced physical or sexual abuse; and, among women incarcerated for a violent crime, those who reported that they had been abused were more likely than other offenders to have victimized a relative or intimate (Greenfeld and Minor-Harper, 1990).

The National Commission on Correctional Health Care (1992 a, b, c) recognizes the need to provide treatment to this special population. The Receiving Screening standard (J-31, P-31, and Y-28 Initial Health Screening) suggests inquiry into current gynecological problems and pregnancy for women and female adolescents; the Health Assessment standard (J-35, P-34, and Y-33 Health Appraisal) suggests pelvic examinations and Pap smears should be considered but are not mandated, except in prisons; the Health Promotion and Disease Prevention standard (J-45, P-45, and Y-47) recommends self-examination for breast cancer and family planning as a subject for health education; and the Dietary Services Y-54, along with Appendix IV Nutrition Guidelines, address the issue of nutritional intake. Standards J-56, P-56, and Y-37 and J-57, P-57, and Y-14 (Family Planning Services) which are used in the Commission's accreditation program for jails, prisons, and juvenile detention and confinement facilities (respectively) include the following:

J-56 & P-56 Pregnant Inmates (important)

Written policy and defined procedures require, and actual practice evidences, that comprehensive counseling and assistance are given to pregnant inmates in keeping with their express desire in planning for their unborn children, whether they desire abortion, adoptive service, or to keep the child.

Y-37 Pregnant Juveniles (essential)

In recognition of the high-risk nature of adolescent pregnancy, juveniles remaining in the facility after pregnancy has been diagnosed receive regular pre-natal and post-natal care, including medical examinations, appropriate activity levels, safety precautions, nutrition, guidance, and counseling.

J-57 & P-57 Prenatal Care (essential)

Inmates remaining in the jail (prison) after pregnancy has been diagnosed receive regular prenatal care, including medical examinations, advice on appropriate levels of activity and safety precautions, nutrition guidance, and counseling.

Y-14 Family Planning Services (important)

Written policy and defined procedure require that comprehensive family planning services, in accordance with states, be available on the premises or by referral.

POSITION STATEMENT

The National Commission on Correctional Health Care recognizes that the number of female inmates is large and is growing annually, and presents unique and increasing health problems for correctional facilities. Therefore, the Commission recommends the following.

1. All correctional institutions should be required to meet recognized community standards for female health services as promoted by standards set by the National Commission on Correctional Health Care.
2. Correctional health services and women's advocacy groups should collaborate to provide leadership for the development of policies and procedures that address women's special health care needs in corrections.
3. Correctional institutions should provide intake procedures that include histories on menstrual cycle, pregnancies, gynecologic problems, and nutritional intake (by conducting a nutritional assessment) (Anno, 1991).
4. Correctional institutions should provide intake examinations that include a breast exam and, depending on the patient's age, sexual history, and past medical history, a pelvic exam, Pap smear, and baseline mammogram (Anno, 1991).

5. Correctional institutions should provide laboratory tests to detect sexually transmitted diseases (STDs) including gonorrhea, syphilis, and chlamydia for all females, especially since many are asymptomatic for STDs. Additionally, females should receive a pregnancy test on admission to correctional facilities (Anno, 1991). Further, since new research has indicated that pregnant women who are infected with HIV are less likely to transmit the virus to their newborn if they are treated with AZT during their pregnancy, women should be educated about this new finding and encouraged to be tested for HIV if they are pregnant.

6. Comprehensive services for women's unique health problems should be provided in prisons, jails, and juvenile detention and confinement facilities:

   A) Considering the special reproductive health needs of women, the frequency of repeating certain tests, exams, and procedures (e.g. Pap smears, mammogram, etc.) should be based on guidelines established by professional groups such as the American Cancer Society and the American College of Obstetricians and Gynecologists, and should take into account age and risk factors of the female correctional population (Anno, 1991).

   B) Considering the high levels of victimization (sexual and physical) within the female inmate population, and considering the circumstances of incarceration of violent female offenders (i.e., they frequently have committed interpersonal altercation violence against a family member or intimate), counseling to resolve issues of victimization and perpetration of violence against intimates (such as conflict resolution skills or parenting skills) should be available.

   C) Considering the large number of women who are incarcerated who have dependent children, counseling on issues of parenting and child custody issues should be available to women in correctional institutions.

   D) Considering the high rates of depression women report upon incarceration, counseling should be available to women in correctional facilities to address this issue.

   E) Considering the high rates of alcohol and/or drug problems women report on incarceration, counseling should be available to women in correctional facilities to address this issue.

   F) Considering the unique developmental needs of female adolescents, special attention should be given to their needs in the provision of the aforementioned services.

G) Considering that many female adolescents who enter the juvenile justice system have unique educational needs, special attention needs to be given to counseling and habilitation in this area.

Adopted by the Board of Directors
September 25, 1994

REFERENCES

ACHSA president testifies before the Senate. (Summer, 1993). *CorHealth—The Newsletter of the American Correctional Health Services Association*, pp. 1–2.

Anno, B. J. (1991). *Prison Health Care: Guidelines for the Management of an Adequate Delivery System*. Chicago: National Commission on Correctional Health Care.

Baunach, P. J. (1985). Mothers in Prison. New Brunswick, New Jersey: Transaction Books.

Greenfeld, L. A. and Minor-Harper S. (March 1990). Women in Prison. Washington D.C.: U.S. Department of Justice, Office of Justice Programs, Bureau of Justice Statistics. (NCJ-127991).

National Commission on Correctional Health Care (1992a). *Standards for Health Services in Jails*. Chicago: Author.

National Commission on Correctional Health Care (1992b). *Standards for Health Services in Juvenile Detention and Confinement Centers*. Chicago: author.

National Commission on Correctional Health Care (1992c). *Standards for Health Services in Prison*. Chicago: Author.

Snell, T. L. (March 1990). Women in Jail, 1989. Washington D.C.: U.S. Department of Justice, Office of Justice Programs, Bureau of Justice Statistics. (NCJ-134732).

Snell, T. L. and Morton, D. C. (March 1994). Women in prison: Survey of state inmates 1991. Washington D.C.: U.S. Department of Justice, Office of Justice Programs, Bureau of Justice Statistics. (NCJ-145321).

National Commission on Correctional Health Care
2105 N. Southport, Chicago, IL 60614-4017
(312) 528-0818

GUIDELINES FOR PERINATAL CARE

Third Edition

American Academy of Pediatrics
American College of Obstetricians and Gynecologists
Supported in part by
March of Dimes
BIRTH DEFECTS FOUNDATION

Guidelines for Perinatal Care was developed through the cooperative efforts of the AAP Committee on Fetus and Newborn and the ACOG Committee on Obstetrics: Maternal and Fetal Medicine. The guidelines should not be viewed as a body of rigid rules. They are general and intended to be adapted to many different situations, taking into account the needs and resources particular to the locality, the institution, or type of practice. Variations and innovations that improve the quality of patient care are to be encouraged rather than restricted. The purpose of these guidelines will be well served if they provide a firm basis on which local norms may be built. The segments related to obstetric practice do not replace the ACOG *Standards for Obstetric— Gynecologic Services,* but rather expand on the principles suggested therein.

SUBSTANCE ABUSE

Recent studies have documented that an increasing number of women of childbearing age are abusing licit and illicit substances. Although statistical data are insufficient, there are indications that approximately 1 in 10 infants may be exposed to illicit drugs during pregnancy. The National Institute on Drug Abuse 1988 National Household Survey revealed that 8.8% of women of childbearing age admitted to having used an illicit drug in the month before questioning. A recent survey of 36 private and public hospitals showed that approximately 11% of women delivering in these hospitals had used illegal drugs at some time during their pregnancies. A preliminary study in Pinellas County, Florida, demonstrated that cocaine and marijuana use during pregnancy were almost equally distributed across racial and socioeconomic lines.

Drug-Exposed Infants

An increasing number of infants are being admitted to special-care nurseries for complications caused by their intrauterine exposure to alcohol and other drugs. It is important to consider that drug-exposed infants often go unrecognized and are discharged from the newborn nursery to homes where they are at increased risk for a complex of medical and social problems, including abuse and neglect.

The Problem

All illicit drugs reach the fetal circulation by crossing the placenta, and they can cause direct toxic effects on the fetus, as well as fetal and maternal dependency. For example, the opiate-exposed fetus may experience withdrawal in utero when drugs are withdrawn from a dependent mother or, after delivery, when the mother's use no longer directly affects her newborn. Although the incidence of breast-feeding by substance-abusing mothers is generally low, it is important to counsel nursing mothers about the hazards of drug use.

Symptoms of neonatal opiate withdrawal are often present at birth but may not reach a peak until 3–4 days or as late as 10–14 days after birth. Evidence of withdrawal from narcotics can persist in a subacute form for 4–6 months after birth. Common features of the neonatal abstinence syndrome mimic those of an adult's withdrawal from narcotics. Significant signs and symptoms for the neonate include a high-pitched cry, sweating, tremulousness, excoriation of the extremities, and gastrointestinal disturbances. Although withdrawal from nonnarcotic substances, such as marijuana, does not appear to result in as severe a syndrome of abstinence as withdrawal from narcotics, the newborn may exhibit irritability and restlessness, poor feeding, crying, and impaired neurobehavioral activity also seen in the neonatal narcotics abstinence syndrome. There is a need for increased research to define the degree of permanent residual in these infants.

Environmental factors also place drug-exposed children at high risk for abuse, neglect, and developmental delay. The long-term effects on learning and school performance of children exposed to illicit drugs in utero have not been well documented. Although some research is in press to study this issue, more emphasis is needed in this area.

Pediatric Implications

Universal neonatal screening for illicit drugs is not recommended. The long-term consequences, i.e., the harms versus the benefits of labeling the infant or the mother (or both), are not known. However, since there are well-documented and potential effects on children exposed to drugs in utero, it is essential that pediatricians recognize drug-exposed infants. Obtaining a thorough maternal history in a nonthreatening, organized manner, from all women, is the key to diagnosis. Screens will surely be negative when drugs were used early in pregnancy and can be negative even when women have taken drugs during the 48 hours before delivery. Because urine toxicology screens may vary among laboratories, pediatricians should be aware that tests for marijuana, its metabolites, and the metabolites of cocaine may not be included unless requested specifically.

Infants and children of substance-abusing parents or guardians are at increased risk for physical, sexual, and emotional abuse. Although all states require physicians to report suspected child abuse or neglect, some states also mandate reporting to child protective services infants with neonatal drug screens positive for illicit drugs. Many of these agencies are overburdened and unprepared to deal appropriately with the potential flood of babies born to substance-abusing mothers. Pediatricians should, therefore, work with their state social service agencies and state legislatures to extend the assistance now available through child protective services. Until that is accomplished, pediatricians should consider recruiting the assistance of the local child protective services agency to provide multidisciplinary treatment and support for the affected mother, child, and family. Local pediatricians should discuss with all professionals and agencies involved how multifaceted problems resulting from drug exposure in utero might best be addressed in their communities. In general, a coordinated multidisciplinary approach in the development of a plan without criminal sanctions has the best chance of helping children and families.

Health Policy

Health policy issues posed by drug-exposed infants can be divided into two components: 1) how to prevent infants from being exposed to potentially harmful drugs before birth and 2) how to address the needs of drug-exposed infants and children.

Prevention of exposure before birth is a vexing problem that has defied solution. At the threshold is a need to explore more effective ways to help people resist the initial and subsequent use of drugs. Until the issue of how to prevent drug exposure appropriately and effectively is resolved, we are left to deal with how to address the needs of drug-exposed infants as children. Although there are some data about the potential for illicit drugs to cause congenital malformations and other health problems in the infant and young child, little is known about subsequent problems confronting drug-exposed infants as they enter their school years and adolescence. Longitudinal studies of these children are crucial.

The following recommendations are offered as a means of dealing with the health policy issues posed by substance abuse:

- Pediatricians can be involved in organizing community-based social service or child protective service systems, designed to provide essential services for drug-abusing women and their children.
- A comprehensive medical and psychosocial history, including specific inquiry regarding maternal drug use, should be a part of every newborn evaluation.
- Newborn urine toxicology should be regarded only as potential adjunct to a thorough maternal drug history. Universal toxicologic screening is not recommended.
- The pediatrician should include maternal drug use in the differential diagnosis of any neonate with suggestive symptomatology.
- The pediatrician should be knowledgeable about state and local child protection reporting requirements.
- In most circumstances, when a drug-exposed infant or drug-abusing mother is identified, the pediatrician should consider recruiting the assistance of local child protective services to provide multidisciplinary treatment and support for the affected mother, child, and family.
- The pediatrician should evaluate the drug-exposed infant for other medical conditions associated with maternal drug use, including the possibility of concurrent sexually transmitted diseases in the mother and infant.
- Since adverse effects of drug exposure may not be evident at birth, the pediatrician should be alert to potential long-term consequences that may become apparent during ongoing care.
- Models of coordinated nultidisciplinary prevention, intervention, and treatment services that improve access to early comprehensive care for all substance-abusing pregnant women and their children should be developed and evaluated. Evaluation of current and new treatment modalities is imperative to determine their effectiveness.
- Funds for research, prevention, and treatment should be made available to address issues of drug-exposed infants.

- The public must be assured of nonpunitive access to comprehensive care that will meet the needs of the substance-abusing pregnant woman and her infant.
- Pediatricians are encouraged to become actively involved in policy issues related to drug-exposed infants and children at the federal, state, and local levels.

Cocaine Abuse in Pregnancy

Cocaine has become a major public health concern as a result of the dramatic increase in its use over the last decade. In the 1970s, cocaine use was primarily limited to the well-to-do because of its expense, with the intranasal route preferred. More recently, there has been a decrease in the street cost and an increasing prevalence of intravenous and smoked routes of administration. This change in the pattern of use has increased the potential for medical complications and for compulsive or addictive use.

Cocaine, with street names of coke, snow, lady, and gold dust, is a local anesthetic derived from the leaves of *Erythroxylon coca,* a tree indigenous to Peru and Bolivia. When administered systemically, cocaine blocks the presynaptic reuptake of sympathomimetic transmitters (norepinephrine and dopamine), allowing for excess transmitter at the postsynaptic receptor sites. The potentiation of norepinephrine results in intense vasoconstriction, an acute rise in arterial pressure, and tachycardia. Both the euphoria and the reinforcing or addictive effects of the drug are thought to be related to the potentiation of dopamine in the central nervous system. Cocaine is commonly used intranasally (snorting), intravenously, orally, and by smoking the free alkaloid form (freebasing). Crack is a highly purified form of the free alkaloid, so named because of the cracking or popping sound made when the crystals are heated in a test tube.

Maternal Implications

The pharmacokinetics of cocaine use during pregnancy has been poorly studied, although cocaine is known to cross the placenta readily. It is thought that urine tests of neonates exposed to transplacental cocaine may be positive for a period of time similar to that for the adult, although benzoylecgonine has been detected in neonatal urine for up to 4 days with an assay sensitive to 10 ng/ml.

Cocaine is degraded by plasma and hepatic cholinesterases to water-soluble metabolites (benzoylecgonine and ecgonine methylester). The most commonly used urine test detects benzoylecgonine at a sensitivity of 300 ng/ml. The elimination half-time is approximately 4.5 hours, allowing detection in urine for 24–48 hours after varying intravenous doses.

Serious medical complications reported in association with cocaine use include the following:

- Acute myocardial infarction, both with and without underlying coronary artery disease
- Cardiac arrhythmias, including life-threatening ventricular arrhythmias
- Rupture of the ascending aorta
- Cerebrovascular accidents
- Seizures
- Bowel ischemia
- Hyperthermia
- Sudden death

These complications are directly or indirectly attributable to the intense sympathomimetic effects of cocaine.

Research in perinatal cocaine abuse is problematic because of a population of patients who tend to have unplanned pregnancies of uncertain gestational age, to seek prenatal care late, to have suboptimal nutrition, to be heavy cigarette smokers and multiple drug abusers, and to fail to keep appointments. For these reasons, data are often incomplete and control groups are difficult to construct.

As in other substance-abusing populations, cocaine-dependent pregnant women have a high incidence of infectious diseases, especially hepatitis, acquired immune deficiency syndrome, and other sexually transmitted diseases. Other problems during pregnancy are anticipated in a population that underutilizes prenatal care. Even so, cocaine-using women often experience an uncomplicated labor and delivery, although they may be at increased risk of abruptio placentae. The outcomes of pregnancies complicated by cocaine abuse have consistently been shown to be worse than those complicated by abuse of other substances.

Neonatal Implications

Cocaine abuse during pregnancy should be considered a major perinatal risk. Cocaine-exposed infants have an increased incidence of premature birth, impaired fetal growth, and neonatal seizures. Although a specific cocaine withdrawal syndrome in the neonate has not been defined clearly, signs of irritability and tremulousness, lethargy, or an inability to respond appropriately to stimulation may occur. Many, however, seem to have specific clinical manifestations in the early neonatal period.

Perinatal cerebral infarctions have occurred in infants whose mothers have used cocaine during the few days before delivery. These perinatal cerebral infarctions exemplify the severe morbidity that may be associated with intrauterine exposure to cocaine. Issues of increased risk of malformations and abnormalities of respiratory control have been raised but await confirmatory studies. Because most published studies of cocaine's effect on pregnancies and infants have focused on recognized substance-abusing populations, little information is a available regarding the effects of low doses of cocaine. In addition, interpretations of clinical studies are complicated by the fact that abuse of multiple drugs often occurs.

A survey of urban hospitals demonstrated positive urine toxicology for cocaine metabolites in 10–25% of pregnancies. The seriousness of perinatal cocaine abuse is underscored by the marked increase in use of the drug by women of childbearing age, by the misconception that cocaine is neither dangerous nor addictive, and by the ability of many cocaine users to hide their habits. Accordingly, the following recommendations are made:

- All pregnant women should be queried regarding past and present drug use at the time of the first prenatal visit.
- A woman acknowledging cocaine use should be carefully counseled regarding the perinatal implications of cocaine use in pregnancy and offered support mechanisms to aid in her abstinence, if appropriate.
- To reinforce and encourage continued abstinence, periodic urine testing for metabolites of cocaine may be desirable in a pregnant woman admitting to cocaine use prior to or during pregnancy. The requirement for consent may vary from state to state.
- Urine testing of the mother or the neonate or both may be useful in some clinical situations, such as in the presence of unexplained intrauterine growth retardation, third-trimester stillbirth, unexpected prematurity, or abruptio placentae in a woman not known to have hypertensive disease, even when cocaine abuse has not been previously suspected.

RESOURCES AND RECOMMENDED READING

American Academy of Pediatrics, Committee on Substance Abuse. Drug-exposed infants. *Pediatrics* 1990; *86*(4):639–642.

American College of Obstetricians and Gynecologists. *Cocaine abuse: Implications for pregnancy.* Committee Opinion 81. Washington, DC: ACOG, 1990.

B

Model Statute of the National Alliance for Model State Drug Laws

Note: Additional information on the Model Statute is available from the National Alliance for Model State Drug Laws. (Formerly the President's Commission on Model State Drug Laws), Alexandria, VA (703) 836-6100.

THE WHITE HOUSE PRESIDENT'S COMMISSION ON MODEL STATE DRUG LAWS

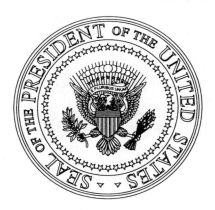

TREATMENT

December 1993

299

MODEL FAMILY PRESERVATION ACT POLICY STATEMENT

Pregnant addicted girls and women and parents with dependent children face many obstacles when seeking treatment for addiction. Although outpatient services are generally available, there is a severe shortage of alcohol and other drug addiction residential treatment programs designed to serve the inpatient treatment needs of this population.

Across the country there are a range of outpatient and inpatient drug and alcohol addiction treatment programs. Although the numbers of programs and geographic accessibility of programs vary widely in the states, some of these programs are available to accommodate the treatment needs of adolescents, adults and pregnant addicted women and girls. However, few inpatient programs are physically constructed or programmatically structured to handle the needs of mothers with newborns and parents with dependent children.

In recognition of the changing roles in society, services developed to address this gap in the continuum of care will want to consider the needs of pregnant girls and women and the needs of men as well as women who have dependent children.

Although gender roles are changing, girls and women still handle the bulk of the responsibility for the care of infants and young children. For this reason, the shortage of facilities also able to accommodate dependent children primarily affects girls and women when there is need for inpatient treatment.

Stigma and negative stereotyping surrounding addiction is intense for both men and women. This leads to delays in seeking help and reinforces the denial of even the existence of the problem. However, stigma for girls and women is generally more intense and is in part, responsible for delaying identification and referral until later in the progression of the disease.

Compounding the problem of stigma, a woman in need of inpatient care is often faced with a decision to give up her children to gain access to treatment. The children often represent her last vestige of self-respect and self-esteem. In addition, once a woman has identified her addiction and sought addiction treatment, she is likely to have trouble maintaining or regaining custody of the children after treatment is concluded. Fearful of losing custody of her children, going to treatment becomes a choice few women are prepared to make.

This primary barrier to care can be averted by the development of residential rehabilitation centers prepared to address the inpatient treatment needs of girls, women and men with dependent children. In addition to addressing the addiction, these programs need to be structured to teach parenting, nutrition, and other life skills as well as to provide preparation and linkage to educational and vocational programs.

The best way to help the drug-exposed child is to help the parent recover from addiction. Treatment must be comprehensive and provided in an environment where the multivariate needs of parents and children can be addressed. A key element of the comprehensive service model is a continuum of family-oriented services directed at numerous risk factors and available at a single site.[1]

Since children of alcoholics and addicts are at high risk of developing addictions themselves, another necessary component of care is age appropriate prevention and education for them. In addition, intervention and counseling for the children is often needed to resolve the problems of living with an untreated alcohol and/or drug addicted parent.

The cost benefits to society are obvious even if measured only in the prevention of fetal alcohol and drug effect and syndrome.[2] For drug-exposed infants, hospital costs alone are 4 times higher than they are for non-exposed infants.[3] Heavy alcohol use during pregnancy is a leading cause of birth defects associated with mental retardation. Fetal alcohol syndrome is the leading known environmental cause of mental retardation in the western world.[4]

In addition to reducing health care costs to society, effective treatment with this population also lessens the social and economic costs of decreased productivity, accidents and crime.

These programs do far more than prevent fetal impairment. They hold out hope of healing the fractured families of addiction and of breaking the multi-generational cycle of alcohol and other drug abuse.

ENDNOTES

1. Kandall S., et al., TREATMENT IMPROVEMENT PROTOCOL (TIP): DRUG-EXPOSED INFANTS, THE RECOMMENDATIONS OF A CONSENSUS PANEL (Center for Substance Abuse Treatment, U.S. Department of Health and Human Services, 1992).
2. Langenbucher, J. W., McCrady, B. S., Brick, J. Esterly, R., *Addictions Treatment with Pregnant Women, Chapter 7,* in SOCIOECONOMIC EVALUATIONS OF ADDICTIONS TREATMENT (Center of Alcohol Studies, Rutgers University, 1993).

3. U.S. General Accounting Office, DRUG EXPOSED INFANTS: A GENER-
    ATION AT RISK (B-238209, June 1990).
4. National Institute on Alcohol Abuse and Alcoholism, 8th SPECIAL
    REPORT TO THE UNITED STATES CONGRESS ON ALCOHOL AND
    HEALTH (U.S. Department of Health and Human Services, Washington,
    DC, 1993).

HIGHLIGHTS OF THE MODEL
FAMILY PRESERVATION ACT

- Encourages the establishment
  of residential addiction treatment programs for pregnant
  addicted girls and women and
  parents with dependent children.
- Establishes program elements
  that are family-centered in focus.
- Establishes program elements
  that are addiction oriented.
- Provides for an array of support
  services attuned to the needs of
  addicted people with dependent children.

- Provides for educational and
  vocational counseling and services geared to re-entry and
  restoring self-sufficiency.
- Requires data collection and
  annual reporting to the governor and legislature.
- Establishes a training program
  for related health and human
  services to enhance identification and referral for help.

MODEL FAMILY PRESERVATION ACT

Section 1. Title

The provisions of this [Act] shall
be known and may be cited as the
"Model Family Preservation Act."

Section 2. Legislative Findings.

(a) An epidemic of alcohol
and other drug abuse among
women of childbearing years is
destroying the lives of count-
less women, young children,
and babies.

(b) In addition to the obligation
of society to protect young
lives, fiscal responsibility alone
requires that the skyrocketing
costs to society of lifetime
care for children and families
affected by alcohol and other
drugs be addressed. To avoid
or reduce these costs, alcohol
and other drug treatment programs for all women of childbearing years and parents in

need of such programs must be provided.

(c) There is a serious shortage of such alcohol and other drug treatment resources for women of childbearing years.

(d) Women with small children and pregnant women are further inhibited from seeking treatment by being forced to give up their children to enter inpatient treatment care and by the threat that they will lose long-term custody of their children if they seek treatment.

(e) Children raised in families with an addicted parent are at a high risk to develop the disease of addiction as they grow older.

(f) Impaired parenting by addicted parents may place the children at risk of developing social, emotional, and scholastic problems.

(g) Treatment of parents which includes the counseling of dependent children allows the parent(s) to maintain custody or contact and increases the likelihood of a successful recovery and the interruption of the cycle of addiction.

(h) Whenever consistent with and appropriate to the recovery of the parent and child in treatment, the noncustodial parent shall be included in parenting skills training, treatment, family counseling and other relevant activities.

COMMENT

The chapter entitled Addictions Treatment with Pregnant Women, from the Rutgers University study SOCIOECONOMIC EVALUATIONS OF ADDICTIONS TREATMENT, provides a sense of the substantial costs to society of fetal alcohol and other drug effect and syndrome. The ongoing costs of not addressing this problem are higher than providing addiction treatment.

Section 3. Residential Alcohol and Other Drug Treatment Programs for Women in Childbearing Years, Pregnant Women, and Parents and Their Dependent Children.

(a) The [single state authority on alcohol and other drugs] shall [provide] [have the power to provide] directly or through grants to residential alcohol and other drug treatment and related services for women in childbearing years, pregnant women, parents and their dependent children and parents who do not have custody of their children where there is a reasonable likelihood that the children will be returned to them if the parent participates satisfactorily in the treatment program. Grant moneys shall be used for treatment and related services provided to residents of this state by alcohol and other drug treatment programs licensed by the [single state authority on alcohol and other drugs] which provide the following services:

(1) Residential treatment services for women and their children, subject to reasonable limitations on the number and ages of the children, provided in a therapeutic community setting and including, but not limited to:

(A) On-site family centered addiction and alcohol and other drug abuse education, counseling and treatment;

(B) On-site individual, group and family counseling including both parents where appropriate;

(C) On-site alcohol and other drug prevention and education activities for children approved by the [single state authority on alcohol and other drugs];

(D) On-site intervention and counseling that is attuned to the developmental and special needs of children of alcoholics and other addicts;

(E) Involvement with Alcoholics Anonymous, Narcotics Anonymous, support groups for children of alcoholics and other addicts, and other family support groups; and

(F) Activities which enhance self-esteem and self-sufficiency for parent and child;

(2) On-site parenting skills counseling and training designed specifically for parents in recovery from alcohol and other drug abuse;

(3) Access to school for children and parents where appropriate, including, but not limited to, securing documents necessary for registration;

(4) Job counseling and referral to existing job training programs;

(5) On-site therapeutic day care for children when the parent is attending counseling, school or a job training program and when the parent is at a job or looking for a job and at other times as appropriate;

(6) Referral and linkage to other needed services including but not limited to health care and special therapy for children;

(7) On-site structured reentry counseling and activities;

(8) Referral to continuing care and treatment upon discharge from the residential program; and

(9) Referral to transitional housing appropriate for the family and its ongoing recovery.

(b) This [single state authority on alcohol and other drugs] shall require programs receiving funds under this section to collect and provide to the department information concerning the number of parents and children denied treatment or placed on waiting lists and may require such data and other information as the agency deems useful. Confidentiality of records regarding identifiable individuals enrolled in treatment programs funded under this section shall be maintained.

(c) The [single state authority on alcohol and other drugs] shall annually convene a meeting of all recipients of funds for programs funded under this section and other interested parties so that the agency may receive input regarding ways to improve and expand treatment services and prevention activities for women in childbearing years, pregnant women, parents and young children.

(d) The [single state authority on alcohol and other drugs] shall report annually to the governor and the general assembly as to its activities and expenditures under this section, the activities of recipients of funds under this section, the number of women and children denied treatment or placed on waiting lists, the recommendations in summary form made at the annual meeting provided for in subsection (c) and the recommendations of the department.

(e) As used in this section, the term "therapeutic community setting" means an alcohol- and other drug-free, residential, non-hospital treatment program using therapeutic community principles as the underlying philosophy.

COMMENT

The goal of this legislation is to foster the growth of these needed residential treatment services. For those unlikely to recover through outpatient and Alcoholics and Narcotics Anonymous alone, inpatient programs that can accommodate pregnancy and the care of infants and children on site need to be made available.

Services delineated in subsection (a) are designed to provide comprehensive prevention, education, treatment and

counseling and to provide for vocational and educational goals as well. Services called for are specifically tailored to the needs of addicted people and their children and are family-oriented in nature. Any cost of service will be offset by savings in reduced need for treatment of fetal alcohol and other drug effect and syndrome and in financial reductions in other areas.

It is crucial that skillful provision of addiction treatment take precedence over other programming until the foundations of recovery are established. Parenting, educational, vocational and other services must be anchored in a solid addiction treatment and recovery program.

Failure to accomplish this primary goal will result in relapse, more suffering and trauma to already distressed families and children and additional wasted resources.

The data gathering discussed in subsection (b) will assist the state in its planning and needs assessment process.

Sharing information with the governor and general assembly through the mechanism provided in subsection (d) will alert policymakers to progress and problems on a routine, annual basis.

Given the high and typi-

cally irretrievable costs of fetal alcohol and drug effect and syndrome and the potential for prevention of addiction in the at risk children, highlighting this issue through the annual reporting process is sensible public policy.

Section 4. Staff Training and Referral Mechanisms.
The [single state authority on alcohol and other drugs] shall have the power, and its duty shall be:

(a) To establish on a demonstration basis, programs to train the staff of child protective services agencies, counseling programs and shelters for victims of domestic violence, recipients of funds under the High Risk Maternity Program or the Federal Maternal and Child Health Block Grant and community or state health care centers in order to identify pregnant women and parents in those programs who are in need of alcohol and other drug treatment. This proposed cross training program will lead to earlier identification and referral of addicted pregnant women and parents and should avert family suffering and disruption while reducing health care costs; and

(b) To establish referral networks and mechanisms

between these agencies and appropriate alcohol and other drug treatment programs.

Section 5. Liberal Construction.
The provisions of this [Act] shall be liberally construed to effectuate the purposes, objectives and policies set forth in Section 2.

Section 6. Severability.
If any provision of this [Act] or application thereof to any person or circumstance is held invalid, the invalidity does not affect other provisions or application of the [Act] which can be given effect without the invalid provision or application, and to this end the provisions of this [Act] are severable.

Section 7. Effective Data.
This [Act] shall be effective on [reference to normal state method of determination of the effective date] [reference to specific date].

C

Resources for Assistance with Program Development

Peter Weilenmann

This list of resources that might be of use to a person, family, friend or an agency involved with a child affected by parental alcohol or drug use has been organized to conform to Maslow's hierarchy of needs, as follows:

> 1st Level: Basic Physiological Needs: Pressing medical or health concerns as well as living arrangements.
> 2nd Level: Safety and Security: These are areas that may be longer in duration.
> 3rd Level: Affection and Social Activity: Most are related to financial issues.
> 4th Level: Esteem and Status: Relate to legal, employment, and advocacy organizations.
> 5th Level: Self-Realization and Fulfillment: Relate to educational issues.

> (It should be noted that, inevitably, there is overlap among these levels.)

FIRST LEVEL: BASIC PHYSIOLOGICAL NEEDS

CDC National AIDS Clearinghouse
CDC National AIDS Hotline

Hemophilia and AIDS/HIV Network for Dissemination of
  Information

US Architectural and Transportation Barriers Compliance
  Board—Access Board

US Department of Housing and Urban Development—HUD

Phoenix Society (Burns)

American Association of Kidney Patients

American Brain Tumor Association

American Diabetes Association

American Kidney Fund

American Liver Foundation

Chronic Fatigue and Immune Dysfunction Syndrome Association

Federal Hill—Burton Free Hospital Care Program

Leukemia Society of America

National Alliance for the Mentally Ill

National Clearinghouse on Family Support and Children's
  Mental Health

Beech-Nut Nutrition Hotline

Gerber Consumer Information

March of Dimes Birth Defects Foundation

Family Survival Projects (Brain Injury)

Association for Brain Tumor Research

Friends of Brain Tumor Research

American Cancer Society

National Cancer Institute

American Academy for Cerebral Palsy and Developmental Medicine

United Cerebral Palsy Association

National Headache Foundation

National Center for Health Statistics

National Health Information Center

US Department of Health and Human Services

  a) Administration for Children
  b) Health Care

    c) Social Security Administration
    d) Public Health Services

The American Academy of Pediatrics
Association for the Care of Children's Health
National Maternal and Child Health Resource Center
Asthma and Allergy Foundation of America (AAFA)
Pharmaceutical Manufacturers Association

SECOND LEVEL: SAFETY AND SECURITY

National Organization for Rare Disorders
Office of Special Education and Rehabilitation—Services (OSERS)
    US Dept of Education
American Lung Association
American—Speech—Language—Hearing Association
American Trauma Society
Children with Attention Deficit Disorders (C.H.A.D.D.)
National Center for Learning Disabled Adults
National Institute on Drug Abuse Helpline
OSAP National Clearinghouse for Alcohol and Drug Information
Clearinghouse on Child Abuse and Neglect/ Family Violence
    Information
National Resource Center on Child Sexual Abuse
National Head Injury
National Spinal Injury Association
National Mental Health Association
Alliance of Genetic Support Groups
National Information Center on Orphan Drugs and Rare Diseases
Attention Deficit Disorder Association
Cleft Palate Foundation
Cooley's Anemia Foundation
Cornelia de Lange Syndrome Foundation
Cystic Fibrosis Foundation

Epilepsy Foundation of America
Little People of America
National Down Syndrome Congress
National Down Syndrome Society

THIRD LEVEL: AFFECTION AND SOCIAL ACTIVITY

National Foundation for Consumer Credit
Social Security Administration
Zebley Implementation Project (SSI)
Sibling Information Network
Community Legal Services (for SSI)

FOURTH LEVEL: ESTEEM AND STATUS

Disability Rights Education and Defense Fund ADA
Equal Employment Opportunity Commission
Job Accommodation Network
Equal Employment Opportunity Commission
National Organization on Disability
American Bar Association Child Advocacy Center
Association for the Care of Children's Health
Children's Defense Fund
Coordinating Council for Handicapped Children
Council for Exceptional Children
Federation for Children with Special Needs
NICHCY (National Information Center for Children and Youth
    with Disabilities)
National Easter Seal Society
National Institute of Child Health and Human Development—NIH
Disability Rights Education and Defense Fund
Higher Education and Adult Training for People with Handicaps
President's Committee on Employment of the Handicapped

FIFTH LEVEL: SELF-REALIZATION AND FULFILLMENT

American Association for Vocational Instructional Materials
Association for Childhood Education International
Health Resource Center (Education)
National Center for Research in Vocational Education
National Center for School Leadership
National Committee for Citizens in Education
US Office of Education Research and Improvement
National Literacy Hotline
Office of Special Education Programs (OSEP)
Head Start (Project) Administration on Children Youth and Families, Office of Human Development Services; US Department of Health and Human Services
Office of Minority Health Resource Center, US Department of Health and Human Services
National Council of La Raza (NCLR)
National Clearinghouse on Literacy Education (NCLE)
National Clearinghouse for Bilingual Education (NCBE)
Department of Vocational Rehabilitation
Americans with Disabilities Act Regional Disability and Business Accommodation Center
Accessible Community Transportation in Our Nation (Project Action)
American Association for Counseling and Development
American Psychological Association

OTHER RESOURCES

CIVIC & COMMUNITY GROUPS

Big Brothers and Big Sisters
Business/professional organizations
Campfire Girls
Chamber of Commerce

Churches and synagogue groups
Eagles
Elks
Four—H Clubs
Jaycees
Kiwanis of Columbus/ Eastern Star
Lions Club
Optimists
Rotary International
Salvation Army
Shriners
United Way Agencies
YMCA/YWCA
American Red Cross

PUBLICLY FUNDED PROGRAMS

Community action agencies
Community Service
Department of Social Services
Extension Services
Free Health Department
Head Start
Infant programs
Medicaid
Public libraries
Public schools

PARENTS' GROUPS

Cultural Organizations
Mother's Morning Out
Parent-to-Parent Networks
Parent Resource Centers

Parents Without Partners
PTA and PTO
Support/advocacy groups

REFERENCES

Abraham, H. Maslow, *Toward a psychology of being.* D. Van Nostrand Co., Princeton, NJ, USA, 1962.

Abraham, H. Maslow, *Motivation and personality.* Harper and Row, New York, USA, 1970.

D

Resources for Professional Education: Universities with Specialized Programs of Health Professions Training in Substance Abuse

University of Southern
  California
Clinical Family Medicine and
  Pediatrics
1975 Zonal Avenue, KAM-500
Los Angeles, CA 90033

University of Southern
  California
Department of Family
  Medicine
1420 San Pablo 8J B205
Los Angeles, CA 90033

University of Denver
Graduate School of Social Work
Spruce Hall South, Room 333
2148 South High Street
Denver, CO 80208

University of Connecticut
School of Nursing, U - 59
147 Courtyard Lane
Storrs, CT 06268

University of Connecticut
School of Social Work
1798 Asylum Avenue
West Hartford, CT 06117-2698

Yale University
School of Medicine
Department of Psychiatry
Substance Abuse Center
34 Park Street, Room S104
New Haven, CT 06519

University of South Florida
College of Nursing
12901 Bruce B. Downs
  Boulevard
MDC-Box 22
Tampa, FL 33612-4799

University of Illinois at Chicago
College of Nursing
845 South Damen Avenue
Chicago, IL 60612

University of Kansas Medical
  Center
Department of Psychiatry
Room 1038 Taylor Building
3901 Rainbow Boulevard
Kansas City, KS 66160-7500

Boston University
School Of Medicine
Director, Division of Psychiatry
Boston City Hospital
Boston, MA 02118

Boston University
School of Social Work
Alcohol and Drug Institute
264 Bay State Road
Boston, MA 02215

University of Massachusetts
  Medical School
55 Lake Avenue, North
Worcester, MA 01655

The Johns Hopkins University
Department of Psychiatry
550 North Broadway, Room
  202
Baltimore, MD 21205

The Johns Hopkins University
School of Medicine
Park Building, Room 307
600 North Wolfe Street
Baltimore, MD 21287-2530

University of Maryland at
  Baltimore
School of Social Work
525 West Redwood Street
Baltimore, MD 21201

Wayne State University School
  of Medicine
Department of Family
  Medicine
University Health Center 4-J
4201 St. Antoine
Detroit, MI 48201

UCLA
Department of Psychiatry
37-384A Neuro Psychiatric
  Institute
760 Westwood Plaza
Los Angeles, CA 90024

Bowman Gray School of
Medicine
Department of Physiology and
  Pharmacology
Medical Center Boulevard
Winston-Salem, NC 27157-1083

University of North Carolina at
  Chapel Hill
School of Medicine
Department of Psychiatry
CB# 7175, Medical School
Building A
Chapel Hill, NC 27599

Rutgers, The State University
School of Social Work
New Brunswick, NJ 08903

University of Nevada - Reno
School of Medicine
Department of Psychiatry and
  Behavioral Sciences
Reno, NV 89557-0046

New York University
SEHNAP, Division of Nursing
50 West 4th Street
New York, NY 10003

Case Western Reserve
    University
Frances Payne Bolton School of
    Nursing
10900 Euclid Avenue
Cleveland, OH 44106-4904

Case Western Reserve
    University
Mandel School of Applied
    Social Sciences
(MSASS)
11235 Bellflower Road
Cleveland, OH 44106-7164

Case Western Reserve
    University
School of Medicine
Department of Family
    Medicine
10900 Euclid Avenue
Cleveland, OH 44106-4950

Ohio State University
College of Medicine
Department of Psychiatry
1670 Uphan Drive
Columbus, OH 43210

University of Cincinnati
College of Nursing and Health
Department Head
Community Health,
    Administrative, and
    Psychiatric Nursing
3110 Vine Street
Cincinnati, OH 45221-0038

Brown University
Center for Alcohol and
Addiction Studies
Box G
Providence, RI 02912

Vanderbilt University
School of Medicine
Department of Medicine
2553 The Vanderbilt Clinic
Nashville, TN 37232-5305

Vanderbilt University
School of Medicine
Department of Psychiatry and
    Pharmacology
A-2205 MCN, 21st Avenue
South
Nashville, TN 37232

University of Texas - Houston
Health Science Center
School of Nursing
1100 Holcombe Boulevard
Suite 5518
Houston, TX 77030

University of Texas Health
    Science Center at San
    Antonio
Audie Murphy VA Hospital
7400 Merton Minter Boulevard
San Antonio, TX 78284

University of Virginia
Health Sciences Center
Department of Psychiatric
    Medicine
Blue Ridge Hospital-Drawer D
Charlottesville, VA 229011

University of Virginia
Health Sciences Center
Medical Education, Box 382
Charlottesville, VA 22908

Virginia Commonwealth
    University
School of Social Work
1001 West Franklin Street
Richmond, VA 23284-2027

University of Washington
School of Nursing
Department of Psychosocial
Nursing, SC - 76
Seattle, WA 98195

University of Wisconsin
    Medical School
Department of Family
    Medicine
777 South Mills Street
Madison, WI 53715

Index

J

K

L

SP *Springer Publishing Company*

Women, Children, And HIV / AIDS

Felissa L. Cohen, RN, PhD, FAAN
Jerry D. Durham, RN, PhD, FAAN, Editors

"This timely text provides nurses with cutting-edge information on HIV disease and explores the various issues specific to these populations. The context is accurate and comprehensive..."

—American Journal of Nursing

"Women, Children, and HIV / AIDS is a landmark publication...Compiled by a dedicated cadre of nursing authorities, it takes a totally realistic, deep look at current conditions and expectations, and blends it with forward-looking clinical advise for helping women and children living with HIV / AIDS."

—Nurse's Book Society

Contents:

I. HIV Infection and AIDS: An Overview • Caring for a Child with AIDS: Views of a Family Member

II. HIV Infections and AIDS in Women. The Epidemiology of HIV Infection and AIDS in Women • Prevention of HIV Infection in Women and Children • Clinical Manifestations and Treatment of HIV Infection and AIDS in Women • Reproductive Issues, Pregnancy, Childbearing in HIV-Infected Women

III. HIV Infection and AIDS in Children and Adolescents. Epidemiology of HIV Infection and AIDS in Children • Epidemiology of Infection in Adolescents • Prevention of HIV Infection in Adolescents • The Clinical Spectrum and Treatment of HIV Infection in Children and Adolescents

IV. Perspectives on Selected Issues Affecting Women and Children. Family and Living Issues for HIV-Infected Children • HIV-Infected Women and Children: Social and Ethical Perspectives • Psychosocial and Economic Concerns of Women Infected by HIV Infection • The Community: Mobilizing and Accessing Resources and Services • The Threat of AIDS for Women in Developing Countries • The Challenge of AIDS for Health Care Workers

1993   328pp   0-8261-7880-4   hardcover

536 Broadway, New York, NY 10012-3955 • (212) 431-4370 • Fax (212) 941-7842

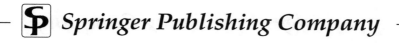 *Springer Publishing Company*

Jonas's **Health Care Delivery in the United States, Fifth Edition**

Anthony R. Kovner, PhD

"The most useful overview of facts and issues in our health care system—a required text in our Administrative Medicine Program."
—**David A. Kinding,** MD, PhD,
Professor of Preventive Medicine,
University of Wisconsin—Madison Medical School

This pre-eminent text provides a well-organized, readable overview of vital information for students in public health, health administration, community health, medicine, nursing, and the allied health sciences. The Fifth Edition presents updated material on the latest public health concerns including drugs, violence, institutionalized living, populace literacy, etc. Also includes coverage on primary prevention, Healthy People 2000, alternative medicine, multicultural issues, hospital organization, managed health care organizations, DSM-IV, OBRA, new ethical issues (such as physician-assisted suicide), plus updated and current statistical information.

Praise for the Earlier Edition:
"An extremely well-documented description of how personal health services are organized and delivered... It is non-technical, very interesting, and well integrated." — **Medical Care**

Partial Contents: What is Health Care? • Nursing • Population Data for Health and Health Care • Ambulatory Care • Financing for Health Care • Long-Term Care • Mental Health Services • The Government's Role in Health Care • Health Care Cost Containment • The Quality of Care • Technology Assessment in Health Care • Governance and Management • Comparative Health Systems • Health Care Ethics

1995   600pp   0-8261-2078-4   *softcover*
0-8261-2079-2   *hardcover*

536 Broadway, New York, NY 10012-3955 • (212) 431-4370 • Fax (212) 941-7842

$ Springer Publishing Company

Nutrition Policy in Public Health
Felix Bronner, PhD, Editor

This is the first book to deal comprehensively with nutrition policy in the public health of the United States. It combines theoretical and practical approaches to integrating nutrition concepts into public health planning with research and intervention strategies.

The book also summarizes international policies, calling attention to what has and hasn't worked, and focuses on what nutritionists can do and the knowledge they need to do it. The many dimensions of the relationship between nutrition and disease (an obvious but complex and controversial topic) and what counsel nutritionists can provide a concerned public are covered in detail. The book stresses the complex interaction among nutrients, lifestyles, genetic makeup, and health.

Contents:
General Aspects of Nutrition Policy. Nutrition Policy in Public Health: Rationale and Approaches • Behavior and Food Intake: What Constitutes Effective Policy • Food-Borne Health Risks: Food Additives, Pesticides and Microbes • Legal Aspects of Food Protection • Food Production, Processing, Distribution and Consumption
Nutrition-Related Conditions and Diseases—Policies and Approaches. Intervention Strategies for Undernutrition • The Obesity Epidemic: Nutrition Policy and Public Health Imperatives • Coronary Heart Disease and Public Health Nutrition • Nutrition in the Etiology, Prevention, Control and Treatment of Cancer • Osteoporosis • Dental Caries Prevention • Selected Disease Entities: AIDS, Alcoholism, Diabetes Mellitus, Lead and Lead Poisoning, Neural Tube Defects, Nutritional Anemia
Nutrition Policies and Approaches Targeted at Populations at Risk. Pregnant Mothers and Their Children • Issues in Development of a Nutrition Policy for Preschool and School-Aged Children • Nutrition Policy for the Elderly **Nutrition Policy Perspective.** Opportunities and Challenges of New Nutrition Environments: International Experiences and Implications for US Policymaking

1997   345pp   0-8261-9660-8   hardcover

536 Broadway, New York, NY 10012-3955 • (212) 431-4370 • Fax (212) 941-7842